HEALTH AND HEALTH CARE IN NORTHERN CANADA

Edited by Rebecca Schiff and Helle Møller

Accounting for almost two-thirds of the country's land mass, northern Canada is a vast region, host to rich natural resources and a diverse cultural heritage shared across Indigenous and non-Indigenous residents. In this book, the authors analyse health and health care in northern Canada from a perspective that acknowledges the unique strengths, resilience, and innovation of northerners, while also addressing the challenges aggravated by contemporary manifestations of colonialism.

Old and new forms of colonial programs and policies continue to create health and health care disparities in the North. Written by individuals who live in and study the region, *Health and Health Care in Northern Canada* utilizes case studies, interviews, photographs, and more, to highlight the lived experiences of northerners and the primary health issues that they face. In order to maintain resilience, improve the positive outcomes of health determinants, and diminish negative stereotypes, we must ensure that northerners – and their cultures, values, strengths, and leadership – are at the centre of the ongoing work to achieve social justice and health equity.

REBECCA SCHIFF is a professor and chair in the Department of Health Sciences at Lakehead University.

HELLE MØLLER is an associate professor in the Department of Health Sciences at Lakehead University.

Health and Health Care in Northern Canada

EDITED BY
REBECCA SCHIFF AND HELLE MØLLER

UNIVERSITY OF TORONTO PRESS
Toronto Buffalo London

Toronto Buffalo London
utorontopress.com

ISBN 978-1-4875-0211-9 (cloth)
ISBN 978-1-4875-2179-0 (paper)
ISBN 978-1-4875-1461-7 (EPUB)
ISBN 978-1-4875-1460-0 (PDF)

Library and Archives Canada Cataloguing in Publication

Title: Health and health care in northern Canada / Rebecca Schiff and Helle Møller.
Names: Schiff, Rebecca (Professor of public health), author. | Møller, Helle, 1962– author.
Identifiers: Canadiana (print) 20210293535 | Canadiana (ebook) 20210293772 | ISBN 9781487502119 (hardcover) | ISBN 9781487521790 (softcover) | ISBN 9781487514617 (EPUB) | ISBN 9781487514600 (PDF)
Subjects: LCSH: Medical care – Canada, Northern. | LCSH: Medicine – Canada, Northern. | LCSH: Indigenous peoples – Health and hygiene – Canada, Northern. | LCSH: Canada, Northern – Social conditions.
Classification: LCC R463.N65 S35 2021 | DDC 362.109719 – dc23

This book has been published with the help of a grant from the Federation for the Humanities and Social Sciences, through the Awards to Scholarly Publications Program, using funds provided by the Social Sciences and Humanities Research Council of Canada.

University of Toronto Press acknowledges the financial assistance to its publishing program of the Canada Council for the Arts and the Ontario Arts Council, an agency of the Government of Ontario.

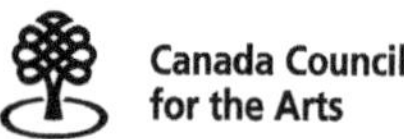

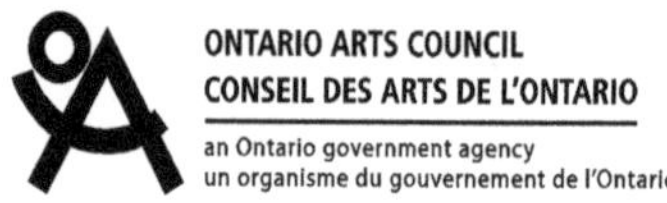

Funded by the Government of Canada | Financé par le gouvernement du Canada | Canada

Contents

List of Figures and Tables

Figures

Tables

Foreword

As a long-time researcher and educator in northern and Indigenous health, I am delighted to learn that, finally, there is now a book devoted to health and health care in northern Canada. I am honoured to have been given a preview of the manuscript and asked to write this Foreword. The absence of a book devoted exclusively to this important topic has long been recognized. This gap has now been admirably filled by Professors Schiff and Møller and their contributors. The many regions that constitute the Canadian North – which will not be defined here as the topic is thoroughly discussed in the book – share many common characteristics but are also diverse in terms of geography, demography, culture, politics, and economy. Few people can claim familiarity with or expertise in all these regions, their populations, and their health issues. The broad perspective adopted by the editors is evident in the wide range of topics selected. They conceive of health and health care holistically, incorporating quantitative and qualitative data sources and embracing the Western and traditional Indigenous world views.

Remote and *northern* are terms that can only be defined relative to somewhere else, such as *urban* and *southern*, which in the Canadian context constitutes the *mainstream*. Using terms such as *remote* and *northern* often exposes the speaker's unconscious bias, which is that of an outsider, perhaps even an external expert, attempting to offer advice or impose solutions on the less privileged who have the misfortune to be living in the periphery or hinterland. I admit to having had such a bias in my academic career, which has taken me years to overcome, if I even succeeded completely. Nevertheless, with that caveat in mind, it is still useful to retain these terms as they can highlight inequities in health outcomes and health care delivery among regions and populations.

Over the years, I have been encouraged by two trends that bode well for health and health care in the North. One trend is the increasing number of northerners – both Indigenous and non-Indigenous – who are seeking advanced training to become health professionals, administrators. and researchers. Many have returned to institutions, agencies, and communities in the North to contribute to improving the health and well-being of northerners. I have also observed that, during their training, which is still predominantly offered by academic centres in the south, northern trainees bring their unique, authentic, lived experiences and expertise to the classrooms, enriching peers and instructors alike. The other trend is the increasing number of southerners – both Canadian-born and recent immigrants – who are eager to learn first-hand about health conditions in the North and seek opportunities to devote part of their training in the North, undertaking projects, practica, courses, and electives of varying duration in northern locations. This two-way flow of ideas and mutually respectful co-learning can only hasten the "decolonization" of education, practice, and research among northern peoples and communities.

One purpose of this book is to document and explain the existence and extent of health inequities. It goes beyond the usual litanies of apparently intractable problems and insurmountable deficits to instead highlight the strengths and resilience that abound among northern people and communities. Throughout, solutions and strategies for improving health and health care are also suggested, though not prescribed.

I am a firm believer that one can learn much from books, which summarize existing knowledge and identify gaps. For the novice, books can excite curiosity in an unfamiliar field. For the already familiar or even expert, there will always be areas that have previously been overlooked or neglected. In this multi-authored book, the editors and contributors have provided the readers with a guide to what is pertinent, relevant, and important. I can predict that this book will play a major role in advancing the field of northern health in Canada.

Kue Young
Professor emeritus
University of Toronto and University of Alberta

Preface

HELLE MØLLER AND REBECCA SCHIFF

We would be remiss not to mention that the novel coronavirus COVID-19 emerged after we had written this book, as we were finalizing for publication, and how "in only a short period of time, the COVID-19 pandemic has unleashed an unprecedented crisis" globally (1 para1) and nationally (2). The pandemic has, as stated in the UN's Sustainable Development Goals COVID-19 report (1) highlighted the plight of the least privileged globally (3) and in Canada (2,4) even further.

As many of the chapters in this book highlight, northerners often face barriers to achieving health equity through inequities in the various dimensions of health, including the northern Indigenous determinants of health/socioecological determinants of health, and in northern health care systems. These barriers are further emphasized during health emergencies, such as those presented by a pandemic.

While we acknowledge that a whole book could be written about the ways in which COVID-19 has impacted health and health care in northern and remote Canada, we wanted to briefly recognize the impacts of some of the highly intertwined determinants of health in this book. These include some of the proximal determinants that have long-lasting implications, such as food security, housing, and income or socio-economic status; the intermediate determinants, such as health care and educational systems; community infrastructure and capacities; environmental stewardship or connections to the land; and cultural and linguistic continuity, kinship, and social ties; and the distal determinants within which all other determinants are constructed (5), including national, institutional, political, legal, and cultural factors (6) and, for Indigenous peoples, colonization, colonialism, "racism, social exclusion [and] … repression of self-determination" (5 p22).

Proximal Determinants

Income and Food Security

As discussed by Schiff and Schembri in this volume (chapter 2), food insecurity is a well-known issue experienced by northern and remote communities in Canada. For many Indigenous peoples and communities, these issues have been exacerbated by lockdown measures and the closure of businesses, followed by layoffs and furloughs, to curb the spread of COVID-19. These measures and the overall impact of the pandemic on the food supply has amplified concerns about already fragile food supply systems and chains, employment, and incomes (7).

Housing

Food security is linked to housing and several other determinants, including "education, adequate employment and … overall health and well-being" (8 para3). COVID-19 has compounded the issue of housing insecurity for many. For people who live in overcrowded housing or are homeless, conventional and sound physical distancing measures implemented during pandemics, like staying at home, are not an option (8–10): "The ability to isolate or social distance hinges on access to stable and adequate housing" (9 para5). Historically, housing and homelessness have been well-known challenges in rural, northern, and remote communities (11), particularly northern fly-in, First Nations reserves, and Inuit communities (9). But while the "unique needs of homeless populations during pandemics has been a major component of the Canadian federal response to the COVID-19 crisis" northern, rural, and remote communities "have received little to no funding to aid in their care of homeless people during the pandemic" (11 para1).

With COVID-19 and the need to isolate in already crowded homes, challenges in areas like mental health and violence against women and children have increased globally (3) and in Canada (12). In rural and remote communities where access to health care and social service options (13), mental health supports, and emergency shelters is very limited, the situation for women – particularly pregnant women – and children may be significantly aggravated (3).

Intermediate Determinants

Health Care Systems

The shortages of health care professionals and well-functioning health care systems have intensified across Canada during COVID-19, nowhere more acutely than in northern and remote communities (14–16). The southern health care systems, where northern residents are sent for anything that cannot be dealt with in a northern health centre or small northern hospital, have faced unprecedented challenges during COVID-19. Planned tests and elective surgery have been cancelled and postponed because of fears of further spread of the disease and of overextending the capacity of the health care system as victims of COVID-19 filled hospitals across the country (17). For northern residents living in fly-in communities, the cancellation of and reduction in flights because of COVID-19 turned to questions of life and death as no flights meant no medical evacuations – whether for having cancer treatment, giving birth, or treating a complicated fracture (18). Strongly urged to do so by Indigenous politicians and organizations alike, the federal government did rise to the occasion and provided the funding needed to enable some airlines to continue operating (19). Leaving a northern community to access medical care in the south has, however, become an even more arduous, and for many, a more frightening experience, than it was already (20) because of the fear of bringing COVID-19 back home and the need to stay in isolation hubs for 14 days before being able to board a homebound flight (19). The fear of spread prompted an increase in the use of the internet in both health care and educational systems everywhere (14,21–23) and made telemedicine and virtual medical appointments essential.

Telemedicine

Canada was fortunate to have an existing telemedicine infrastructure, which was significantly expanded early in the pandemic (21). The expansion has, unfortunately, not benefited many northern and remote communities. COVID-19 has drawn further attention to the stark disparities in access to high-speed internet between northern, rural, and remote communities and their southern counterparts (14,22). Many northern and remote communities were already hugely underserved before the pandemic hit, and COVID-19 challenged the federal government to follow through on promises to bring high-speed internet to northern, rural, and remote communities (21). These promises were not realized for many northern communities, and fear of them never being realized moving forward has been expressed (23). The disparity in connectivity between northern and southern communities has instead been exacerbated during COVID-19; consequently, disparity in access to health care has also been exacerbated. The opportunity that existed before COVID-19 to make an appointment with a physician or specialist from a southern hospital has, for some northerners, been impossible during the pandemic. Taking into consideration the health and safety of the individuals, families, and communities in their care, while also considering their own health and safety, many providers have chosen to conduct their appointments online (4,12). This change has meant that people who live in a northern and or remote community with no or limited connectivity or no or limited access to a computer or phone simply won't see a care provider until their concern has intensified and may require hospitalization (4,23).

Women's and Maternal Health

Pregnancy and postpartum checkups with midwives or physicians have, for many women, changed to being virtual appointments. This change has led to increasing uncertainty, anxiety, and depression among pregnant and postpartum women (24). Anxiety and depression have been three to four times higher than usual since the advent of COVID-19 (25). Women who live in northern communities have probably felt the isolation more deeply than other women in Canada; many northern communities are characterized by no or few health care facilities, no or extremely limited space to isolate individuals if infected, and little or no access to the protective personal equipment available in other communities (26–28). For women in Indigenous fly-in communities, this has intensified the stress associated with being evacuated to give birth in urban hubs (29), where COVID-19 infection rates are higher than in the birthing women's home communities, resulting in concern for babies' health and for bringing home infection (25,30).

For many Indigenous peoples and communities, the birth of a child is normally a time for family and community gatherings and celebration (29) and holds particular significance for the Elders of the family, as they come to give the baby the name with which the child "enters … the tribe" (31 para2). Such traditions have been difficult to honour with the prohibitions against larger gatherings and with COVID-19-related morbidity and mortality statistics very high among older people. As a result, older people, for their own health and safety, have been encouraged to self-isolate if living independently or been forced into isolation if living in long-term-care facilities (32). Indigenous communities' fear of losing traditional and cultural knowledge and Knowledge Keepers has, during COVID-19 been more present than ever, as older people in northern, rural, remote, and Indigenous communities typically "are forced to leave their communities" to access health and long-term care "when they grow older" (33 para13). The tradition in many Indigenous communities of keeping Elders in the community, rather than encouraging a move to a long-term-care facility outside the community, may have been lifesaving for Indigenous Elders during COVID-19 (34).

Mental Health, Addiction, and Suicide

It is not surprising that mental health issues and addiction during COVID-19 have increased globally (35) and in Canada (36,37). Similarly, while people everywhere may be physiologically impacted by COVID-19, some may be particularly affected, such as pregnant and postpartum women; children and young people; seniors and their families, especially seniors living in long-term-care facilities; people who are precariously employed or unemployed; people who are precariously housed or homeless; and people living in communities that are underserved in relation to health care, social services, and education (e.g., northern and remote communities) (38). The population groups and communities that have least access to care are unfortunately also among the population groups and communities in Canada that generally see the highest rates of suicide and suicide attempts (39). And although Mara Grunau, the executive director of the Centre for Suicide Prevention in Alberta, posits that suicide attempts and suicide rates generally go down at the beginning of a crisis, she also notes that "the cumulative effect spikes after 12 to 18 months" (37 para20). That means that the real or long-lasting impact of COVID-19 on mental health has yet to be seen, just like the real or long-lasting impacts of COVID-19 on education (40).

Education and the Overall Health of Youth and Children

COVID-19 has underscored the inequity in access to education and the tools necessary for access, particularly for northern and Indigenous communities, where connectivity is a challenge and far from all students have computers (22,41,42). Moreover, as schools and day cares have closed in an attempt to maintain health and safety, some children have been without a safe place, access to food from breakfast and lunch programs, and other supports (2), increasing the risks to their health and of food insecurity rather than lowering them.

Distal Determinants

In addition to highlighting the plight of the least privileged in nations and societies, and the ways in which histories, current politics, and policies perpetuate inequities and disparities, COVID-19 has also brought to light the strength and resilience of Indigenous communities despite these communities (particularly northern Indigenous communities) living with many inequities in relation to dimensions and determinants of health. Indigenous communities had, on average, only 25 percent of the infection rates of Canada, and the death toll has been even smaller (43). Indigenous communities initially had successfully limited the spread of the infection by, among other things, "articulating and enforcing rules on who can enter their communities, often implementing far stricter measures than those enacted by local municipalities, such as closures and checkpoints" (44 para12). In addition, many Indigenous communities used traditional means to maintain and improve health and immune responses and to overcome the anxiety and depression that followed in the wake of COVID-19

(14,45). In response to the challenges imposed by COVID-19, many northern Indigenous communities found strength in returning to and or increasing focus on more traditional land-based food systems and developed "new ways to exercise their food self-determination to meet the changing needs of their communities" (14,46 para14). Not only Indigenous peoples and communities but also people living in northern Canadian communities generally returned to or started growing their own gardens/vegetables and making food from scratch (47).

Throughout 2020, COVID-19 exacerbated existing disparities in the dimensions of health, including the northern Indigenous determinants of health/socioecological determinants of health, and in northern health care systems. However, COVID-19 has also demonstrated that it is possible for local, provincial and territorial, and federal governments to act decisively and quickly to implement needed supports and make changes in systems affecting population health and well-being (whether or not the support has been enough for the northern and remote areas of Canada notwithstanding), with the federal government, in the 2020 throne speech, offering further support to the populations most severely impacted (48).

We are hopeful that the increasing focus on disparities between northern and southern communities in Canada and how disparities among and between populations impact the health and well-being of us all, will have a positive impact on addressing inequities in dimensions and determinants of health and well-being moving forward, of people living in Canada generally and in northern Canada specifically. Research to document the outcomes of this increased focus, however, is essential. At the time we wrote this preface, little research centring on COVID-19 in a northern context has been published (49). An increased focus on the effects of pandemics such as COVID-19 on northern communities and regions in Canada is needed as a tool for advocacy and for crucial changes in health and health care disparities.

REFERENCES

1. United Nations Department of Economic and Social Affairs [Internet]. New York (NY): United Nations; c2020. UN report finds COVID-19 is reversing decades of progress on poverty, healthcare and education; 2020 Jul 7 [cited 2020 Oct 15]. Available from: http://www.un.org/development/desa/en/news/sustainable/sustainable-development-goals-report-2020.html
2. Canadian Human Rights Commission [Internet]. Ottawa (ON): Canadian Human Rights Commission; c2020. Statement – inequality amplified by COVID-19 crisis; [cited 2020 Sep 1]. Available from: http://www.chrc-ccdp.gc.ca/eng/content/statement-inequality-amplified-covid-19-crisis

3. Human Rights Watch [Internet]. New York (NY): Human Rights Watch; c2020. Submission to the UN special rapporteur on violence against women, its causes and consequences regarding COVID-19 and the increase of domestic violence against women; 2020 Jul 3 [cited 2020 Sep 2]. Available from: http://www.hrw.org/news/2020/07/03/submission-un-special-rapporteur-violence-against-women-its-causes-and-consequences
4. Jones AM. Northern Sask. outbreak reveals plight of Indigenous communities during COVID-19. CTV News [Internet]. 2020 May 10 [cited 2020 Sep 8]. Available from: http://www.ctvnews.ca/canada/northern-sask-outbreak-reveals-plight-of-indigenous-communities-during-covid-19-1.4933431
5. Reading C, Wien F. Health inequalities and social determinants of Aboriginal Peoples' Health [Internet]. Prince George (BC): National Collaborating Centre for Aboriginal Health; 2009 [cited 2020 Oct 20]. Available from: http://www.nccih.ca/docs/determinants/RPT-HealthInequalities-Reading-Wien-EN.pdf
6. Arah OA, Westert GP, Delnoij DM, Klazinga NS. Health system outcomes and determinants amenable to public health in industrialized countries: a pooled, cross-sectional time series analysis. BMC Public Health [Internet]. 2005 Dec;5(1):81. Available from: https://doi.org/10.1186/1471-2458-5-81
7. Wirzba S. COVID-19 is worsening food insecurity in Nunavut. McGill Int Rev [Internet]. 2020 Jun 23 [cited 2020 Sep 20]. Available from: http://www.mironline.ca/covid-19-is-worsening-food-insecurity-in-nunavut/
8. Perri M, Dosani N. COVID-19 highlights the plight of the homeless [Internet]. [place unknown]: Healthy Debate; 2020 May 18 [cited 2020 Sep 17]. Available from: https://healthydebate.ca/opinions/covid-19-highlights-homeless
9. Labelle M. Can the government help Canada's most vulnerable population amid a pandemic? [Internet]. Thunder Bay (ON): Northern Policy Institute; c2020 [cited 2020 Sep 1]. Available from: http://www.northernpolicy.ca/indigenous-peoples-covid-19
10. Buccieri K, Schiff R. Pandemic preparedness and homelessness: Lessons from H1N1 in Canada. Toronto (ON): Canadian Observatory on Homelessness Press; 2016.
11. Schiff R, Buccieri K, Schiff JW, Kauppi C, Riva M. COVID-19 and pandemic planning in the context of rural and remote homelessness. Can J Public Health [Internet]. 2020 Sep 24 [cited 2020 Oct 20];111:967–70. Available from: http://link.springer.com/10.17269/s41997-020-00415-1
12. Shields R. Mental health in Canada: Covid-19 and beyond – CAMH policy advice [Internet]. Toronto (ON): Centre for Addiction and Mental Health; 2020 Jul [cited 2020 Oct 12]. Available from: https://www.camh.ca/-/media/files/pdfs---public-policy-submissions/covid-and-mh-policy-paper-pdf.pdf
13. Kyas M. Northern Ontario's state of mental health and why [Internet]. Thunder Bay (ON): Northern Policy Institute; c2020 [cited 2020 Oct 12]. Available from: http://www.northernpolicy.ca/northern-ontario-mental-health

14. Fournier S. Responding to COVID-19 – Indigenous communities can't be expected to do more with less. 2020 May 1 [cited 2020 Oct 12]. In: Insights Blog [Internet]. Ottawa (ON): Conference Board of Canada; c2020. Available from: http://www.conferenceboard.ca/insights/blogs/responding-to-covid-19-indigenous-communities-can-t-be-expected-to-do-more-with-less
15. George J. Nunavut spends nearly $3M annually on security at health centres. Nunatsiaq News [Internet]. 2020 Sep 23 [cited 2020 Oct 12]. Available from: https://nunatsiaq.com/stories/article/nunavut-spends-nearly-3m-annually-on-security-at-health-centres/
16. Ready E. "We were already short nurses": State of northern nursing amidst COVID-19 [Internet]. CKPGToday.ca [Internet]. 2020 Apr 20 [cited 2020 Oct 12]. Available from: https://ckpgtoday.ca/2020/04/20/we-were-already-short-nurses-state-of-northern-nursing-amidst covid-19/
17. Wiseman SM, Crump T, Sutherland JM. Surgical wait list management in Canada during a pandemic: many challenges ahead. Can J Surg [Internet]. 2020 May 8;63(3):E226–8. Available from: http://canjsurg.ca/63-3-e226/ doi: 10.1503/cjs.006620
18. Colleta A. Canada's Nunavut: A vast territory with few people – and no coronavirus. Washington Post [Internet]. 2020 Jun 2 [cited 2020 Oct 12]. Available from: http://www.washingtonpost.com/world/the_americas/coronavirus-canada-nunavut-inuit-first-nations/2020/05/31/5bd6aeec-9f74-11ea-be06-af5514ee0385_story.html
19. Brown B. Nunavut health-care system needs steady flight schedules during pandemic, minister says. CBC News North [Internet]. 2020 Apr 17 [cited 2020 Oct 12]. Available from: http://www.cbc.ca/news/canada/north/airlines-need-money-for-pandemic-nunavut-government-says-1.5535264
20. Møller H. Tuberculosis and colonialism: current tales about tuberculosis and colonialism in Nunavut. Int J Indig Health [Internet]. 2013 Jun 4;6(1):38. Available from: https://journals.uvic.ca/index.php/ijih/article/view/12344 doi: 10.18357/ijih61201012344
21. Stewart B. How COVID-19 worsens Canada's digital divide. CBC News [Internet]. 2020 Sep 23 [cited 2020 Oct 15]. Available from: http://www.cbc.ca/news/canada/british-columbia/covid-19-highlights-urban-rural-digital-divide-1.5734167
22. Flanagan R. Without broadband access, online learning not viable in rural, remote Canada. CTV News [Internet]. 2020 Sep 3 [cited 2020 Oct 12]. Available from: http://www.ctvnews.ca/canada/without-broadband-access-online-learning-not-viable-in-rural-remote-canada-1.5090861
23. Knight E. If a crisis like COVID-19 hasn't pushed government to take action to improve broadband access, what can? CBC News [Internet]. 2020 Aug 23 [cited 2020 Oct 14]. Available from: http://www.cbc.ca/news/opinion/opinion-erin-knight-internet-access-1.5682217
24. Bascaramurty D. For women waiting to give birth COVID-19 adds several other issues to worry about. Globe and Mail [Internet]. 2020 Apr 5 [cited 2020 Oct 14].

Available from: http://www.theglobeandmail.com/canada/article-for-women-waiting-to-give-birth-covid-19-adds-several-other-issues-to/

25. Thomas M. Pregnancy and the pandemic: "Giving birth anywhere is a risk now." CTV News [Internet]. 2020 May 28 [cited 2020 Sep 8]. Available from: http://www.ctvnews.ca/health/coronavirus/pregnancy-and-the-pandemic-giving-birth-anywhere-is-a-risk-now-1.4959752
26. Indigenous Services Canada [Internet]. Ottawa (ON): Government of Canada; c2020. Press release, Update on COVID-19 in Indigenous communities; 2020 Jul 17 [cited 2020 Oct 14]. Available from: http://www.newswire.ca/news-releases/update-on-covid-19-in-indigenous-communities-883077011.html
27. Malatzky DC, Gillespie J, Couch DDL, Cosgrave DC. Why place matters: a rurally-orientated analysis of COVID-19's differential impacts. Soc Sci Humanit Open [Internet]. 2020;2(1):100063. Available from: https://linkinghub.elsevier.com/retrieve/pii/S2590291120300528 doi: 10.1016/j.ssaho.2020.100063
28. Sokic N. Indigenous communities face an urgent need for PPE. Healthing.ca [Internet]. 2020 Apr 27 [cited 2020 Oct 15]. Available from: http://www.healthing.ca/diseases-and-conditions/coronavirus/on-the-urgency-of-ppe-in-indigenous-communities
29. Lawford KM, Giles AR, Bourgeault IL. Canada's evacuation policy for pregnant First Nations women: resignation, resilience, and resistance. Women Birth [Internet]. 2018 Dec 1;31(6):479–88. https://linkinghub.elsevier.com/retrieve/pii/S1871519217302019 doi: 10.1016/j.wombi.2018.01.009
30. Toth K. This Nunavut mom came to Yellowknife to give birth. Now, her family's stuck and self-isolating. CBC News [Internet]. 2020 [cited 2020 Oct 12]. Available from: http://www.cbc.ca/news/canada/north/nunavut-couple-baby-stuck-yellowknife-covid19-1.5511641
31. Talaga T. The power of Indigenous kinship. Walrus [Internet]. 2018 Dec 21 [cited 2020 Sep 15]. Available from: https://thewalrus.ca/the-power-of-indigenous-kinship/
32. Welsh M. Isolated and lonely, "caged" seniors driven to despair – and defiance. The Star [Internet]. 2020 May 18 [cited 2020 Oct 20]. Available from: http://www.thestar.com/news/canada/2020/05/18/isolated-and-lonely-caged-seniors-driven-to-despair-and-defiance.html
33. Graham J. Loss of Canada elders to coronavirus threatens Indigenous culture. Reuters [Internet]. 2020 Jun 1 [cited 2020 Sep 15]. Available from: http://www.reuters.com/article/us-health-coronavirus-canada-indigenous-idUSKBN2382D4
34. Banning J. Why are Indigenous communities seeing so few cases of COVID-19? Can Med Assoc J [Internet]. 2020 Aug 24;192(34):E993–4. Available from: http://www.cmaj.ca/lookup/doi/10.1503/cmaj.1095891 doi: 10.1503/cmaj.1095891
35. Dubey MJ, Ghosh R, Chatterjee S, Biswas P, Chatterjee S, Dubey S. COVID-19 and addiction. Diabetes Metab Syndr Clin Res Rev [Internet]. 2020 Sep;14(5):817–23. Available from: https://linkinghub.elsevier.com/retrieve/pii/S1871402120301776 doi: 10.1016/j.dsx.2020.06.008

36. D'Andrea A. COVID-19 sees 750 per cent spike in virtual mental health calls at CAMH. The Star [Internet]. 2020 May 4 [cited 2020 Oct 14]. Available from: http://www.thestar.com/news/gta/2020/05/04/covid-19-causes-750-per-cent-spike-in-virtual-mental-health-calls-at-camh.html
37. Wright T. Crisis lines in Canada face volunteer, cash crunch even as COVID-19 drives surge in calls. The Star [Internet]. 2020 Apr 27 [cited 2020 Sep 26]. Available from: http://www.thestar.com/news/canada/2020/04/27/crisis-lines-in-canada-face-volunteer-cash-crunch-even-as-covid-19-drives-surge-in-calls.html
38. Mental Health Commission of Canada. COVID-19 and mental health: policy responses and emerging issues [Internet]. Ottawa (ON): Mental Health Commission of Canada; 2020 [cited 2020 Oct 3]. Available from: http://www.mentalhealthcommission.ca/sites/default/files/2020-06/COVID_19_policy_responses_emerging_issues_eng.pdf
39. Government of Canada [Internet]. Ottawa (ON): Government of Canada; c2019. Suicide in Canada; [updated 2019 Jul 22; cited 2020 Oct 15]. Available from: http://www.canada.ca/en/public-health/services/suicide-prevention/suicide-canada.html#a2
40. Organisation for Economic Co-operation and Development [Internet]. Paris (FR): Organisation for Economic Co-operation and Development; c2020. Education and COVID-19: Focusing on the long-term impact of school closures; 2020 Jun 29 [cited 2020 Oct 15]. Available from: http://www.oecd.org/coronavirus/policy-responses/education-and-covid-19-focusing-on-the-long-term-impact-of-school-closures-2cea926e/
41. Fowler D. We need to get all Canadian students online quickly in the face of pandemic uncertainty. CBC News [Internet]. 2020 Jun 2 [cited 2020 Sep 4]. Available from: http://www.cbc.ca/news/opinion/opinion-children-students-internet-access-1.5583321
42. Porter J. Schools in northern Ontario First Nations resort to phone and fax machine to restart classes. CBC News [Internet]. 2020 Aug 27 [cited 2020 Sep 15]. Available from: http://www.cbc.ca/news/canada/thunder-bay/phone-fax-school-1.5701272
43. Indigneous Services Canada [Internet]. Ottawa (ON): Government of Canada; c2020. Coronavirus (COVID-19) and Indigenous communities; [cited 2020 Sep 15]. Available from: http://www.sac-isc.gc.ca/eng/1581964230816/1581964277298
44. Richardson L, Crawford A. COVID-19 and the decolonization of Indigenous public health. Can Med Assoc J [Internet]. 2020 Sep 21;192(38):E1098–100. Available from: http://www.cmaj.ca/lookup/doi/10.1503/cmaj.200852 doi: 10.1503/cmaj.200852
45. Kennedy-Kish B, Longboat KD. Indigenous wellbeing in the times of COVID-19: Four directions virtual support hub [Internet]. Toronto (ON): Women's College Hospital; 2020 [cited 2020 Oct 12]. Available from: https://www.womenscollegehospital.ca/assets/pdf/IndigenousHealth/8.5X11-RGB.pdf

46. Decembrini AD. Indigenous food sovereignty and COVID-19 [Internet]. Vancouver (BC): First Peoples Law Corporation; 2020 Aug 26 [cited 2020 Sep 4]. Available from: http://www.firstpeopleslaw.com/public-education/blog/indigenous-food-sovereignty-and-covid-19
47. Mullins L, Charlebois S, Music J, Finch E. Home food gardening in response to the Covid-19 pandemic [Internet]. Halifax (NS): Agri-food Analytics Lab, Dalhousie University, Faculty of Agriculture; 2020 Oct 7 [cited 2020 Oct 18]. Available from: https://cdn.dal.ca/content/dam/dalhousie/pdf/sites/agri-food/Home%20Food%20Gardening%20EN.pdf
48. Harris K. Liberals promise to extend emergency COVID-19 supports, build national child-care program in throne speech. CBC News [Internet]. 2020 Sep 23 [cited 2020 Oct 20]. Available from: http://www.cbc.ca/news/politics/throne-speech-trudeau-address-2020-1.5735325
49. Savage D, Fisher A, Choudhury S, Ohle R, Strasser R, Orkin A, Mago V. Investigating the implications of COVID-19 for the rural and remote population of Northern Ontario using a mathematical model. [cited 2020 Oct 20]. In: medRxiv: The Preprint Server for Health Sciences [Internet]. Cold Spring Harbor (NY): Cold Spring Harbor Laboratory. c2020. Available from: http://medrxiv.org/lookup/doi/10.1101/2020.09.17.20196949 doi: 10.1101/2020.09.17.20196949

Acknowledgments

Dr. Rebecca Schiff and Dr. Helle Møller would like to acknowledge the patience, dedication, and work of all the authors who contributed to this volume. We also acknowledge the Department of Health Sciences and Faculty of Health and Behavioural Sciences at Lakehead University, which provided material support and allowance for the time to complete this volume. We want to thank the Awards to Scholarly Publications Program of the Federation of the Humanities and Social Sciences for its financial support. We would also like to acknowledge Dr. Kue Young, for his generous contribution of a map of northern Canada and foreword for the volume. Finally, thanks to our editor at University of Toronto Press for her ongoing support and encouragement throughout the creation of this book.

HEALTH AND HEALTH CARE IN NORTHERN CANADA

Introduction: Health and Health Care in Northern Canada

REBECCA SCHIFF AND HELLE MØLLER

The Canadian North is a vast region. Canada's northern and remote geographies (encompassing both the Arctic territories and remote, subarctic areas of seven provinces) account for almost two-thirds of the country's land mass. Northern Canada is home to abundant natural resources and a diversity of rich cultural heritage shared across Indigenous and non-Indigenous residents of this extensive region. Indeed, the geographical and cultural significance of the region is reflected in Canada's national identity, which is closely tied to imagery and narratives of northern peoples and lands (1). This book is about health and health care in northern Canada. It is written from a perspective that acknowledges the unique strengths, resilience, and innovation of northerners in addressing the challenges of northern living and northern health care systems, challenges often imposed and aggravated by histories and contemporary manifestations of colonialism.

Who Are We and Why Did We Create This Book?

The idea for a book on this topic initially emerged out of a common recognition by the editors (Rebecca and Helle) that there were no volumes that brought together an overview of the unique health and health care challenges and innovative solutions being developed in the North. As such, we set out on a path to begin to bring together some of this knowledge. However, before delving further into this, we feel that it is imperative to begin this book by introducing ourselves and situating our interest in this topic. A book on the North is inherently connected with Indigenous peoples and, as a result, we begin by naming our privilege here as non-Indigenous, white researchers to identify our positionality in this work and our understanding that the information shared here is filtered through our own personal and professional lenses and interpretations:

> REBECCA: I descend from first- and third-generation immigrants with a mix of European origins – Dutch and Belgian on my mother's side and Ashkenazi Jewish

(from Germany and Russia) on my father's side. Through my relationships with Indigenous family and friends, I feel privileged to have had opportunities to be involved in ceremony and learn about contemporary life in some First Nations and Inuit communities and about Cree, Nakoda, Blackfoot, and Cherokee traditions and spirituality. In my 20s I was also gifted the name White Bear Woman by a Cree Elder and take it quite seriously to honour this name through the way that I live and work. I came to work professionally with Indigenous communities shortly after finishing my doctoral work on sustainable food systems. I had the opportunity to become involved with several research projects, mostly related to housing and homelessness in Calgary and Regina, in which Indigenous organisations were key partners. After several years of postdoctoral work, I took a position with Memorial University, based at the Labrador Institute in Happy Valley-Goose Bay. That position included a mandate focused on community-engaged research with the northern and remote Inuit and First Nations communities in Labrador. Living in Labrador, I developed an awareness of the beauty and strengths of the North. I also developed a deep appreciation for the innovation of northerners in addressing the challenges of northern living, challenges to health and wellness that are often aggravated by experiences of racism, colonial pasts, and neocolonialism. This fostered an ongoing interest in offering what I could to northern communities to support their work towards health and sustainability. My approach to my work with Indigenous individuals and communities is affected by this complexity of professional and personal experiences. It is through these lenses, as well as a passion for social justice, that I approach my work.

HELLE: I am of Danish origin and grew up in what was perceived to be a very homogenous Denmark in a working-/middle-class family. I have lived in Canada since 1996. I was educated as a nurse and an anthropologist in both Denmark and Canada. From 1997 to 2015, I worked and lived in several communities in Nunavut and Greenland, in Nunavut as a nurse, an educator of medical interpreters, a tuberculosis consultant for the government, and a researcher on the sociocultural aspects of tuberculosis. I have worked as an educator of nurses at Ilisimatusarfik (University of Greenland) and as an editor of a book focusing on Greenlandic nurses in Greenland. I have also worked as a researcher on what it means to be an Inuk (Greenlandic and Canadian) educated as a nurse in a Danish/Euro-Canadian culture and language caring for people of Inuit background in both Nunavut and Greenland. I am currently involved in research focusing on marginalized Greenlanders and how to improve the living conditions of this population. I carry out this work as a faculty member in the Department of Health Sciences at Lakehead University, where I have been employed since 2011. Through work, study, research, and friendships I have gained insight into the impact of colonization and settler presence in Indigenous communities, particularly in relation to health, health care, and health education. As a consequence, I attempt in my work to shine a light on these issues and advocate for change and social justice. However, despite any experiences I have working and living on Indigenous territory among Indigenous people and the connections and friendships I have forged through these, I am a fairly recent Danish immigrant to Canada and as such a non-Indigenous, white settler – with all the unearned privilege that come with this position – who is researching northern and Indigenous issues.

What Is "the North"?

In the literature the North is described in several different ways by different disciplines and organizations. These definitions can have political, social, and financial implications. In some contexts, "the North" in Canada is limited to the circumpolar north or "Far North," that is, north of 55° or 60° latitude depending on the source. Frequently, the "North" of Canada is defined politically by the boundary of the three territories (Territorial North). In other contexts, northern Canada is understood to encompass the Territorial North and the northern parts of provinces, otherwise known as the Provincial North(s). The Provincial North is sometimes referred to as the "Forgotten North" as described by Coates and colleagues (2 p6):

> The Provincial Norths in Canada are among the most marginalized, externally controlled and impoverished regions in the country, a reality largely obscured by the country's long-time preoccupation with conditions in the Territorial North.

We acknowledge that what are often perceived to be "northern conditions" prevail in areas of the Provincial North. In this book, the North is therefore conceptualized broadly to include both the Territorial and Provincial Norths (see Figure 1.1). We follow a description proposed by du Plessis and colleagues (3), a definition published by Statistics Canada. They use a US classification system for non-metropolitan analysis ("Beale codes") which they modify ("modified Beale codes") for a Canadian context.

The modified Beale codes provide 10 distinct categories for metropolitan and non-metropolitan analysis based on the relative weighting of parameters of population size, density, and context and include consideration of the size of a territorial unit: local, community, or regional. Code 10 is the classification for "northern hinterland," which includes all three territories and a breakdown by province of the southernmost latitude for consideration within this code. This approach to defining the North is valuable since it includes the Provincial North and provides a concise definition for that region. We acknowledge that there are multiple approaches to defining the Provincial Norths, including each province's own definition of their northern administrative region (NAR). We specifically chose not to use provincial administrative divisions since for some provinces (e.g., Ontario), the NAR encompasses communities and areas that

Figure I.1 Map of northern Canada

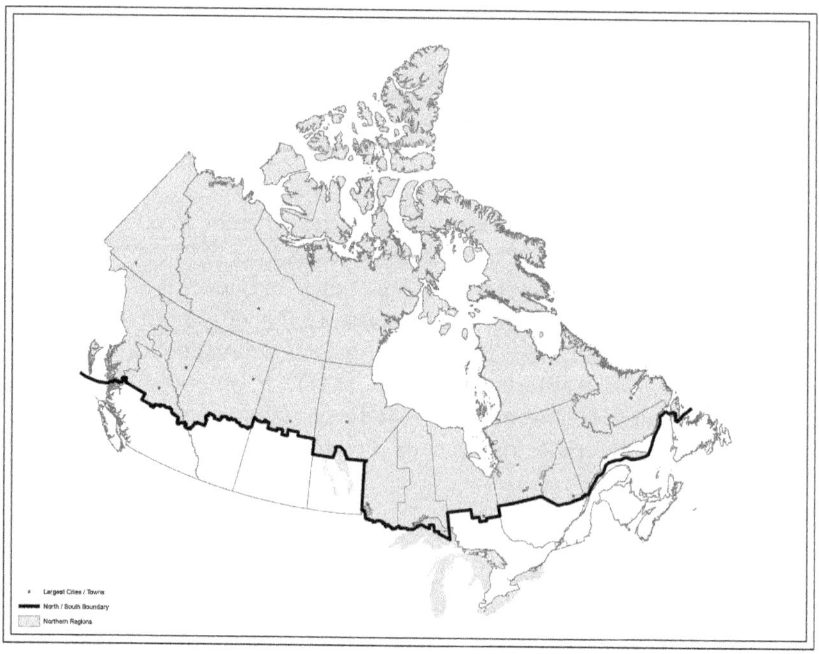

Map reprinted by permission of Dr. Kue Young. Regional boundaries are those of health regions as defined by Statistics Canada.

would not be considered northern or remote when compared with the climatic, geographic, and transport accessibility features of other provinces' NARs. The definition provided by du Plessis and colleagues (3) provides greater consistency in these areas and aligns well with what could generally be agreed upon as northern (despite provincial variations) according to climatic conditions, ecological profile, and relative remoteness (i.e., more limited transport accessibility), and for these reasons is the chosen definition of reference for this volume.

While the definition of du Plessis and colleagues (3) provides what we feel to be the best current proximation for the Provincial North (as part of the wider North), it comes with certain challenges. One of the most significant of these is a lack of data aggregated across this region. Most data for the northern parts of provinces are reported according to the NARs. Some NARs contain cities and towns (e.g., Sudbury and Thunder Bay), which in other contexts (and by comparison with the other NARs) might not be considered northern and whose data can obfuscate findings about more northern and remote regions. While there is a lack of current demographic information for the Provincial North, as Coates and colleagues (2) describe, this region is generally acknowledged as encompassing disproportionately geographically large areas of the provinces that are sparsely populated. They are also home to larger proportions of First Nations and Métis residents, who face different challenges in terms of social determinants and health care access when compared with their southern counterparts.

In contrast to the Provincial North, basic demographic information about the territories is quite readily available. The three northern territories in Canada, Yukon (pop. = 35,874), the Northwest Territories (pop. = 41,785), and Nunavut (pop. = 37,500) account for approximately 0.3 per cent of Canada's total population. With only 115,000 inhabitants spread over about 40 per cent of Canada's land mass, the Territorial North is very sparsely populated (4). As with the Provincial North, Indigenous peoples constitute large proportions of the population. In Yukon, Indigenous people (First Nations, Inuit, and Métis) constitute approximately 25 per cent of the population (4), most of whom are First Nations (85 per cent). In the Northwest Territories, Indigenous people account for 52 per cent of the population, of whom approximately 64 per cent are First Nations, 15 per cent are Métis, and 21 per cent are Inuit (5). In Nunavut, 85 per cent of the population identifies as Indigenous, almost all of whom are Inuit (6).

Despite the availability of demographic information about the territories, other challenges related to data limit our ability to understand health determinants and address health inequities in the North. As noted by Young and colleagues (7) the tendency to report territory-wide health data, rather than disaggregating them into Indigenous (First Nation, Métis, Inuit) and Non-Indigenous sub-populations, and into northern and southern areas within the provinces, obfuscates significant inequities and disparities between Indigenous and non-Indigenous populations and between northern and southern populations documented in the research literature. This edited volume is conceptualized from an equity perspective, with the whole of Canada representing what is achievable (7) but, as is evident from the chapters in this book, is far from the norm in most northern communities and regions.

Any book about northern Canada would be remiss not to recognize that while the demographic profile of people who live in northern Canada is heterogeneous, Canada's northern regions are home to a significant Indigenous "collective made up of many, separate, sovereign, unique, and wonderful Nations" (8, para. 9). As such, many of the chapters in this book focus on Indigenous issues, which are often complicated through policy and systems that fail to differentiate between northern and southern (as well as rural and urban) experiences (see chapter 20 by Lavoie, Kornelsen, and Boyer). In northern Canada, Inuit primarily inhabit Arctic regions of Inuit Nunangat,[1] which includes each of the four Inuit land claims regions: Nunatsiavut, in Labrador; Nunavik, in

Quebec; the territory of Nunavut; and Inuvialuit, in the Northwest Territories. The Provincial North and many parts of the territories are home to large number of First Nations who represent a diversity of language groups and cultures. Métis communities also play a significant role in the North, where they make up a notable proportion of the population across most of the Provincial Norths and territories.

The North also comprises generations of settlers who immigrated to these regions initially from different European nations. The colonization of Canada occurred through several missionary, sovereignty, whaling, fur trade, and gold rush bust and boom waves. While Labrador and many parts of the Provincial North experienced early waves of settler groups, many parts of the Territorial North experienced much more recent colonization. Colonization is woven throughout the chapters as a significant element affecting health and health outcomes throughout the North. When the North was colonized, it was with the aim of establishing Canadian sovereignty over those vast territories. Perfunctory health care, education, and policing were established, but not much effort was put into them or into attempts at equity with southern Canada; we are dealing with the legacy of that, and it is evident in people's health statuses that they have not had access to same education, infrastructure, health care, or economic development opportunities.

Of the total populations of the three territories, about 45 per cent reside in Whitehorse, Yellowknife, and Iqaluit, and although proportions vary significantly, approximately 75 per cent of the combined populations in these cities are non-Indigenous (9). This distribution has important implications since urban centres are where the majority of jobs, services, and political institutions are concentrated. This is not dissimilar to the Provincial North, where power and services are also concentrated in a few regional centres.

Why "Northern Health and Health Care"?

This book, in part, responds to the question, why focus on northern health and health care? Part of this response involves what we feel is a necessary recognition of the health and health care inequities experienced in the North; that is, part of coming up with solutions is recognizing challenges, as well as the strengths and resilience that exist to respond to those challenges (and this is woven throughout the organization of this book, as detailed below). Remote and northern communities in Canada demonstrate both unique and significantly worse health outcomes than less isolated "southern" Canadian populations. When we note this, we also need to note that these health outcomes are closely tied to social and ecological determinants of health (SEDoH). We posit that northerners experience challenges related to some SEDoH (such as education, food, and housing) to a much greater extent than their southern counterparts do and that these challenges are aggravated by historical and ongoing experiences of colonialism. We also suggest that there are some SEDoH that are unique to or much more visible in the North – such as the impact of resource extraction on health and wellness and the effects of climate change on health care in northern (and particularly northern Indigenous) communities (see sections I and II of this volume). The SEDoH are aggravated not only by geographic factors (e.g., climate and distance) but perhaps more so by colonial attitudes towards northern policy development and lack of attention from southern policymakers. These issues are largely responsible for health inequities, which the World Health Organization (WHO) (10) defines as "the unfair and avoidable differences in health status seen within and between countries" (10, para5). Rather than differences between countries, in the Canadian context this manifests as differences in health status between different regions within the country and specifically across a north-south divide.

In this sense, place is intimately tied to the SEDoH and subsequently to health status and health outcomes. As noted by Kulig and Williams in the introduction to their edited volume *Health in Rural Canada* (11), where you live has a big influence on the quality and variety of educational institutions you have easy access to. Whether medical professionals are educated within your community and through curriculum that is geared to the particular circumstances of the people living there also has an impact on the quality of health care available. Whether health care providers are educated or have placements in your community in turn influences whether they seek employment there and thus whether there are more or less vacancies. Where you live will also influence how easy or challenging it is to gain employment and, if you do, whether you will be able to secure day care for your child or children. As you grow older it will influence your ability to continue getting around if you are no longer able to drive yourself as public transportation varies according to where you live.

Thus, northern communities experience unique challenges related to SEDoH, both social and otherwise, that do not affect southern communities in the same ways or to the same extent. This includes limitations in terms of education, infrastructure, food, housing, energy/heating sources, water, waste management, and economic development, among others. Compared to the south, health care is also significantly limited in terms of the quantity, quality, variety, and cultural appropriateness of services. Much of this can be attributed to a uniquely northern situation, which is characterized by challenging geographies, climate, unequal economic opportunities, ongoing effects of colonization, and concentration of power and decision making in southern capitals and urban centres.

At the same time, and again as observed by Kulig and Williams (11), while place matters to health, so too do gender or sexuality, culture, and, we would add, differing histories and sociopolitical contexts. These all help to clarify the variations in health status and outcomes experienced by Inuit, First Nations, and Métis peoples (11). Indigenous peoples in the Canadian North experience particularly unfavourable health outcomes when compared to settler populations (12), and there are SEDoH that affect Indigenous peoples in particular, such as colonization and colonialism (13,14) and the legacy of residential schools and forced relocations. These further complicate and compound the already distinct health-related challenges of northern living.

Despite these barriers, northerners demonstrate incredible resilience and innovation in the face of significant adversity. Over time, research and practice in the Canadian North has evolved to provide significant innovation in processes, technology, and approaches to health and social service provision. These approaches provide a groundwork for supporting wellness and addressing inequities, and grounds for ongoing discovery and innovation.

With this book, we add to previously published volumes that focus on health and health care either more generally in rural Canada (such as *Health in Rural Canada* by Kulig and Williams (11)) or broadly across the entire Arctic and circumpolar North (such as *Health Transitions in Arctic Populations* by Young and Bjerregaard (15) and *Circumpolar Health Atlas* by Young, Rawat, Winifried, Chatwood, and Bjerregaard (16)). No known volume provides an overview of current issues and innovations in health and health care specific to the Canadian North. Our interest in producing this manuscript was to provide a new contribution that can begin to synthesize the issues and emerging knowledge, based on the most current information, on northern health and health care in Canada.

Organization of This Book

The purpose of this book is to deepen our knowledge about health determinants and challenges in health care delivery for communities in northern Canada, as well as northern strengths and innovation for the improvement of health and health care for remote populations. This volume includes a particular focus on the situation and needs of Indigenous people as the original inhabitants of northern Canada, but also addresses the diversity of communities and experiences across the North. Of particular importance, this book pays specific attention (particularly in Section III) to future needs and innovation to achieve health equity for northern communities.

It would be beyond the scope or capacity of a single volume to provide a completely comprehensive discussion of every issue and solution in northern health and health care. This book attempts to provide a broad overview, based on current information and data, of what we have identified as some of the current and important topics in northern health and health care. Therefore, we have included chapters that focus on certain select, significant issues to begin this discussion. Numerous other topics and approaches would complement this picture of northern health. Because of the interrelatedness of health issues for northern and Indigenous communities, many chapters reference other health issues outside the main focus of that chapter; these references refer readers to other chapters and other resources outside this volume that focus on related issues.

We have organized the book into three sections. Each section begins with an introduction, summarizing themes that are woven throughout the chapters in that section. The section introductions discuss other issues that may not be covered by individual chapters but are nevertheless important. The chapters in each section paint a broad picture of primary issues that northern peoples face regarding health and health care, as well as draw on occasional case studies to illustrate these issues. Many chapters are written by northerners and some use quotations, photographs, and other materials to highlight voices and perspectives of people living in northern Canada (see, for example, Kauppi et al., chapter 3; Healey Akearok et al., chapter 5, and Cunsolo et al., chapter 12). This book intentionally includes many authors across chapters to provide insight into the many voices and perspectives in northern Canadian health and health care.

Each section responds to that earlier question: why a focus on northern health and health care? Having both lived in the North and spent many years considering these factors, we feel that it would be a disservice to write a book that did not begin with an explicit acknowledgment not only of the inequities in SEDoH (including health care inequities) but also the ways in which ongoing manifestations of colonialism continue to impede work towards equity and wellness for northerners and northern communities. Discussing colonialism and neocolonialism is an important part of the response to that question – and this is reflected in many, though not all, of the chapters. Although an important and significant topic in this book, (neo)colonialism is not the sole focus, and many chapters concentrate on other important structural inequities which impact northern health.

Reflecting again on that earlier question, another critical part of the response is what others (southerners) have to learn about strength, resilience, and innovation from the North. We feel that it would also be an incredible disservice not to recognize these assets and the innovative approaches to creating health solutions in the North. There is a focus on these strengths throughout many of the chapters; however, we chose to privilege this theme with the last word on this topic – as the final section of this book.

Section I sets the groundwork, establishing a picture of the SEDoH, including colonialism and other factors that aggravate these determinants, as well as some of the health inequities that have resulted from this. In Section II, we take a closer look at one very significant health determinant, health care systems, which are particularly limited by northern geography, climate, cultural indifference, and other challenges. The final segment, Section III, takes a look to the future, to resilience, assets, and the inherent capacity of northern communities and their allies to address the challenges presented in the previous sections. Here authors discuss innovative approaches to health promotion and health care that hold promise for the future in relation to supporting determinants, health, and health care in northern communities in the best way possible. Section III serves as our conclusion – pointing to innovations and approaches that require further consideration in our work towards northern and northern Indigenous health equity.

NOTE

1 Inuit Nunangat is an Inuktitut term used to describe traditional Inuit homelands in Canada, encompassing land, water, and ice; the term is often used to refer to the four Inuit land claims regions described above.

REFERENCES

1. Saul JR. A fair country: telling truths about Canada. Toronto (ON): Viking Canada; 2008.
2. Coates K, Holroyd C, Leader J. Managing the Forgotten North: governance structures and administrative operations of Canada's Provincial Norths. North Rev. 2015;38:6–54.
3. du Plessis V, Beshiri R, Bollman RD, Clemenson H. Definitions of rural [Internet]. Rural and Small-Town Canada Analysis Bulletin. Ottawa (ON): Statistics Canada; 2001 [cited 2018 May 1]. Catalogue No.: 21-006-XIE. Available from: http://www.statcan.gc.ca/pub/21-006-x/21-006-x2001003-eng.pdf
4. Statistics Canada [Internet]. Ottawa (ON): Statistics Canada; [modified 2016 Mar 29]. Aboriginal peoples: fact sheet for Yukon; [modified 2016 Mar 29; cited 2017 Jul 1]. Available from: http://www.statcan.gc.ca/pub/89-656-x/89-656-x2016012-eng.htm
5. Statistics Canada [Internet]. Ottawa (ON): Statistics Canada; [modified 2016 Mar 29]. Aboriginal peoples: fact sheet for Northwest Territories; [modified 2016 Mar 29; cited 2017 Jul 1]. Available from: http://www.statcan.gc.ca/pub/89-656-x/89-656-x2016013-eng.htm
6. Statistics, Canada [Internet]. Ottawa (ON): Statistics Canada; [modified 2016 Mar 29]. Aboriginal peoples: fact sheet for Nunavut [modified 2016 Mar 29; cited 2017 Jul 1]. Available from: http://www.statcan.gc.ca/pub/89-656-x/89-656-x2016017-eng.htm

7. Young, KT, Chatwood S, Marchildon GP. Healthcare in Canada's North: are we getting value for money? Healthc Policy. 2016;12(1):59–70.
8. Animkii Inc. Why we use Indigenous instead of Aboriginal. Muskrat Magazine [Internet]. 2017 Jun 7 [cited 2017 Jul 1]. Available from: http://muskratmagazine.com/why-we-use-indigenous-instead-of-aboriginal/
9. Statistics Canada [Internet]. Ottawa (ON): Statistics Canada; [modified 2018 May 24]. 2011 National Household Survey profile, 2011; 2016 Nov 23 [cited 2018 May 1]. Catalogue No.: 99-004-XWE. Available from: http://www12.statcan.gc.ca/nhs-enm/2011/dp-pd/prof/index.cfm?Lang=E
10. World Health Organization [Internet]. Geneva (CH): World Health Organization; c2021. Social determinants of health, [cited 2018 May 1]. Available from: http://www.who.int/social_determinants/sdh_definition/en/
11. Kulig JC, Williams A, editors. Health in rural Canada. Toronto (ON): UBC Press; 2011.
12. Young K, Chatwood S. Comparing the health of circumpolar populations: patterns, determinants, and systems. In: Evengard B, Nymand Larsen J, Paasche O, editors. The new Arctic. Cham (CH): Springer; 2015. p. 203–11.
13. Kelm ME. Colonizing bodies: Aboriginal health and healing in British Columbia, 1900–50. Vancouver (BC): UBC Press; 1998.
14. Mowbray M. Social determinants and Indigenous health: the international experience and its policy implications. Geneva (CH): World Health Organization Commission on Social Determinants of Health; 2007.
15. Young T, Bjerregaard P, editors. Health transitions in Arctic populations. Toronto (ON): University of Toronto Press; 2008.
16. Young K, Rawat R, Winifried D, Chatwood S, Bjerregaard P, editors. Circumpolar health atlas. Toronto (ON): University of Toronto Press; 2012.

SECTION I

Social and Ecological Dimensions of Health and Wellness in the North

REBECCA SCHIFF AND HELLE MØLLER

Health and wellness in the Canadian North are, as elsewhere, closely tied to a variety of social, economic, cultural, and environmental factors that both influence and are influenced by health. The first section of this book deals with some of these factors, which we broadly define as *dimensions of health and wellness*. The dimensions of health and wellness account for various *domains* of health (physical, emotional, social, mental, spiritual) and for the *iterative and dynamic interactions* between these domains, as well as between health and its *determinants*. Health determinants are a key component of the dimensions of health and wellness, and a focus of many chapters in this section. Determinants of health are biological, social, ecological, and economic factors that collectively affect and determine the health status of individuals and communities. The Public Health Agency of Canada defines 12 health determinants in the Canadian context: income and social status, social support networks, education and literacy, employment and working conditions, social and physical environments, personal health practices, child development, biological factors, health service, gender, culture, and race and racism (1). Some of these factors play out at an individual level while others are generated at societal levels.

Social Determinants of Health and Ecological Determinants of Health

Social determinants of health (SDoH) are a category of health determinants that are specific to social and economic conditions. While some of the broader health determinants are described as individual risk factors (such as biological factors) the SDoH originate at a community or societal level. SDoH are largely responsible for global health inequities, which the World Health Organization (2) defines as "the unfair and avoidable differences in health status seen within and between countries" (2 para5). They are shaped by the "inequitable distribution of power, money and resources" (3).

Various authors have described the SDoH within a specifically Canadian context, where the impacts of SDoH have been identified as "much stronger than the ones associated with behaviors such as diet, physical activity, and even tobacco and excessive alcohol use" (4 p5). Bryant et al. (5) identify a number of SDoH that are particularly relevant to communities in Canada:

1. Income and income distribution
2. Education
3. Unemployment and job security
4. Employment and working conditions
5. Early childhood development
6. Food insecurity
7. Housing
8. Social exclusion
9. Social safety network
10. Health services
11. Indigenous status
12. Gender
13. Race
14. Disability

The SDoH concept can be expanded to also recognize the impact of environmental conditions on health; the ecological determinants of health (EDoH). EDoH recognize the ways in which issues such as climate change, resource extraction, pollution, and ecotoxicity affect individual and collective health and overall wellness (6). The impact of ecological conditions on health is undeniable (in 2017, *The Lancet* launched a new journal – *The Lancet Planetary Health* – that is devoted to discussion on the topic of ecology–human health interactions). In this section, we also recognize the undeniable links between society and ecology and as such propose an integrated examination of social and ecological determinants of health (SEDoH).

An Indigenous Rejoinder to Determinants Frameworks: Indigenous Social Determinants of Health

In Canada, general health determinants frameworks (such as that proposed by Bryant et al. (5)) have been challenged by new frameworks that are specific to the experiences of Indigenous (First Nations, Inuit, and Métis) peoples. The need for frameworks specifically for Indigenous peoples is grounded in evidence that First Nations, Inuit, and Métis peoples conceptualize health in different ways than some of their non-Indigenous counterparts (i.e., holistic, wellness-based interpretations as opposed to biomedical models of health[1]) and have experiences that are distinct from non-Indigenous Canadians; therefore, Indigenous peoples experience distinct health determinants (such as colonialism) and experience health determinants in different ways, than non-Indigenous peoples (7–8). In general, these have come to be referred to as Indigenous social determinants of health (ISDoH). Reading and Wien (9) provided one of the earliest ISDoH frameworks. Their conceptualization challenged the previous Western-based frameworks, was rooted in Indigenous conceptualizations of wellness (including the importance of community for wellness), and posited that each determinant occurred at one of three levels: proximal, intermediate, or distal. Within this framework, proximal determinants are those that directly affect an individual's health, such as housing and food security. Intermediate determinants occur at a community level and include factors such as health care systems, community infrastructure, and cultural continuity. The distal determinants are the "political, social, and economic contexts that construct both intermediate and proximal determinants" (9 p20). Distal determinants include issues that have had serious and long-lasting impact on Indigenous peoples' health, such as colonialism and neocolonialism, racism, and social exclusion.

SEDoH and ISDoH in the North

The general population of northern Canada, and Indigenous peoples in the North, also experience SEDoH in unique ways and are impacted by factors that might be considered significant enough to exist as determinants that are specific to the northern context – northern SEDoH/ISDoH. People living in the Canadian North (Indigenous and non-Indigenous) experience significant barriers with respect to SEDoH that are uniquely tied to northern geographies and health care systems. Northern residents also experience determinants differently than those living in southern regions. In northern Canada, factors such as food security, housing, climate, economic development, and access to health services are affected by elements that are less prevalent in southern regions – the influences of a distinct climate and geography that impacts social, political, and economic structures and opportunities. Northern communities might include additional SEDoH such as geography, transportation, and infrastructure. Indigenous peoples of the Canadian North experience particularly unfavourable health outcomes when compared to non-Indigenous populations (10–14). They experience not only the unique northern SEDoH but also the ISDoH, with distal determinants playing a particularly significant role for many individuals and communities.

This section of the book focuses specifically on various dimensions of health and wellness, with particular attention to the SEDoH and ISDoH as experienced in northern contexts. Specific attention is paid to the SEDoH and ISDoH experiences of Indigenous peoples in northern Canada. The chapters introduce some health dimensions and determinants that are unique to or are felt more acutely in northern contexts. There is a particular focus on determinants where northerners experience significant disparities when compared, in general, to their southern counterparts. Some of the issues that are felt acutely in the North include mining and industrial development, food security, housing, access to education, climate change, and colonialism, among others. Authors touch upon many related health dimensions in various domains of health and various northern determinants of health, including infrastructure, transportation, geography, and economic development. The issue of access to health services, which is also a critical determinant of health, is given special consideration in Section II of this book.

This section begins with a consideration of three well-documented proximal determinants that are felt quite acutely in northern Canada: education, food, and housing. Chapter 1 by Walton considers the significance of education as an intermediate determinant of health for northerners. Specific consideration is given to the historic lack of access to secondary and postsecondary education and the ways that this limitation impacts diverse dimensions of well-being in the North. Walton considers the particular impacts of colonization processes on educational systems and educational outcomes for Inuit in northern Canada. She also considers some of the promising developments in secondary and postsecondary education in Inuit communities, developments that recognize and value Inuit culture and leadership.

In chapter 2, Schiff and Schembri provide an overview of the food-related challenges of northern communities, along with critical analysis of some past approaches to addressing food security in the North. They suggest the need to consider comprehensive approaches to food security in the North – three-pronged solutions that can simultaneously address challenges related to store-bought food, northern agriculture and fisheries, and traditional food systems. They also suggest the need for strengths- and asset-based approaches that value food sovereignty and community-led solutions to northern food security. In chapter 3, Kauppi, Faries, Montgomery, Mossey, and Pallard consider the significant lack of adequate housing in northern Canada and its substantial impact on the health of northerners. They consider the impact of federal policy on northern housing and health-related issues. Their findings point to the need for the national housing strategy to recognize the significant effects of poor housing on the health of northerners.

The section then turns to some less conventional examinations of northern health and SEDoH – in particular, and as described below, the role of health determinants in driving infectious disease, the significance of gender equity and women's health in the SEDoH spectrum, and a final issue that has had far-reaching impact across the north: resource extraction and mining.

The collective health of northern peoples and communities – whether children, young people, adults, elders, men, or women – is affected by infectious diseases. As noted in chapter 4 by Orr and Larcombe, although mortality from infectious diseases has significantly decreased in northern communities, morbidity (particularly compared to southern communities) remains high. Orr and Larcombe describe the determinants of the prevalence of infectious diseases such as tuberculosis, gastrointestinal infections, and sexually transmitted infections and their relation to SEDoH. Among other determinants, they identify adverse socio-economic conditions as contributing factors – with poverty, malnutrition, social distress, and exclusion having a substantial impact.

A stronger focus on the health and well-being of women would likely improve the health and well-being of the children and youth in northern Canada. As Healey Akearok, Meadows, Koonoo, and Michael explain in chapter 5, women's health has the potential to affect the complex and interconnected health of the whole community. Healey Akearok et al. highlight the key factors that are important for women's health and wellness, such as Inuit identity, culture, and community support. They also stress factors that strain the health and well-being of women, including family and personal relationships, substance abuse, and the ways in which women cope with these issues. The authors stress the significance of viewing health and wellness from a holistic and inclusive approach and the need to engage Nunavummiut in the development of strategies to support health and well-being for women and for community members generally.

The final chapter in this section, chapter 6 by Jones and Johnston, considers one issue that has affected health and wellness across the North yet has not been previously identified as a determinant of health: the impact of mining and resource development on the health of northerners. While not identified in other literature as a determinant of health, we assert that the significant impact of resource development in Northern Canada demands consideration in a determinants of health context. Economic dependence on natural resource development, particularly mining, has become a common experience in many northern communities. Experiences with mining have created both positive and negative economic, social, cultural, and environmental impacts; impacts that are accompanied by dramatic changes in health status and ripple effects on a broad range of SEDoH. Jones and Johnston consider these effects and the processes that have been used to assess the potential impacts of proposed resource developments in northern communities. They offer suggestions for expansion and improvement of impact assessment processes to address the wide range of social, economic, health, cultural, and environmental effects of northern mining and resource development.

NOTE

1 Biomedical models tend to focus on the absence of illness as an indicator of health, separate health into different components – physical, mental, emotional – and separate health from the rest of a person's experience. In contrast, many North American Indigenous worldviews use wellness frameworks that are not focused on the absence of disease but rather on the concept of "living well" and that recognize an interconnection between all aspects of health and lifestyle.

REFERENCES

1. Public Health Agency of Canada [Internet]. Ottawa (ON): Public Health Agency of Canada; [modified 2020 Oct 7]. What determines health? [cited 2017 Mar 23]. Available from: https://www.canada.ca/en/public-health/services/health-promotion/population-health/what-determines-health.html
2. World Health Organization [Internet]. Geneva (CH): World Health Organization; c2019. What are social determinants of health? [cited 2019 Dec 10]. Available from: http://www.who.int/social_determinants/sdh_definition/en/
3. World Health Organization. Rio political declaration on social determinants of health [Internet]. Geneva (CH): World Health Organization; 2011 Oct 21 [cited 2019 Dec 10]. Available from: https://www.who.int/sdhconference/declaration/Rio_political_declaration.pdf
4. Mikkonen J, Raphael D. Social determinants of health: the Canadian facts. Toronto (ON): York University School of Health Policy and Management; 2010.
5. Bryant T, Raphael D, Schrecker T, Labonte R. Canada: a land of missed opportunity for addressing the social determinants of health. Health Policy. 2011 Jun;101(1):44–58. doi:10.1016/j.healthpol.2010.08.022
6. Parkes MW, Poland B, Allison S, Cole DC, Culbert I, Gislason MK, Hancock T, Howard C, Papadopoulos A, Waheed F. Preparing for the future of public health: ecological determinants of health and the call for an eco-social approach to public health education. Can J Public Health. 2020 Feb;111(1):60–4.
7. Greenwood M, de Leeuw S, Lindsay N. Challenges in health equity for Indigenous peoples in Canada. Lancet. 2018 Apr 28;391(10131):1645–8.
8. Reading C. Structural determinants of Aboriginal peoples' health. In: Greenwood M, de Leeuw S, Lindsay NM, editors. Determinants of Indigenous Peoples' health: beyond the social. Toronto (ON): Canadian Scholars; 2018. p. 3–18.
9. Reading CL, Wien F. Health inequalities and the social determinants of Aboriginal peoples' health. Prince George (BC): National Collaborating Centre for Aboriginal Health; 2009.
10. Inuit Tapiriit Kanatami. 2014. Social determinants of Inuit health in Canada. Ottawa (ON): Inuit Tapiriit Kanatami.

11. Young K, Chatwood S. Comparing the health of circumpolar populations: patterns, determinants, and systems. In: Evengard B, Nymand Larsen J, Paasche Ø, editors. The new Arctic. Cham (CH): Springer; 2015. p. 203–11.
12. Devine C. Contemporary circumpolar health issues and innovative responses in the Anthropocene. In: O'Donnell B, Gruenig M, Riedel A, editors. Arctic summer college yearbook: an interdisciplinary look into arctic sustainable development. Cham (CH): Springer; 2018. p. 131–42.
13. Cohen SA, Talamas AX, Sabik NJ. Disparities in social determinants of health outcomes and behaviours between older adults in Alaska and the contiguous US: evidence from a national survey. Int J Circumpolar Health. 2019 Jan 1;78(1):1557980.
14. Baron M, Riva M, Fletcher C. The social determinants of healthy ageing in the Canadian Arctic. Int J Circumpolar Health. 2019 Jan 1;78(1):1630234.

1 Education and Health: Education as a Social Determinant of Health for Inuit in Nunavut

FIONA WALTON

Introduction

Education and educational qualifications are a key determinant of health closely tied to socio-economic levels. Nunavut communities face a number of challenges related to education, including the limited availability of qualified and culturally competent educators, high levels of staff turnover, lack of access to a range of educational facilities, and lack of postsecondary options and programs. Considering the factors that contribute to improving education has far-reaching value for the future of Nunavut communities.

The educational levels of Inuit in Canada's Arctic are determined by measures that include high school completion and postsecondary success based largely on expectations established in Canadian mainstream contexts. In Inuit Nunangat, the four northern regions composing the Inuit homeland in Canada, the National Strategy on Inuit Education 2011 noted that "roughly 75% of children are not completing high school" (1 p7). Consequently, postsecondary opportunities for young Inuit, particularly at a professional level, continue to be a challenge. Lacking postsecondary education qualifications, Inuit are not eligible for well-paid employment, even in their own communities. In Nunavut, qualified individuals, often from southern Canada, continue to fill vacant professional positions in schools, health centres, and government departments, maintaining longstanding inequities that prevent many Inuit from accessing higher paying positions. In spite of the creation of Nunavut in 1999, which established a public government committed to creating employment geared to the 85 per cent of Inuit in the population at that time, persistent inequities continue to reflect the colonial history.

One exception to this pattern is significant. In the late 1970s, Inuit started enrolling in teacher education programs offered in Nunavut by McGill University, and more recently by the University of Prince Edward Island, which offered two iterations of a master of education. Inuit graduates of these teacher education programs have moved into leadership positions in schools and within government departments. Successful teacher education programs provide striking examples of what is possible when bilingual (Inuktut/English) postsecondary programs are accessible to Inuit in their own region and communities. Also, when education is delivered in a way that reflects Inuit values, beliefs, and ways of being, educational success results (2–10). When students are actively supported and encouraged to pursue an education by their families, teachers, friends, and community, they can do very well educationally, which provides them with access to a far wider variety of options in terms of career and life choices (3,6,10–11). The more Inuit access postsecondary education and the higher their levels of qualifications, the more education can act as a positive influence as a key determinant of health.

To share some examples of positive changes that have taken place in the largest Inuit region in Canada, this chapter examines educational challenges and opportunities specific to Nunavut through a focus on Inuit experiences with education. These examples bring hope for the future of Inuit education and can positively influence the overall health of Inuit. The chapter concludes with a section dedicated to Inuit educational leadership and its importance within education programs that serve Inuit. Inuit role models in communities, schools, and postsecondary contexts act as catalysts and change agents to inspire younger Inuit to strive for better lives by completing high school and postsecondary programs. Leaders in any society act as agents of change by using their knowledge, power, and voices to raise awareness of issues that impact their own people. This is vital in any Indigenous context in Canada.

Situating the Author

Just before the creation of Nunavut, for 15 years from 1982 to 1997, I lived in Iqaluit and travelled across Nunavut in a variety of roles in education, including as a special education consultant, supervisor of schools, and instructor at the Eastern Arctic Teacher Education Program (EATEP), based in Iqaluit at that time. EATEP later became the Nunavut Teacher Education Program (NTEP). I finished my career in the North with two additional years in Yellowknife, from 1997 to 1999, where I was the director of curriculum and school services in the Department of Education. After moving south in 1999 to teach and conduct research at the University of Prince Edward Island, I continued to maintain close ties with Nunavut, particularly while acting as the coordinator of two iterations of the Nunavut master of education (MEd) program developed and offered between 2006 and 2013.

From 2010 to 2015, I also acted as the principal investigator of an ArcticNet grant entitled “Inuit Qaujimajatuqangit and the Transformation of High School Education in Nunavut” (2–3). Over the same period, I worked as a member of a second ArcticNet research team on a project with Thierry Rodon as the principal investigator. "Improving Access to University Education in the Eastern Arctic" considered the successes and challenges facing Inuit involved in postsecondary education (12).

Inuit Nunangat Educational Statistics and Strategies

In 2016, Statistics Canada reported that "47.8% of people aged 25 to 64 in Nunavut had a high school diploma or equivalency certificate, compared with 86.3% in [the rest of] Canada" (13), and 33.6% had a postsecondary certificate, diploma, or degree (13). This compares to a rate of approximately 65 per cent for postsecondary school graduation in the rest of Canada (14). These lower levels of qualifications, as previously mentioned, reduce the capacity of Inuit to apply for postsecondary education and employment opportunities that would enable them to shape the future of Nunavut and the other three Inuit regions of Canada.

When Mary Simon was the president of the National Inuit organization, Inuit Tapiriit Kanatami (ITK), and Chairperson of the National Committee on Inuit Education (NCIE), she stated that "the reality of Inuit Education in Canada is that too many of our children are not attending school, too few are graduating, and even some of our graduates are not equipped with an education that fully meets the Canadian Standard." She describes this situation as the "greatest policy challenge of our time. Some 56% of our population is under the age of 25, so improving educational outcomes is imperative" (1 p3). Guided by Simon's leadership, the NCIE, representing all four regions of Inuit Nunangat, published *First Canadians, Canadians First: National Strategy on Inuit Education 2011*, which provides 10 ambitious recommendations for improving education (1 p9): mobilizing parents, developing leaders in Inuit education, increasing the number of bilingual educators and programs, investing in the early years, strengthening Inuit-centred curriculum and language resources, improving services to students who require additional support, increasing success in postsecondary education, establishing a university in Inuit Nunangat, developing a standardized Inuit language system, and measuring and assessing educational success. These recommendations were to be implemented in the educational systems across all four Inuit regions through the leadership provided by the representatives on the NCIE. An update to the National Strategy is available in an *Interim Report on Milestones, 2012–2014* released by the Amaujaq National Centre for Inuit Education at ITK (15). The document certainly provides a hopeful blueprint for change in Inuit education.

Implementing educational change successfully takes a great deal of time and effort, as Michael Fullan has argued (16). Plans for changes in education fail because of the complexities involved in ensuring system-wide changes take place; however, Fullan is optimistic about the ability of small groups of educators to work collaboratively to effect significant change at the school or community level, especially when a leader shares the vision and goals of the particular group (16). He also outlines the possibilities for longer-term change at a systemic level, but this requires strategically focused leadership that is shared and maintained across schools or school districts (16).

A Colonial Legacy Shapes Education in an Inuit Context

The impact of colonization on education in Inuit contexts in Canada frames educational statistics as disheartening when, in fact, they are improving gradually as the educational issues of Indigenous people in Canada, including Inuit, are addressed.

Like First Nations children in the past, Inuit children in the early 1950s were taken from their parents who were living in remote camps on the land and sent to residential schools. One of these schools was the Roman Catholic Chesterfield Inlet Indian Residential School known as the Joseph Bernier Federal Day School, which opened in 1929 and closed in 1970. The school-residence was called Turquetil Hall. The Grey Nuns of Montreal operated the school and residence. The Truth and Reconciliation Commission gathered testimony from survivors who attended the school. Their stories described a punitive environment that taught Inuit children English and denigrated their Inuit identity and background (17).

Inuit children and young people came home from residential schools speaking English, wearing southern-style clothing, and behaving in ways that seemed quite different from their parents' ways. As a result, alienation sometimes took place between parents and their children, and this impacted the intergenerational transmission of Inuit cultural knowledge and skills in Inuktut. The long-term effects include difficulties associated with completing schooling and postsecondary education programs. Colonizing forces embedded in institutional contexts and teaching practices within community schools continued to impact the ability of Inuit to succeed even when education was available at the local level. This history is documented in more detail by McGregor (18 p55):

> The formal education system … was culturally assimilative and the most significantly disempowering colonial practice imposed upon Inuit. Moreover, economic development did not coincide with educational development, and the jobs promised to Inuit who did finish their education or practical training did not materialize. Therefore, the educational system did not facilitate self-determination, a positive self-identity, or economic self-sufficiency.

McGregor also noted that the experiences in residential school "embedded in many Inuit youth a sense of shame about their own culture and language" (18 p66).

Young men and women who had attended residential schools may have suffered physical, sexual, or psychological abuses; unresolved pain sometimes led to discord in families that negatively impacted children and created intergenerational health effects.

By the early to mid-1950s, children were required to attend federal schools built in the communities, and after the formation of the Northwest Territories on 1 April 1970, territorial schools were managed by the Department of Education in Yellowknife. During the first 15 years of federal and territorial schooling, teachers from southern Canada, or from places like England, Scotland, and the United States, taught Inuit children to speak, read, and write in English. In the early 1970s, two enlightened handbooks focused on curriculum for elementary and middle schools were produced (19,20). The first, *Elementary Education in the Northwest Territories: A Handbook for Curriculum Development*, known as the Red Book, argued that because students come to school speaking in their own language, "the learning program in the kindergarten through grade three levels is to be carried on in the mother tongue with English being gradually and specifically taught as a second language" (19 p3). The middle-school document, *Learning in the Middle Years: A Handbook for Curriculum Development*, known as the Green Book, pointed out that "to be a young Indian, Eskimo or Metis person is to live in a society that is almost completely dominated by non-native people" (20 p1). While the language used in the handbooks may seem dated now, many of the ideas are as relevant today as they were then. Regrettably, in spite of the availability of such forward-looking ideas for teaching and learning in a way that "has meaning in the local situation" (20 p7), it often proved difficult to maintain these approaches in the small schools in Inuit communities. Most teachers and principals eventually returned to southern Canada, and the high turnover made it difficult to sustain consistency in approaches to teaching and school management.

One very important result of the distribution of these curriculum handbooks was that Inuit in the eastern Arctic started to take on roles as classroom assistants to help teachers to communicate with children who spoke Inuktut. By the late 1970s, some of these classroom assistants had started courses at EATEP in Iqaluit so that qualified Inuit teachers could offer an education to Inuit children and young people in Inuktut. Seventeen-year-old Naullaq Arnaquq was a classroom assistant at that time. She taught a kindergarten class on her own, with guidance from qualified teachers from southern Canada (18). While a few Inuit classroom assistants from the eastern Arctic had already completed their teacher education programs at Fort Smith in the western Arctic, the EATEP classroom assistant program enabled the schools to offer instruction in Inuktut in the early grades and, eventually, for some schools to extend this instruction into junior high and high school.

In 1979, Naullaq Arnaquq (18) and 11 other classroom assistants became the first full-time students in the teacher education program in the eastern Arctic. In 1984, certified by McGill University, the first bachelor of education (BEd) program was made available and welcomed Inuit teachers. Since then, over 450 Inuit teachers have graduated from the NTEP. Increasing the number of Inuit teachers in the school system is critical for the development of a strong Inuit identity in future generations (21).

In March 1982, a groundbreaking special committee on education in the Northwest Territories was created to address issues that included "high drop-out rates, poor comprehension, poor parent/teacher relationship, low recruitment of Native teachers and foreign curriculum for northern lifestyle, lack of proper high school facilities, and lack of continuing and special education facilities" (22 p6). This visionary report, *Learning, Tradition and Change in the Northwest Territories* (22), led to the creation of 10 divisional boards of education across the Northwest Territories and Nunavut Arctic College in the eastern Arctic. The boards included representatives from each community education council and enabled coordinated services to be delivered to schools at the community level. Created in 1985, the Baffin Divisional Board of Education was the first board to be created in the Northwest Territories, and others were soon established.

Over the next 15 years, many of the recommendations in *Learning, Tradition and Change* (22) were implemented. This included the creation of high schools in communities, the establishment of inclusive education services in schools, and the development of teaching and learning centres staffed by Inuit educators and focused on developing curriculum materials and books in Inuktut. It was a time of promise and hope for the future based on the belief that if the recommendations were implemented, positive changes for education in communities would result. Students no longer needed to leave their own communities to complete high school; services and supports were provided to students with learning challenges; and a program of studies based on Inuit themes, Piniaqtavut: Integrated Program (23), was created to provide some relevant teaching units and learning materials written in Inuktut and English. In 1996, *Inuuqatigiit: The Curriculum from an Inuit Perspective* (24) was completed by a committee of experienced Inuit educators and leaders working with the Northwest Territories Department of Education. This crucial, groundbreaking document provided a foundational guide for Inuit teachers. Inuit embraced *Inuuqatigiit* as a document that reflected their knowledge and culture and affirmed their identity and the value of Inuktut (10).

The creation of the divisional boards and the teaching and learning centres led to a new and very promising era of change for Inuit education in the eastern Arctic. Though the majority of teachers and principals in most Nunavut schools continued to be hired from southern Canada, culturally based learning could now be delivered in Inuktut by Inuit teachers and classroom assistants to Inuit students. This valuable change depended on maintaining high numbers of bilingual Inuit teachers, classroom assistants, and Elders in the schools, as well as on ensuring that the teaching and learning centres were well resourced to produce and distribute materials in Inuktut.

In May 2000, just a year after the creation of Nunavut, the three Nunavut education councils collaboratively published *Tuqqatarviunirmut Katimajiit – The Nunavut Educational Leadership Project Report* (25). Its purpose was "to counteract the effects of history and colonization and to create a school system that is northern in character" (25 p2). This history needed to be counteracted because "the system requires Inuit leadership … to provide Inuit role models for students … [who] speak the language of the community … relate better to parents … [and] ensure inherent, automatic use of Inuit values, beliefs, attitudes" (25 p2). A bulleted summary addressed the impact of the colonial legacy on the Inuit participants whose testimony provided the basis for the report. The Inuit participants believed that colonization had contributed to the following:

- low self-esteem and lack of confidence on the part of many Inuit
- a yearning to be able to be themselves, to let their guard down, to be an Inuk
- the need to tell the painful stories of the past and the present and for healing to take place to enable people to move forward with their lives
- an attitude that silence is survival
- exhaustion from training and re-training Qallunaat (southern) educators about how to live in the North and understand Inuit culture
- a feeling of powerlessness among many Inuit
- a feeling of being second class in their own home
- a sense of anomie, which results from low self-esteem, alcohol or drug abuse, and physical, psychological, and sexual abuse
- unemployment (particularly for men) and poverty
- a complex bureaucracy that operates mostly in English
- decision makers who don't understand the culture or context
- institutions that don't reflect Inuit beliefs and values, or ways of knowing, being, or doing (25 pp1–2)

The findings were immensely important. They clearly identified some of the reasons that Inuit learners, and teachers, regardless of the level in the educational system, continued to have difficulty succeeding educationally. It was clear that in spite of the positive changes taking place, education remained largely colonial in its structures, approaches, teaching methods, and ways of organizing schools. Sufficient numbers of Inuit teachers were not finding the conditions in the school system conducive to the emergence of Inuit leadership. Adequate supports were needed for the school system to become more solidly founded on Inuit ways of knowing, doing, and being, as *Inuqatigiit* had suggested. Addressing the very deep-rooted and hidden issues related to colonization was evidently going to be necessary if the school system was to become more Inuit based; however, achieving this across the entire educational system in Nunavut was a significant challenge in 2000 and continues to require ongoing strategic support.

Even in Nunavut, where there is a settled land claim and an 84 per cent Inuit majority, and in spite of the gradual improvements, having supports for Inuit fully implemented is held back by many factors, including the persistence of lower educational levels. The Northwest Territories Land Claims Commission captured this pervasive and ongoing influence when it wrote, "Self-determination and the perpetuation of colonialism are mutually exclusive" (26 p21). In spite of the best efforts of many individuals and the divisional boards of education, as well as the ongoing efforts of the Nunavut Department of Education to develop Inuit educational leaders, the negative impact of colonizing influences in the school system seems to be a perennial issue. For deeper change to take place, Inuit identity, ways of being, and Inuktut need to be a central focus in the school system. Addressing these foundational issues in a systemic way over time is challenging but necessary if substantive change is to take place. It is clear that changes cannot be implemented without ensuring that strong and fully supported Inuit leadership is actively encouraged across the educational system.

In early 2017, a Nunavut government review of the 2008 Education Act proposed a 10-year extension to implementing the teaching of Inuktut in Nunavut schools, from 2020 to 2030. The review also proposed changes to the 2008 Inuit Language Protection Act that gave every parent or guardian "the right to have his or her child receive Inuit language instruction" to "the right to receive the majority of the child's school instruction in the Inuit language" (27). The proposal weakens the support for Inuktut in Nunavut and threatens the survival of one of the three strongest Indigenous languages in Canada. This change received significant criticism. Ensuring that Inuktut survives as a vibrant language depends a great deal on having the language taught in the schools (28). However, in July 2019, Statistics Canada published a study related to the evolution of Inuktut in Nunavut (29). While it reported that "a growing percentage of the Inuit population do not have Inuktut as their mother tongue," it also reported that the number of people "who used Inuktut at work increased from 58% to 61%" (29). These data indicate that the policies related to increasing the use of Inuktut in Nunavut are starting to have a positive impact on the retention of the language.

In spite of successful efforts to develop a strong teacher education program in Nunavut and offering many successful community-based teacher education programs and the two iterations of the Nunavut MEd program offered by the University of Prince Edward Island, transforming the educational system in Nunavut from one dominated by Euro-Canadian languages and culture to one that is more Inuit based, with Inuktut being taught on an equal footing with English, is an ongoing process. It is difficult to maintain high numbers of Inuit teachers in schools when the Nunavut government needs highly qualified Inuit in many positions. The formation of the Nunavut government on 1 April 1999 drew and continues to draw many degree-holding Inuit from teaching positions into other positions in the Nunavut government and in non-government Inuit organizations.

Education is a complex process in any society. Educators in Nunavut are called upon to teach children and young people in ways that help them to learn, think, speak, read, write, compute, and fully express themselves in two languages across a range of traditional and non-traditional subject areas and curriculum topics established primarily in and by mainstream, Eurocentric school systems, particularly at the secondary-school level. In an online publication in *Inuit Studies* in 2009, and based on a survey of teachers at the secondary level, Lynn Alyward concludes that "Nunavut schooling is a deeply intercultural process for all. The cultural crossings are unique to each participant's perspective. Inuit and non-Inuit educators and students must stretch their approaches in ways unfamiliar to themselves, and in ways that cause great discomfort and, in some cases, tremendous stress" (30 para32).

Many creative and forward-looking initiatives, including the development of culturally based education programs and the publication of books in Inuktut, continue to take place. Students are involved in activities on the land, sea, ice, and snow. However, education is delivered to groups of students, sometimes large groups of students with multiple and challenging needs that prove to be difficult to address consistently over time. This makes it hard to move graduation levels closer to national levels. Maintaining order and discipline in a classroom based on expectations drawn from southern educational systems can create misunderstandings. Teachers may use counterproductive disciplinary measures, resulting in behaviour issues in the classroom (31). Discipline involves the use of power. Michel Foucault refers to the "point where power reaches into the very grain of individuals, touches their bodies and inserts itself into their actions and attitudes, their discourses, learning processes and everyday lives" (32 p39). It is within the "regime of its exercise *within* the social body" (32 p39) that the power of colonialism is felt, is enacted, and exerts control over any colonized population. In an Inuit context in the Canadian Arctic, this influence can be felt as a biopsychosocial form of violence. It seeks to shape identity, voice, and subjectivity, but it can also be named and resisted within anti-colonial educational experiences, such as the Nunavut MEd program, and in the classrooms of teachers committed to decolonizing educational practices (33).

Research Findings Related to High Schools in Nunavut

Funding from ArcticNet from 2010 to 2015 enabled a team of researchers to complete case studies of two high schools in Nunavut. Attagoyuk School in Pangnirtung and Quluaq School in Clyde River were selected. Experienced Inuit principals were guiding each of these schools when the research took place, and in Pangnirtung a co-principalship allowed for a close and collaborative relationship between an Inuk and non-Inuit principal. The research team completed a documentary video to disseminate the results of the research more widely than is possible through academic publications. The documentary video allowed participants to share their stories from their own perspectives in their own language. *Going Places: Preparing Inuit High School Students for a Changing, Wider World* (34) was created in Inuktut with English subtitles. Both schools were places where bilingual education was clearly evident up to the high school level. High numbers of Inuit staff worked in both these schools, enabling Inuktut and English to be used interchangeably in a way that reflected the bilingual and bicultural vision that was clearly laid out at the start of the Nunavut 2008 Education Act (35), which states:

1. The public education system in Nunavut shall be based on Inuit societal values and the principles and concepts of Inuit Qaujimajatuqangit …
2. The following guiding principles and concepts of Inuit Qaujimajatuqangit apply under this Act:

    a. Inuuqatigiitsiarniq (respecting others, relationships and caring for people);
    b. Tunnganarniq (fostering good spirit by being open, welcoming and inclusive);
    c. Pijitsirniq (serving and providing for family or community, or both);
    d. Aajiiqatigiinniq (decision making through discussion and consensus);
    e. Pilimmaksarniq or Pijariuqsarniq (development of skills through practice, effort and action);
    f. Piliriqatigiinniq or Ikajuqtigiinniq (working together for a common cause);
    g. Qanuqtuurniq (being innovative and resourceful); and
    h. Avatittinnik Kamatsiarniq (respect and care for the land, animals and the environment) …

3. It is the responsibility of the Minister, the district education authorities and the education staff to ensure that Inuit societal values and the principles and concepts of Inuit Qaujimajatuqangit are incorporated throughout, and fostered by, the public education system.

While there is no reference to Inuktut in this section of the Act, Inuit values are shared and transmitted intergenerationally between and among Inuit as they use their own language to interact and live their lives. When the language is actively used, the *Inuit Qaujimajatuqangit* values are maintained. Many Inuit educators and Elders who speak Inuktut are needed in schools in order to achieve these goals.

The schools in Pangnirtung and Clyde River were selected for this research because they were led by Inuit principals who based their leadership practices on Inuit values in committed and effective ways that were deeply compelling. Using the approach of "a day in the life" of a student in each school, videotaped interviews with students, the school principals, staff, the district education authority (DEA) members, and Elders reveal remarkable congruence between the *Inuit Qaujimajatuqangit* vision and educational practices. Eva, a 19-year-old student in Pangnirtung, told the researchers that she is "trying to finish school for my son's sake" (34).

Attagoyuk School provided a daycare right in the school so that Eva can visit her son at lunchtime and during breaks. Lena Metuq, the co-principal in Attagoyuk School and at that time the longest-serving Inuit principal in Nunavut, stated, "We try to incorporate *Inuit Qaujimajatuqangit* into everything we do" (34). She mentions that positive relations are encouraged at the school and that a "welcoming" environment is modelled. Positive relationships mirror the kind of experiences desired by the students who wanted kindness and safety in their schools. At Quluaq School in Clyde River, 19-year-old Shawn tells the researchers that he is determined to finish school and travel the world. He says that "people in the community, including my parents and friends, encourage me. This has been tremendous support for me" (34). Shawn continues to comment on the number of people who offer him support and encouragement. Once again, the positive relationships evident in Shawn's comment were visible in Quluaq School, which offers kindergarten to grade 12 programs and provides a gathering centre for the community. The school offers a breakfast program every day, and parents bring their children early so that they can start their school days with a warm meal in a welcoming place. Practising *Pijitsirniq* by serving and providing for family or community, students serve lunch to Elders in the community once a week with food hunted through the school's on-the-land program. Elders are visible in the school, and more than half the staff is Inuit. Jukeepa Hainnu, the principal at the time of the research, grew up in the community and started her career as an educator in 1982. The variety of roles she had held in the school had provided her with a wide range of experience and had earned her the respect of the community and the DEA. Strong evidence of a shared vision for the school is visible between the Elders, DEA members, parents, Inuit staff, the principal, and students and is recorded in the documentary. The chair of the DEA in Clyde River, Jacob Jaypoody, noted that Jukeepa "follows Inuit traditional methods, the Inuit way in the school" (34). Jukeepa herself sees this as central because she uses traditional Inuit discipline to resolve issues. Bobby Joanas, a language specialist who teaches the high school classes in Inuktut, purports that practising *Inuit Qaujimajatuqangit* involves "a way of being that incorporates respect for everything" (34). Igah Hainnu, another language specialist, stresses that "if we really love them (the students) they will learn Inuit values" (34). This love is needed by the students and helps them to succeed and feel special, as suggested by Joanne Tompkins in her work as a visionary principal (36). In the documentary video made in Clyde River, Geela Paniloo, a high school student, spoke positively about the values she learns through "advice" from the Elders who teach the students (34).

Meeka Arnaquq, a highly respected Elder and DEA member in Pangnirtung comments on the impact of suicide on the spirit and well-being of the students: "These losses of family members and friends really stunted the growth of our young people, I mean emotionally. They should be exuberant and positive, and instead, they are beaten by grief and shell-shocked from losing family and friends. It has drastically changed their outlook on life. The happiest years in their lives have been taken away from them" (34). Students who are affected by suicides, grief, colonial impacts, high rates of pregnancy, food insecurity, and the worries related to low socio-economic levels found in many overcrowded homes do not need to encounter teachers who are punitive and harsh. Instead, they need to be understood and supported.

The ArcticNet research project enabled the creation of a second research-based documentary video *Alluriarniq/Stepping Forward: Youth Perspectives on High School Education in Nunavut* (3). Young people from Pangnirtung, Rankin Inlet, and Kugluktuk, as well as some attending an award-winning program in Ottawa called Nunavut Sivuniksavut, participated in interviews focused on what had helped them succeed in school (11). The young people who were interviewed expressed passionate beliefs about the importance of Inuit culture, language loss, peer pressure, teachers, postsecondary education, feelings after leaving high school, and hopes for the future. A theme in *Alluriarniq*, identity, reveals one of the most pervasive issues in Inuit education. The testimony stresses the importance of being Inuit and embracing an Inuit identity. Students mentioned the influence of their grandparents, who helped the students understand their Inuit history. They believed that having Inuit content in many subject areas strengthens their sense of who they are in the world as Inuit. Providing opportunities for Inuit students to learn about their own culture, throat sing, and perform drum dances, as has taken place at the Nunavut Sivuniksavut program since 1985, enables students to share and generate pride in their Inuit identity.

A clear example of how to reach and teach Inuit students is provided by Joanne Tompkins (6). The educational approaches that were used in Anurapaktuq

School include the use of planning teams to create units that were shared across the school to teach skills at different levels in the curriculum. The unit themes were relevant to students, making the learning real and interesting. Supports with planning and teaching were provided to all teachers, teaching assistants, and Inuit staff who worked together as equal partners in the planning and teaching process. Small-group instruction was provided to students to work on specific skills. A large number of Inuit worked at the school. The principal, teachers, and teaching assistants worked closely with the members of the community education council, and parents were welcomed to the school to participate in support groups offered by the teachers. Inuktut was used extensively throughout the school to ensure that balanced bilingualism was practised. Tompkins provided a concrete example of what is possible for all schools in Nunavut. The minister of education visited this school and was so pleased with what he witnessed that he commissioned a documentary video, *Together We Can Make a Difference* (37), to ensure that the practices used at the school could be widely disseminated. Unfortunately, this video is now very hard to locate, but Tompkins's book (6) is still available.

In spite of the successes documented in Clyde River, Pangnirtung, and the school program described by Tompkins, implementing systemic educational change in Nunavut has proven difficult. Exceptionally successful schools, teachers, and programs are found every year in Nunavut, but maintaining long-term success requires that capable and skilled educational leaders and teachers, both Inuit and non-Inuit, stay in the communities and continue to offer interesting, innovative, creative, and relevant programs to students.

We know from the examples documented in this chapter that success is unquestionably possible. What we also understand is that leadership, particularly Inuit leadership, is needed at all levels in the school system, but most of all within the schools. Successful principals and teachers need to be supported and encouraged. Inuit teachers in particular need opportunities to develop and gain confidence in leadership roles and to be guided when they take on those roles. They also need access to resources and ongoing professional education if they are to make and sustain the changes that will enable them to stay in challenging leadership roles and help students in their schools to succeed.

Conclusion

Examples of best practices that enable and facilitate educational success in Inuit Nunangat are available in books and documentary videos. These and other educational successes achieved in any Inuit Nunangat context need to be documented and shared widely. Ongoing teacher education and professional learning opportunities offered to educators across Inuit Nunangat need to incorporate these successful approaches and methods into courses, workshops, conferences, and professional development sessions. Then, when Inuit educators start their careers or take on leadership roles or when southern teachers arrive in Nunavut, they already know about the examples of success, which will enable them to understand the kind of teaching and leadership that can reach members of Inuit communities. Promising Inuit teachers can visit communities where successful school leaders are creating positive change that leads to higher numbers of Inuit graduates. In addition, providing time and space for educators in schools to discuss, think about, and improve practice is vital. Teaching skills develop over years of practice and through processes of trial and error. Reflecting on successes and challenges in safe spaces and sharing with colleagues is critical, particularly for teachers new to the profession.

To take on leadership roles, Inuit educators need consistent and genuine support and encouragement from other experienced Inuit leaders. This must be part of the educational leadership opportunities provided in partnership with the Department of Education. "Low education levels are linked with poor health, more stress and lower self-confidence" (38 para4). The National Strategy on Inuit Education provided a template for change, hope, and ongoing success in education across Inuit Nunangat. This success is necessary for Inuit, as for any other people, to thrive emotionally, mentally, and physically. The strategy addresses the support that is needed from schools, families, educators, and communities to achieve this success. Education gives people access to employment and to higher levels of education, which provides graduates with access to employment in which the employee has more autonomy. Employment generally results in higher income and social status, all of which improve the likelihood of better health (38). However, the benefit of social support has a far wider reach: "Social support networks, and greater support from families, friends and communities is linked to better health, [as is] a strong cultural connection" (38 para4).

REFERENCES

1. National Coalition on Inuit Education. First Canadians, Canadians first: national strategy on Inuit education 2011. Ottawa (ON): Inuit Tapiriit Kanatami; 2011.
2. McGregor HE. Inuit Qaujimajatuqangit and the transformation of high school education in Nunavut: history, context and statistical profiles of Attagoyuk and Quluaq schools. Iqaluit (NU): Government of Nunavut; 2011.
3. Walton F, Wheatley K, Sandiford, M. Alluriarniq/stepping forward: Youth perspectives on high school education in Nunavut [Internet]. Charlottetown (PE): University of Prince Edward Island; 2012 [cited 2017 Nov 10]. Video: 32 min. Available from: http://www.isuma.tv/es/nunavut-education/alluriarniq-stepping-forward-english

4. Berger P. Eurocentric roadblocks to school change in Nunavut. Inuit Studies. 2009;33(1/2):55–76.
5. Berger P, Epp JR. Practices against culture that "work" in Nunavut schools: problematizing two common practices. McGill J Educ. 2006 Jan 1;41(1):9–27.
6. Tompkins J. Teaching in a cold and windy place: change in an Inuit school. Toronto (ON): University of Toronto Press; 1998.
7. Tompkins J. Tuqqatarviunirmut katimajiit. Geese flying in a northern sky. Paper presented at: American Educational Research Association Annual Meeting; 1999 April 19–23; Montreal, Canada.
8. Tompkins J, Orr J. "It could take 40 minutes – It could take three days": authentic small group learning for Aboriginal education. In: Craig JC, Deretchin FL, editors. The teacher education handbook XVII: teacher learning in small group settings. Lantham (MD): Scarecrow Education; 2009. p. 261–77.
9. Tompkins J, McAuley A, Walton F. Protecting embers to light the qulliit of Inuit learning in Nunavut communities. Inuit Studies. 2009 Jan;33(1/2):95–113.
10. Arnaquq N. Uqaujjuusiat: gifts of words of advice: schooling, education, and leadership in Baffin Island. In: Walton F, O'Leary D, editors. Sivumut – towards the future together: Inuit women educational leaders in Nunavut and Nunavik. Toronto (ON): Women's Press; 2015. p. 11–28.
11. Hanson M. Inuit youth and ethnic identity change: the Nunavut Sivuniksavut experience. Ottawa (ON): University of Ottawa; 2003.
12. Rodon T, Lévesque, F, Kennedy-Dalseg, S. Qallunaaliaqtut: Inuit students experiences of postsecondary education in the south. McGill J Educ. 2015;50(1):1–16.
13. Statistics Canada. Focus on geography series, 2016 Census. Ottawa (ON): Statistics Canada; 2017. Catalogue No.: 98-404-X2016001.
14. Statistics Canada [Internet]. Ottawa (ON): Statistics Canada; [updated 2017 Nov]. Education highlight tables, 2016 Census; [updated 2017 Nov; cited 2020 Jan 16]. Available from: https://www12.statcan.gc.ca/census-recensement/2016/dp-pd/hlt-fst/edu-sco/Table.cfm?Lang=E&T=11&Geo=00&View=2&Age=2
15. Milestone report: national strategy on Inuit education – interim report on milestones 2012–2014. Ottawa (ON): Amaujaq National Centre for Inuit Education; 2014.
16. Fullan M. Freedom to change: four strategies to put your inner drive into overdrive. San Francisco (CA): Jossey-Bass; 2015.
17. The Truth and Reconciliation Commission of Canada. Honouring the truth, reconciling for the future: final report truth and reconciliation commission of Canada. Winnipeg (MB): University of Manitoba; 2015.
18. McGregor HE. Inuit education and schools in the eastern Arctic. Vancouver (BC): UBC Press; 2010.
19. Government of Northwest Territories, Department of Education, Curriculum Division. Elementary education in the Northwest Territories: a handbook for

curriculum development. Yellowknife (NT): Northwest Territories Department of Education, Curriculum Division; 1972.
20. Department of Education, Government of Northwest Territories. Learning in the middle years: a handbook for curriculum development. Yellowknife (NT): Canarctic Publishing; 1973.
21. Snow, K, O'Gorman, M, Tulloch, S, Ochalski, H. Supporting professional development and resilience for Inuit teachers in the Canadian Arctic. Educ North. 2018;25(1–2):108–34.
22. Northwest Territories Legislative Assembly, Special Committee on Education. Learning: tradition and change in the Northwest Territories. Yellowknife (NT): Northwest Territories Legislative Assembly; 1981.
23. Baffin Divisional Board of Education. Piniaqtavut: integrated program. Yellowknife (NT): Government of Northwest Territories; 1989.
24. Government of Northwest Territories, Department of Education, Culture and Employment. Inuuqatigiit: the curriculum from the Inuit perspective. Yellowknife (NT): Government of Northwest Territories; 1996.
25. Tompkins J. Tuqqatarviunirmut katimajiit: the Nunavut educational leadership project report. Iqaluit (NU): Nunavut Department of Education; 2000 May.
26. Northwest Territories Inuit Land Claims Commission. Inuit Nunangat – the people's land: A struggle for survival. Ottawa (ON): Northwest Territories Inuit Land Claims Commission; 1978.
27. Zerehi, SS. Nunavut's Education Act report a step backwards, says languages commissioner. CBC News [Internet]. 2015 Nov 16 [cited 2017 Nov 10]. Available from: https://www.cbc.ca/news/canada/north/nunavut-education-act-review-sandra-inutiq-1.3321035
28. Minogue, S. Facing Inuit teacher shortages, Nunavut education minister wants to move deadlines on bilingual instruction. CBC News [Internet]. 2017 Mar 13 [updated 2017 Mar 14; cited 2017 Nov 10]. Available from: http://www.cbc.ca/news/canada/north/bill-37-nunavut-education-act-language-protection-act-1.4020945
29. Lepage JF, Langlois S, Turcotte M. Evolution of the language situation in Nunavut, 2001 to 2016 [Internet]. Ottawa (ON): Statistics Canada; 2019 Jul 9 [updated 2019 Sep 3; cited 2019 Nov 10]. Available from: https://www150.statcan.gc.ca/n1/pub/89-657-x/89-657-x2019010-eng.htm
30. Aylward ML. Culturally relevant schooling in Nunavut: Views of secondary school educators. Inuit Studies. 2010 Nov 19;33(1–2):77–93.
31. Brody H. The people's land: Eskimos and whites in the eastern Arctic. Harmondsworth (GB): Penguin Books; 1975.
32. Foucault M. Power/knowledge: selected interviews and other writings, 1972–1977. Gordon C, editor. New York (NY): Pantheon Books; 1980.
33. McGregor HE. An Arctic encounter with Indigenous and non-Indigenous youth as pedagogy for historical consciousness and decolonizing. Hist Encount. 2018 Jun 28;5(1):90–101.

34. Sandiford M. Going places: preparing Inuit high school students for a changing, wider world [Internet]. Charlottetown (PE): University of Prince Edward Island, Faculty of Education; 2011 [cited 2017 Nov 10]. Video: 28:18 min. Available from: http://www.youtube.com/watch?v=E9m4GsbkGyc
35. Government of Nunavut. Chapter 15: Education Act [Internet]. Iqaluit (NU): Government of Nunavut; 2008 Sept 18 [cited 2017 Nov 10]. Available from: https://www.gov.nu.ca/sites/default/files/e2008snc15.pdf
36. Tompkins J. Sivuniksamut ilinniarniq: Nunavut student survey. Iqaluit (NU): Nunavut Department of Education; 2003.
37. Baffin Divisional Board of Education. Together we can make a difference. Iqaluit (NU): Baffin Divisional Board of Education; 1992.
38. World Health Organization [Internet]. Geneva (CH): World Health Organization; 2017. The determinants of health; [updated 2017; cited 2017 June 11]. Available from: https://www.who.int/hia/evidence/doh/en/

2 Food and Health: Food Security, Food Systems, and Health in Northern Canada

REBECCA SCHIFF AND VICTORIA SCHEMBRI

Introduction

Food insecurity has become increasingly recognized as a significant issue in northern health research and policy. Over the past decade, numerous government and academic reports have emerged, documenting the severity of this issue for people living in the Canadian North, especially for northern Indigenous communities. These include comprehensive reports documenting considerable issues in northern food systems, such as those published by the Council of Canadian Academies (CCA) (1) and Canada's Public Policy Forum (2). While the federal government has attempted to alleviate food insecurity in the North, for example, through the Nutrition North program, reports produced by the auditor general (3) and a statement by the United Nations (UN) special rapporteur on the right to food (4) have identified faults with those programs. Others have noted that not only are there faults within these programs but that they have also failed to provide a comprehensive response to food security concerns (1,5).

This chapter begins with an examination of the current state of northern food security and the health effects of food issues for northern residents. The chapter then examines some of the proposed approaches to solving the crisis of northern food insecurity, including a review and critical analysis of the discourse of food sovereignty as an approach to resolving northern food issues.

Before venturing into this discussion, however, we want to situate ourselves, to present our positionality in our approach to this issue, the surrounding discourse, and the source of our involvement (as non-Indigenous researchers) in research with Indigenous communities.

We are two non-Indigenous researchers writing on Indigenous issues. We are both of non-Indigenous descent. We both live and work in northern Canada and have lived and worked in remote communities; a bit more information about our personal stories can be found at the end of this chapter. We share an awareness of the beauty and strengths of the North, as well as a deep appreciation for the innovation of northerners in addressing the challenges of northern living, challenges often imposed and aggravated by histories of colonization and contemporary manifestations of colonialism. We name our privilege here as non-Indigenous white researchers to identify our positionality in this work and our understanding that the information shared here is filtered through our lenses and interpretations as researchers of non-Indigenous descent.

Prevalence of Food (In)Security among Northern and Northern Indigenous Communities in Canada

For decades, researchers have been documenting the disproportionately high rates of food insecurity experienced by northerners and particularly the extreme circumstances in northern First Nations and Inuit communities. Since there has been no consistent measurement and reporting of food insecurity rates across the North (i.e., including the Provincial and Territorial Norths), we present a compilation of different studies that have attempted to measure northern food insecurity in different locations. Early studies, such as those by Lawn and Harvey in 2003 (6), found that 83 per cent of households in Kugaaruk (Nunavut) experienced food insecurity; a staggering 10 times the rate experienced by the general Canadian population in 2004 (7). The Inuit Health Survey (8) conducted in 2007 and 2008 (which included 36 communities from the Inuvialuit Settlement Region in the western Arctic, Nunavut, and Nunatsiavut) revealed similar high rates of food insecurity: 62.6 per cent of households were food insecure. Reports from this survey also described different levels of food insecurity, including measurements for marginal, moderate, and severe food insecurity.[1] Among the 62.6 per cent of food insecure households in the Inuit Health Survey, 33.6 per cent were moderately food insecure and 29.1 per cent were severely food insecure. Compared to the 2004 rates for the general Canadian population of 5.1 per cent (moderate food insecurity) and 2.7 per cent (severe), these findings indicated that moderate and severe food insecurity in the Arctic were 8–10 times the Canadian average. While the data on food insecurity in the Provincial North are more limited, research on food insecurity among First Nations households in northern Manitoba and northern Ontario also identified extremely high rates: 75 per cent and 70 per cent of households, respectively, were found to be food insecure (9,10). Other reports such as those produced by the CCA (1) and PROOF[2] (11) confirm the inordinately high rates of food insecurity and, particularly, moderate and severe food insecurity experienced in the North and by households in northern Indigenous communities.

Food Insecurity Impacts on Health for Northern Communities

Food is recognized as a determinant of health for Canadians, in a general context (12) and as an important proximal determinant of health for Indigenous peoples (13). The CCA report points to the serious and adverse health impacts of food insecurity in northern Indigenous communities, linking the lack of fresh, healthy, and affordable food of good quality in the North to rising rates of chronic illnesses, such as cardiovascular disease, diabetes, and some cancers (1). Numerous other studies have documented the relationship between food insecurity among Indigenous people and health behaviours and outcomes, such as obesity, (14) poor general health, (15) high stress (15,16), poor diet, (8) and smoking (16). Moreover, studies point out that severe food insecurity experienced during childhood could have lasting effects on health outcomes later in life (17). Food insecurity has been clearly documented as leading to poor nutritional health and related physical health risks for northern Indigenous communities (1). While food security is documented as a significant proximal determinant of health for Indigenous people in Canada, (13) there is also clear evidence that food insecurity negatively impacts other determinants of health, including economic, social, and mental health domains (1,16).

Factors Limiting Food Security for Northern and Northern Indigenous Communities

The circumstances contributing to higher rates of food security in the North are many and complex. Northern communities experience food security issues that are unique and specific to their locations. Northerners often use a combination of store-bought foods, foods grown within or near communities, and hunted or harvested foods (which some Indigenous communities refer to as *country foods* or *traditional foods*) to meet their needs. Numerous factors limit northerners' access to each of these sources of foods, seriously affecting food security. In the following section, we examine these limiting factors.

Issues in Accessibility, Availability, and Quality of Store-Bought Food

One factor affecting access to safe, healthy, and adequate food for northerners is transportation. Particularly for remote communities, long-distance transportation has a significant impact on the availability, quality, and cost of store-bought foods. Fuel and other costs associated with transportation contribute to food costs that are substantially higher than in Canada's urban centres (18–21). While food costs are higher in northern communities when compared to their southern counterparts, costs in less accessible northern communities are even higher. In other words, food costs are inconsistent across the North such that more remote communities (such as Old Crow, Nain, Pangnirtung, and Resolute) experience much higher costs than those found in northern urban centres such as Yellowknife and Whitehorse. The high cost of retail foods is compounded by low incomes for a considerable number of households in the north; these households face additional economic pressures in affording healthy foods (20–21).

A number of reports over the past 20 years have documented significant concerns related to the quality and availability of fresh foods (1,20–22). Poor quality and availability of fresh foods is mainly linked to challenges in keeping foods fresh during long-distance transportation and adverse weather conditions, which can lead to freezing in cold periods and spoilage in warmer periods (23). Many remote Indigenous communities depend entirely on ferry and plane services to transport food. As a result, the quality and availability of food is frequently compromised. During summer, availability is more reliable in some communities where food can be transported via seasonal roads. However, residents report that the quality of food is poorer since transport by road leads to lengthier transportation times (23).

Issues Impacting Community-Based Food Production

Northern climates and ecologies create challenges for community-based food production. Several factors limit the ability to produce or acquire food through gardening, farming, and fishing in northern communities. Short growing seasons, light levels, permafrost, and poor soil quality impact the capacity to grow food (24,25). Despite an abundance of water, some communities face irrigation challenges because of water quality issues caused by lack of water treatment infrastructure (26). Other communities experience difficulty in accessing safe water for irrigation because of other issues, such as the impact of industrial development, mining, and hydroelectric projects on water quality (21,27). Access to agricultural and fishing supplies is also limited (in terms of cost and selection) because of the same issues that affect store-bought food prices and selection (25,28).

Traditional or Country Foods and Food Security in Northern Canada

For many Indigenous peoples in the North, *traditional* or *country* foods play critical nutritional and cultural roles. Traditional and country foods include foods acquired through hunting, fishing, trapping, and gathering. Access to, consumption of, and sharing of traditional food, such as caribou, moose, fish, and wild berries, have been shown to improve food security and provide social benefits (1). Activities associated with traditional food acquisition preparation also provide spiritual connection to the land, the community, and the past (29).

They have important effects on emotional, mental, and spiritual health (23,30). Moreover, activities related to the procurement, processing, and consumption of traditional food reinforce cultural expressions of identity and pride (30).

CHANGES IN TRADITIONAL AND COUNTRY FOOD PROCUREMENT SYSTEMS OVER THE PAST CENTURY

Colonial activities, including the residential school system, among others, have had a significant impact on traditional food systems. Among the numerous adverse impacts, resettlement and residential schools impaired the transmission of knowledge about traditional food systems and traditional ways of living.

Over the past century, government legislation imposed restrictions on hunting and fishing practices, which diminished communities' control over their lands. Changes in the abundance and distribution of food species because of human-induced environmental changes affected availability of and access to country foods. Through industrialization and globalization, store-bought foods began to appear in northern communities, creating an increased reliance on imported market foods alongside a decrease in the consumption of traditional foods (30,31). From a traditional food diet rich in nutrients, Indigenous peoples in northern Canada have undergone a shift to a diet relying heavily on store-bought foods high in carbohydrates, such as starches and sugar. This has led to dietary issues because of the poor quality, variety, and high cost of market foods (23). With this shift, several diet-related diseases appeared. Poor dental health, chronic constipation, and vitamin deficiencies emerged as early as the middle of the nineteenth century (32.) More recently, chronic diseases such as type 2 diabetes, high blood pressure, and dyslipidemia have significantly affected health for Indigenous communities in the North (1).

Nonetheless, amid these tremendous changes, traditional and country food systems have continued to play a crucial role in the lives of people living in northern Canada generally and Indigenous peoples specifically. The harvest of country foods is still vital to community and individual well-being (33). It strengthens social networks; fosters cultural pride and continuity; connects people to the land and with the past; promotes emotional, mental, and spiritual health; enables the transmission of cultural values, skills, and spirituality; and contributes to the economies of communities.

Strategies to Address Food Security in Northern Canadian Indigenous Communities

Much of the research on food strategies in the North has focused on store-bought and country foods. Several public health nutrition programs have attempted to address food insecurity and associated nutritional inadequacies in northern and northern Indigenous communities. These include strategies such as Healthy Foods North, the Ontario Diabetes Prevention program, and the federal Nutrition North program (34–39). These strategies have attempted to improve food security by addressing the issue of store-bought foods with some, although quite limited, attention to traditional food access. Reports by the CCA and Auditor General of Canada (30,32) have indicated concerns over the effectiveness of the federal Nutrition North program and other market-based approaches. There are other problems with programs focused primarily on nutritional outcomes and market foods. These concerns include the inadequacy of programs that fail to attend to other structural factors (geopolitical issues, neocolonialism) contributing to northern food insecurity.

A focus on market activities often ignores the important historical and current roles of country foods and community-based food production for many northern communities (40,41). The focus on market activities and nutritional outcomes also often fails to recognize the impacts of colonialism on food security in northern Indigenous communities. Neocolonialism has manifested through exclusion in resource and policy discussions and ignored ongoing issues related to Indigenous land rights and private property ownership, which affect traditional food production and procurement practices (42–44). This exclusion, and resulting policy and resource development decisions, have impacted the ability of Indigenous communities to transfer knowledge of traditional methods across generations, including the ability to produce, acquire, and use food resources in culturally relevant ways. The downstream effect has had a significant impact on food insecurity.

More recently, some promising approaches to supporting community-based food production and country food systems have been documented. In the North, many communities are indeed reviving traditional gardening practices and experimenting with new practices and technologies (e.g., greenhouses) to mitigate climatic limitations on growing seasons (41,44–47). There are emerging examples of northern greenhouse projects contributing to food security and a range of health and other community benefits. In Inuvik, Northwest Territories, a greenhouse has shown very promising results: it has increased civic pride, increased tourism, strengthened a sense of community, encouraged community development, and increased food security. Similarly, a greenhouse project in Fort Albany, Ontario, had positive effects on those directly and indirectly involved in the garden (i.e., it provided seeds to home gardeners, and the compost system reduced community waste) (45).

In addition to community-based food production and fishing, innovative programs are emerging that address some of the barriers to accessing and consuming country foods. Community freezer and harvest support programs have been implemented in many northern, primarily Indigenous, communities, and they have demonstrated success in fostering food security, as well as contributing to other determinants of health (1). Community freezer programs help to preserve country foods (e.g., fish, game, and berries) donated by community hunters and are made available to Elders in communities or other community members who have limited capacity to fish, hunt, trap, and gather. Other community hunting/fishing programs financially support individuals with hunting and fishing skills to gather fish and game that can be shared with other community members. Some programs, such as Going Off, Growing Strong in Nunatsiavut, have combined freezers and community hunter programs with skill sharing programs (aimed at transfer of traditional knowledge to younger generations) and demonstrated promising food security and other health-related outcomes (48).

While there are promising developments in terms of community gardening and country food strategies, more work is needed in this area. As well, it is necessary to adopt an approach that recognizes that these communities represent a diversity of cultures and circumstances. This diversity, we suggest, indicates a need for a three-pronged approach that considers the roles of country, store-bought, and community-produced foods within community food systems. Schiff and Brunger (40) examined the potential of community-led planning processes, using a "whole of food system" lens, for creating effective three-pronged approaches to foster healthier northern food systems. Food planning efforts will need to be attentive to the experiences of the people on the ground – experiences that are integral to truly addressing and understanding northern food insecurity. Most significantly, these approaches need to also focus on goals of decolonization and reconciliation for northern Indigenous peoples.

Decolonizing Food Security Strategies in the North: Considering Food Sovereignty in the Context of Self-Determination for Northern Communities

Some academics and advocates argue that a politicized conversation is essential when discussing northern food issues and that the terms *food security* and even *community food security* fall short of understanding (and, subsequently, can even propagate) the imbalanced power relations and historical injustice that produce food insecurity (42,45,49,50). They propose the concept of *food sovereignty* as a means and a goal to achieving healthy and sustainable food systems. The term *food sovereignty* can be interpreted as "the right of peoples to healthy and culturally appropriate food produced through ecologically sound and sustainable methods, and their right to define their own food and agriculture systems" (36, p47). Food sovereignty embraces collective self-determination and as such, it has resonated with and been embraced by Indigenous communities and is echoed in the literature (44,49–52).

Food sovereignty calls attention to the crucial roles that disenfranchisement, colonization, and a lack of community agency have played in undermining northern food systems. Past and current colonial policy and practice has produced and reproduced food insecurity both historically and through contemporary actions and policy. Historically, the production of food insecurity in the North was seen through colonial actions, such as the forced relocation of Nunavik Inuit in the 1950s from traditional hunting and harvesting lands to unfamiliar, less hospitable lands in present-day Nunavut (53). In contemporary terms, neocolonial policy and actions have continued to drive food insecurity (e.g., the federal government of Canada, without consent of affected First Nations communities, proposed plans for a hydroelectric dam in northern British Columbia that will flood agricultural and Indigenous land in the Peace River valley) (54). Government action, or inaction, has also undermined interventions aimed at improving food security. For example, not only does Nutrition North Canada fail to reduce northern food prices to affordable rates, but a lack of transparency and disclosure of how the subsidy reaches northern consumers also inhibits the ability to understand and assess how the program actually functions (54–57).

Food sovereignty highlights the fact that food and the ability to produce and harvest food are highly politicized. Future programs and policy development must recognize that food security for northern communities and northern Indigenous peoples depends on decolonization and self-determination (58). However, while food sovereignty can provide some guidance for future efforts towards the development of policy and processes that protect the rights of northern Indigenous peoples, it must not be regarded as a singular conceptual solution. Since the collective action proposed by food sovereignty discourse can undermine minority voices, we suggest a need to reconsider food sovereignty as a complement rather than a challenge to the dialogue on (community) food security.

Reconsidering Food Sovereignty

Food sovereignty aims to destabilize the colonial foundations of food insecurity that are pertinent to the experiences of northern communities, namely, environmental degradation, dispossession, and political marginalization. But a critical analysis of the food sovereignty discourse reveals some concepts that require further attention. First, scrutiny should be directed towards the "peoples" who define "their own" food systems, seemingly united against an international food system. Across and within Inuit, Métis, and First Nations communities, we must "prob[e] lingering issues of solidarity in food politics across Indigenous-Settler divides" (57, p433) and avoid adopting a framework that "represent[s] culture as a fixed, reified entity, with cultural groups existing in a binary vis-à-vis mainstream culture" (54, p46).

The "self" in self-determination must be deconstructed and cannot be assumed; especially when the cultures, economies, environments, and demographics of the communities of interest are so dynamic. For example, in terms of commodifying country foods, Gombay (59) could not find consensus among the Inuit surveyed in Puvirnituq as to whether country foods should or should not be sold inside and outside the community marketplace because prioritizations of economic and cultural values differed. Selling country foods could encourage traditional hunting and harvesting practices with economic incentives and subsequently promote community livelihoods, but adding economic value could diminish the spiritual value of traditional foods and discourage sharing. This illuminates the tensions in deeming food and practices culturally appropriate or not. Culture and wellness can be interpreted differently by people of the same ethnicity and, as demonstrated, also within the same community, and they can be both barriers to and facilitators of food security (60). Calls for solidarity as proposed through food sovereignty discourse do not necessarily represent democratic approaches to decision making; a focus on democratic processes and Indigenous and marginalized peoples' rights however is certainly warranted.

Assuming that every action against food insecurity needs to be politicized, as food sovereignty frameworks suggest, can also exclude actions and technologies that could hold great potential but do not necessarily possess a political bearing. For example, a partial solution for preserving traditional harvesting and preparation practices could involve interviewing Elders and creating a record of their instructions. Such a solution has been mentioned by Nishnawbe Aski Nation (NAN) at their Food Strategy Collaborative Table Meeting (61). At this meeting, an interest in creating a NAN-Specific Traditional Food Book to "support the preservation and transfer of traditional and local knowledge" (p7) was also identified. A partial solution to high transportation costs of food could involve the use of cargo airships. These can carry bulk loads using less fuel than airplanes, they do not require runways for takeoff and landing (infrastructure that some remote communities lack), and they could lower the cost of transporting food to northern communities by 18 to 55 per cent (1). Though these solutions may not shake the foundations of food insecurity, they can definitely be used in conjunction with larger, transformative projects to provide very tangible (albeit partial) solutions to some of the concerns (i.e., traditional knowledge transfer and cost of food) that pertain to northern Indigenous communities. A staunch food sovereignty framework could potentially overlook these solutions. A descriptive and comprehensive framework, grounded in principles of social justice, sustainability, democratic decision making, and the amplification of the voices of the marginalized, may be the most appropriate way to understand community experiences and possible solutions.

Conclusion: Valuing Individual Identities, Collective Goals, and Community-Led Solutions

Across the North, a lack of agency and community consultation produced food insecurity in the past, continues to do so, and undermines the very interventions aimed at solving these issues. Recognizing the role that disenfranchisement and colonization have played in the history and lives of northern communities has led to calls for self-determination in northern food systems. This advocates for people to determine their own means of acquiring healthy and culturally appropriate foods. However, addressing food security from either a top-down approach or a food sovereignty perspective runs the risk of adopting a framework that cannot address diversity within communities and cultures. Therefore, the elusive "self" that does the determining needs to be explored. Northern lifestyles are dynamic, and their food systems combine modern and traditional modalities. Community-led and bottom-up three-pronged solutions aimed at decolonization and self-determination are necessary for any comprehensive approach to creating healthy and sustainable food systems in the North.

ABOUT REBECCA AND VICTORIA

Rebecca

My introduction at the beginning of this book provides an overview of my interest, in general, in supporting work related to social justice and health equity for northern and Indigenous communities. In addition to this, I have a long history of working on food issues with Indigenous and non-Indigenous communities. My work on food justice and sustainability began almost 20 years ago with a project on urban agriculture and organic food production in Montreal, Quebec. I followed this with a doctoral thesis focused on food policy councils and their role in supporting the development of/transition to sustainable food systems. For many years following my doctoral studies, I was a steering committee member for Food Secure Canada and supported the People's Food Policy Project. I also served on provincial associations such as Food Secure Saskatchewan and local associations such as the Upper Lake Melville Community Food Hub in Labrador, which worked in partnership with Inuit and First Nations organizations and communities in the region. In 2012, I helped write and coordinate the civil society submission to the UN rapporteur on the right to food in advance of his mission to Canada. I spent several years as a board member on the Canadian Association for Food Studies and from 2016 to 2018 served as its president.

Victoria

My name is Victoria (though I prefer to go by Vikki). I am in my mid-20s, a woman, and a second-generation Canadian. I grew up eating meals mostly with grocery store-bought food, with occasional trips to Nono and Nuna's for a freshly hunted moose meal, and daily family dinners. My grandparents came from Europe, although I would say my upbringing and subsequent world view have been influenced most by my membership in a southern Ontario (Milton), urban, Catholic-leaning, middle-income family with two working, post-secondary-educated parents. While completing my degree at the University of Toronto, I spent summers working in Pickle Lake (northern Ontario) as a forest firefighter. When I drove to Pickle, it was the first time I had been north of Barrie, Ontario. I immediately fell in love with the North; but I also noticed some things that were "normal" in the North would be deemed completely unacceptable in the south, particularly, when it came to food: food showed up at the Pickle Lake Northern in less than ideal conditions (i.e., bruised or rotting) and was sold at expensive prices. Plus, it was at least a three-hour drive (one way) to get to the nearest town with a grocery store. I understand food insecurity exists in the south, but it was an experience I had been sheltered against by my parents or had heard about but never really experienced when living in Toronto. Moreover, the severity and normalization of it in the North astounded me. In my studies and (non-academic) travels across Canada, I have learned more about challenges and opportunities for procuring food in the North. I learned more about the role of growing, foraging, hunting, and fishing in northern food systems; the concept of cultural food security; the indelible connection between land sovereignty and food sovereignty that is constantly being fought for by Indigenous communities; and the vicious cycle of food insecurity begetting food-related illnesses, which then begets food insecurity, which disproportionately and more severely impacts Indigenous communities. Most of all, I have spent a lot of time deconstructing "truths" I grew up with to open myself up to relearning what food can mean to different people. I have been pursuing my relearning process through various activities, including but not limited to reading articles, presenting and participating in academic workshops, participating in food ceremonies, sharing meals and stories, conducting interviews, going hunting and fishing, and getting my hands dirty in various gardens.

NOTES

1 The different levels of food insecurity are described by PROOF (11 p4) as "marginal food insecurity: Worry about running out of food and/or limited food selection because of a lack of money for food; moderate food insecurity: Compromise in quality and/or quantity of food due to a lack of money for food; severe food

insecurity: Miss meals, reduce food intake, and at the most extreme go day(s) without food."

2 PROOF (not an acronym) is a team of researchers based at the University of Toronto who research and publish nationwide information on household-level food insecurity in Canada.

REFERENCES

1. Council of Canadian Academies. Aboriginal food security in Northern Canada: an assessment of the state of knowledge [Internet]. Ottawa (ON): Expert Panel on the State of Knowledge of Food Security in Northern Canada; 2014 [cited 2019 Mar 12]. Available from: https://foodsecurecanada.org/sites/foodsecurecanada.org/files/foodsecurity_fullreporten.pdf
2. Canada's Public Policy Forum. Toward food security in Canada's North. Summary report [Internet]. Ottawa (ON): Public Policy Forum; 2015 [cited 2019 Mar 10]. Available from: https://ppforum.ca/wp-content/uploads/2018/05/Toward-Food-Security-in-Canadas-North-PPF-report.pdf
3. Auditor General of Canada. Nutrition North Canada—Aboriginal Affairs and Northern Development Canada. In: 2014 fall report of the auditor general of Canada [Internet]. Ottawa (ON): Office of the Auditor General of Canada; 2014 Nov 6 [cited 2019 Mar 12]. Chapter 6. Available from: http://www.oag-bvg.gc.ca/internet/English/parl_oag_201411_06_e_39964.html
4. De Schutter, O. Report of the special rapporteur on the right to food, Olivier De Schutter: Mission to Canada [Internet]. Geneva (CH): Office of the High Commissioner for Human Rights; 2012 Dec 24 [cited 2019 Mar 12]. Available from: http://www.ohchr.org/Documents/HRBodies/HRCouncil/RegularSession/Session22/AHRC2250Add.1_English.PDF
5. Schiff R, Bernard K. Food systems and Indigenous Peoples in Labrador: issues and new directions. St. John's (NL): Iser Press; 2018.
6. Lawn J, Harvey D. Nutrition and food security in Kugaaruk, Nunavut: baseline survey for the food mail pilot project. Ottawa (ON): Indian and Northern Affairs Canada; 2003.
7. Health Canada. Canadian community health survey, cycle 2.2, nutrition (2004): income-related household food security in Canada. Ottawa (ON): Health Canada; 2007. Catalogue No.: H164-42/2007E-PDF.
8. Huet C, Rosol R, Egeland GM. The prevalence of food insecurity is high and the diet quality poor in Inuit communities. J Nutr. 2012 Mar 1;142(3):541–7
9. Skinner K, Hanning RM, Desjardins E, Tsuji L. Giving voice to food insecurity in a remote Indigenous community in subarctic Ontario, Canada: traditional ways, ways to cope, ways forward. BMC Public Health. 2013 May 2;13(1):427.

10. Thompson S, Kamal AG, Ballard M, Beardy B, Islam D, Lozeznik V, Wong K. Is community economic development putting healthy food on the table? Food Sovereignty in northern Manitoba's Aboriginal communities. J Aborig Econ Dev. 2011;7(2):14–39.
11. Tarasuk V, Mitchell A, Dachner N. Household food insecurity in Canada, 2014 [Internet]. Toronto (ON): Research to identify policy options to reduce food insecurity (PROOF); 2016 [cited 2019 Mar 12]. Available from: http://proof.utoronto.ca/wp-content/uploads/2016/04/Household-Food-Insecurity-in-Canada-2014.pdf
12. Raphael D, editor. Social determinants of health: Canadian perspectives. Toronto (ON): Canadian Scholars' Press; 2009.
13. Reading CL, Wien F. Health inequalities and the social determinants of Aboriginal peoples' health [Internet]. Prince George (BC): National Collaborating Centre for Aboriginal Health; 2009 [cited 2019 Mar 12]. Available from: http://www.ccnsa-nccah.ca/docs/determinants/RPT-HealthInequalities-Reading-Wien-EN.pdf
14. Atikessé L, deGrosbois SB, St-Jean M, Penashue B, Benuen M. Innu food consumption patterns: traditional food and body mass index. Can J Diet Pract Res. 2010 Aug 18;71(3):e41–9.
15. Vozoris NT, Tarasuk VS. Household food insufficiency is associated with poorer health. J Nutr. 2003 Jan 1;133(1):120–6.
16. Willows N, Veugelers P, Raine K, Kuhle S. Associations between household food insecurity and health outcomes in the Aboriginal population (excluding reserves). Health Rep. 2011 Jun; 22(2):15.
17. Pirkle CM, Lucas M, Dallaire R, Ayotte P, Jacobson JL, Jacobson SW, Dewailly E, Muckle G. Food insecurity and nutritional biomarkers in relation to stature in Inuit children from Nunavik. Can J Public Health. 2014;105(4):e233–8.
18. Wendimu MA, Desmarais AA, Martens TR. Access and affordability of "healthy" foods in northern Manitoba? The need for Indigenous food sovereignty. Can Food Stud. 2018 May 23;5(2):44–72.
19. Aboriginal and Northern Affairs [Internet]. Ottawa (ON): Government of Canada; [modified 2010 Sep 15]. Regional results of price surveys [tables]; 2008 [cited 2021 Feb 18]. Available from: https://web.archive.org/web/20120714093300/http://www.aadnc-aandc.gc.ca/eng/1100100035986
20. Boult D. Hunger in the Arctic: food (in)security in Inuit communities: a discussion paper [Internet]. Ottawa (ON): National Aboriginal Health Organization; 2004 Oct [cited 2012 Dec 12]. Available from: https://foodsecurecanada.org/sites/foodsecurecanada.org/files/2004_inuit_food_security.pdf
21. Myers H, Powell S, Duhaime G. Setting the table for food security: policy impacts in Nunavut. Can J Native Stud. 2004;24(2):425–45.
22. Ford JD, Beaumier M. Feeding the family during times of stress: Experience and determinants of food insecurity in an Inuit community. Geogr J. 2011;177(1):44–61.

23. Martin DH, Valcour JE, Bull JR, Graham JR, Paul M, Wall D. NunatuKavut community health needs assessment: A community-based research project – final report [Internet]. Happy Valley-Goose Bay (NL): NunatuKavut Community Council Inc.; 2012 [cited 2012 Dec 8]. Available from: https://www.researchgate.net/profile/Julie-Bull/publication/304998512_NunatuKavut_Community_Health_Needs_Assessment_A_Community-Based_Research_Project/links/592b5cef458515e3d46c9824/NunatuKavut-Community-Health-Needs-Assessment-A-Community-Based-Research-Project.pdf
24. Jóhannesson T. Arctic-quality certification [Internet]. Hvanneyri (IS): Agricultural University of Iceland; 2012 [cited 2017 Apr 10]. Available from: http://www.bioforsk.no/ikbViewer/Content/75386/Torfi%20Proposal_english_revised.pdf
25. Juday G, Barber V, Duffy P, Linderholm H, Rupp S, Sparrow S, Vaganov E, Yarie, J. Agriculture in the Arctic. In: Draggan S, editor. The encyclopedia of the Earth [Internet]. Washington (DC): Environmental Information Coalition and the National Council for Science and the Environment; 2010 [last modified 2012 May 7; cited 2017 Apr 10]. Available from: http://editors.eol.org/eoearth/wiki/Agriculture_in_the_Arctic
26. Sarkar A, Hanrahan M, Hudson A. Water insecurity in Canadian Indigenous communities: some inconvenient truths. Rural Remote Health [Internet]. 2015 [cited 2017 Jan 7];15(3354). Available from: http://www.rrh.org.au
27. Thompson S. Sustainability and vulnerability: Aboriginal Arctic food security in a toxic world. In: Berkes F, Huebert R, Fast H, Manseau M, Diduck A, editors. Breaking ice: renewable resource and ocean management in the Canadian North. Calgary (AB): University of Calgary Press; 2005. p. 47–69.
28. Airhart J, Janes K, Jameson K. Food security – Upper Lake Melville: community-led food assessment, 2010–2011. St. John's (NL): Food Security Network of Newfoundland and Labrador; 2011.
29. Pufall E, Jones AQ, McEwan SA, Lyall C, Peregrine AS, Edge V. Perception of the importance of traditional country foods to the physical, mental, and spiritual health of Labrador Inuit. Arctic. 2011 Jun;64(2):242–50.
30. Martin DH. Food stories: a Labrador Inuit-Métis community speaks about global change [dissertation]. Halifax (NS): Dalhousie University; 2009.
31. Hanrahan M, Sarkar A, Hudson A. Exploring water insecurity in a northern Indigenous community in Canada: The "never-ending job" of the southern Inuit of Black Tickle, Labrador. Arctic Anthropol. 2014;51(2): 9–22. doi: 10.3368/aa.51.2.9
32. Hanrahan M. Tracing social change among the Labrador Inuit and Inuit-Métis: What does the nutrition literature tell us? Food Cult Soc. 2008 Sep 1;11(3):315–33.
33. Nain Research Centre Kaujisapvinga. 2015. Hopedale: Hopedale radar site clean-up; [cited 2017 Apr 10]. Available from: http://nainresearchcentre.com/hopedale/
34. Ober Allen J, Alaimo K, Elam D, Perry E. Growing vegetables and values: benefits of neighborhood-based community gardens for youth development and nutrition. J Hunger Environ Nutr. 2008 Dec 11;3(4):418–39.

35. Pothukuchi K, Kaufman J. The food system: a stranger to the planning field. J Am Plann Assoc. 2000;66(2):113–24.
36. Flowers J, Nochasak S, Jameson K. NiKigijavut Hopedalimi: "Our food in Hopedale" [Internet]. St. John's (NL): The Food Security Network of Newfoundland and Labrador; 2010 Apr 26[2017 Apr 10]. Available from: https://static1.squarespace.com/static/54d9128be4b0de7874ec9a82/t/562d60cce4b0be3276003c49/1445814476631/NiKigijavutHopedalimiReportFINAL.pdf
37. Bennett S, Frank S. Labrador West: community-led food assessment, 2010–2011 [Internet]. St. John's (NL): Food Security Network of Newfoundland and Labrador; 2011 Jun [cited 2017 Apr 10]. Available from: http://www.foodsecuritynews.com/Publications/Labrador_West_CLFA_Final_Report.pdf
38. Appleby T, Armstrong K, Nolan D, Jameson K. Burin Peninsula: community led food assessment, 2010–2011 [Internet]. St. John's (NL): Food Security Network of Newfoundland and Labrador; 2011 Jun [cited 2017 Apr 10]. Available from: https://static1.squarespace.com/static/54d9128be4b0de7874ec9a82/t/562d60ffe4b0be3276003dd6/1445814527577/Burin_Peninsula_CLFA_Final_Report.pdf
39. Markey S, Pierce J, Vodden K, Roseland M. Second growth: community economic development in rural British Columbia. Vancouver (BC): UBC Press; 2005.
40. Schiff R, Brunger F. Northern food networks: building collaborative efforts for food security in remote Canadian Aboriginal communities. J Agric Food Syst Community Dev. 2013 Jun 21;3(3):31–45.
41. Shukla S, Alfaro J, Cochrane C, Garson C, Mason G, Dyck J, Beudin-Reimer B, Barkman J. Nimíciwinán, nipimátisiwinán – "Our food is our way of life": on-reserve First Nation perspectives on community food security and sovereignty through oral history in Fisher River Cree Nation, Manitoba. Can Food Stud. 2019 May 30;6(2):73–100.
42. Kepkiewicz L, Dale B. Keeping "our" land: property, agriculture and tensions between Indigenous and settler visions of food sovereignty in Canada. J Peasant Stud. 2019 Jul 29;46(5):983–1002.
43. Hanrahan M. The lasting breach: the omission of Aboriginal people from the Terms of Union between Newfoundland and Canada and its ongoing impacts. Royal Commission on Renewing and Strengthening Our Place in Canada. St. John's (NL): Government of Newfoundland and Labrador; 2003.
44. Coates K, Poelzer G, Exner-Pirot H, Garcea J, Rodon T, Schiff R, White G, Wilson G. The role of the public sector in northern governance. Ottawa (ON): Conference Board of Canada; 2014.
45. Rudolph KR, McLachlan SM. Seeking Indigenous food sovereignty: origins of and responses to the food crisis in northern Manitoba, Canada. Local Environ. 2013 Oct;18(9):1079–98.
46. Smith A. Decolonizing food literacy: co-creating a curriculum at Lach Klan School with Gitxaala Nation (North Coast, British Columbia, Canada) [abstract] [Internet]. Am Geophys Union, Fall Meeting 2018, abstract #ED11C-0735;

2018 Dec [cited 2019 Apr 10]. Available from: https://ui.adsabs.harvard.edu/abs/2018AGUFMED11C0735S/abstract

47. Daigle M. Tracing the terrain of Indigenous food sovereignties. J Peasant Stud. 2019 Feb 23;46(2):297–315.
48. Skinner K, Hanning RM, Metatawabin J, Tsuji LJS. Implementation of a community greenhouse in a remote, sub-Arctic First Nations community in Ontario, Canada: a descriptive case study. Rural Remote Health. 2014 Apr;14(2):1–18.
49. Organ J, Castleden H, Furgal C, Sheldon T, Hart C. Contemporary programs in support of traditional ways: Inuit perspectives on community freezers as a mechanism to alleviate pressures on wild food access in Nain, Nunatsiavut. Health Place. 2014 Nov;30:251–9.
50. Ray L, Burnett K, Cameron A, Joseph S, LeBlanc J, Parker B, Recollet A, Sergerie C. Examining Indigenous food sovereignty as a conceptual framework for health in two urban communities in Northern Ontario, Canada. Glob Health Promot. 2019 Apr;26(3_suppl):54–63.
51. Martens T, Cidro J, Hart MA, McLachlan S. Understanding Indigenous food sovereignty through an Indigenous research paradigm. J Indig Soc Dev [Internet]. 2016 [cited 2016 Nov 1];5(1): 18–37. Available from: https://umanitoba.ca/faculties/social_work/media/V5i1-02martens_cidro_hart_mclachlan.pdf
52. Thompson S, Kamal AG, Alam MA, Wiebe J. Community development to feed the family in northern Manitoba communities: evaluating food activities based on their food sovereignty, food security, and sustainable livelihood outcomes. Can J Nonprofit Soc Econ Res. 2012;3(2):43.
53. Kamal AG, Linklater R, Thompson S, Dipple J, Ithinto Mechisowin Committee. A recipe for change: reclamation of Indigenous food sovereignty in O-Pipon-Na-Piwin Cree Nation for Decolonization, resource sharing, and cultural restoration. Globalizations. 2015 Jul 4;12(4):559–75.
54. Vowel C. Indigenous writes: a guide to First Nations, Métis, & Inuit issues in Canada. Winnipeg (MB): HighWater Press; 2016.
55. Lavoie J. Site C not subject to "rigorous scrutiny," fails First Nations, Royal Society of Canada warns Trudeau. Narwhal [Internet]. 2016 May 24 [cited 2019 Mar 12]. Available from: https://thenarwhal.ca/site-c-not-subject-rigorous-scrutiny-fails-first-nations-royal-society-canada-warns-trudeau/
56. Burnett K, Skinner K, LeBlanc J. From food mail to Nutrition North Canada: reconsidering federal food subsidy programs for northern Ontario. Can Food Stud Rev. 2015 May 15;2(1):141.
57. Levkoe C, Ray L, Mclaughlin J. The Indigenous food circle: reconciliation and resurgence through food in Northwestern Ontario. J Agric Food Syst Community Dev. 2019 Oct 15;9(B):1–4.
58. Galloway T. Is the Nutrition North Canada retail subsidy program meeting the goal of making nutritious and perishable food more accessible and affordable in the North? Can J Public Health. 2014 Aug 21;105(5):e395–7.

59. Gombay N. Making a living: Place, food, and economy in an Inuit community. Saskatoon (SK): Purich Pub; 2010.
60. Damman S, Eide WB, Kuhnlein HV. Indigenous peoples' nutrition transition in a right to food perspective. Food Policy. 2008 Apr;33(2):135–55.
61. Chin-Yee M, Chin-Yee BH. Nutrition North Canada: failure and facade within the northern strategy. Univ Tor Med J [Internet]. 2015 [cited 2016 Nov 1];92(3). Available from: https://utmj.org/index.php/UTMJ/article/download/215/321/435

3 Housing and Health: Housing and Health Challenges in Rural and Remote Communities

CAROL KAUPPI, EMILY FARIES, PHYLLIS MONTGOMERY, SHAROLYN MOSSEY, AND HENRI PALLARD

We situate ourselves as learners, not experts, regarding Indigenous perspectives on housing and homelessness. Four co-authors are members of groups whose ancestors came to Canada from Europe over 100 years ago as settler/colonizers – and therefore experience white privilege. One co-author, Emily Faries, is a Cree woman from Moose Cree First Nation. She is an educator and a scholar who grew up in a northern remote First Nation and has shared Cree understandings and knowledge on housing and homelessness. Another Cree researcher, Wayne Neegan, engaged with participants to gather information for the photo-voice project. Several Cree, Oji-Cree, Algonquin, and Ojibway graduate students have been central to our projects and shared their views on interpretation. As part of a research team on the project Poverty, Homelessness and Migration for the Centre for Research in Social Justice and Policy, we have been learning with and from Indigenous colleagues, students, and participants about how to engage in anti-oppressive, decolonizing community-based research. Working with northern, rural, and remote communities, we sought to generate knowledge to address injustices that reinforce inequalities in fundamental aspects of life such as housing. Through critical self-consciousness, non-Indigenous collaborators and allies have sought mutual understanding with Indigenous people to work towards equality and social justice. Similar to a view expressed by Jones and Jenkins (1 p474) and consonant with the stated goal of community leadership in participating communities, the work aims to "[give] voice to the oppressed indigenous person enabling a direct and sympathetic hearing from others." Beyond giving voice, a broader objective is to work towards change.

The Realities of Housing and Homelessness in Northern Ontario

The United Nations recognizes that shelter is a basic human need and that adequate housing should be acknowledged as a human right by all countries. In his 2007 visit to Canada, Miloon Kothari, United Nations special rapporteur on adequate housing, concluded that Canadian laws do not "include any explicit recognition of the right to adequate housing – as an enforceable right or as a policy commitment" (2 p5). In spite of this, Canada has participated in the ratification of several human rights instruments, which include the right to adequate housing. Kothari asserted that the ratification of these instruments creates an obligation for Canada to implement strategies to realize this right. The situation has not changed significantly in the years since Kothari's visit although, as a wealthy country, Canada is well positioned to take steps toward legal recognition of the right to housing. Kothari reinforced his concerns in 2011 and 2017, noting that the crisis was ongoing (3,4). In November 2017, the federal government released a policy document outlining a new National Housing Strategy (5); however, concerns have been raised that it will deliver only modest improvements rather than the ambitious statements of claim made in the policy (6,7).

The interconnectedness of housing and homelessness contributes to high rates of Indigenous homelessness, as was noted by Schiff, Turner, and Waegemakers Schiff (8). Several studies in northern Ontario have indicated that the rate of homelessness is high and that forms of hidden homelessness are prevalent (9). In a study in the Cochrane District in northeastern Ontario with a sample of 1224 people who were homeless, Kauppi, Pallard, Hankard, Faries, and Montgomery (10,11) reported that over half (64.7 per cent) were Indigenous people, while less than a third (27.7 per cent) were either anglophones or francophones of European origins. These findings indicate that northern residents, and particularly Indigenous persons living in the North, are not immune to trends in homelessness within Canada that are linked to systemic causes and changes in social policies, as well as pervasive racism against Indigenous people. Those who are identified as Indigenous are too often denied access to housing in the rental market when landlords refuse to rent to them.

Housing and Health

Within the last decade much literature has addressed the substantive relationship between precarious housing and adverse health outcomes (12,15–25). Within diverse populations and settings, precariously housed individuals experience multiple health vulnerabilities. Physical disrepair in housing has been linked to varied health issues, including asthma, respiratory infections, injuries, and mental health challenges (15,16,26). Moreover, children have been found to be more negatively affected, with long-term impacts on their development (15,27,28). Homeless persons and those occupying substandard housing are at great risk of experiencing mental health challenges (16,23,24). In his report on housing in Canada the UN special rapporteur asserted that "adequate housing is increasingly recognized in Canada as a critical social determinant of health" (2 p8). Based on research in Yellowknife, Northwest Territories, and Inuvik, Nunavut, Julia Christensen (29) noted that culturally safe housing policies are required to promote Indigenous health and address homelessness.

Hidden Homelessness

The association between homelessness, housing, and health is a concern (13–22,30). The magnitude of homelessness in rural and northern Canada is not fully known as much of it remains hidden. Yet it has been established that rates of homelessness and hidden homelessness are higher in rural and northern areas compared with urban centres (18).

In addition to substandard housing and overcrowding, hidden homelessness takes many forms in northern and rural communities, including living in tents, bush camps or RVs, motels, hotels; couch surfing; and using other time-limited shelter within informal familial or social networks (9). Hidden homelessness is not publicly visible and remains outside the scrutiny of formal services, with an absence of alternative accommodations despite exposure to violence within a residence or housing costs that consume meagre financial resources to the detriment of meeting other basic needs, such as food and heat.

The understanding that hidden homelessness can fundamentally impact people's lives was underscored by Reach[3] – the Research Alliance for Canadian Homelessness, Housing and Health (22) – which reported that the severe health problems of vulnerably housed individuals and homeless individuals are the same. It stated that "the division between these two groups is false … Instead of two distinct groups, this is one large, severely disadvantaged group that transitions between the two housing states [vulnerable housing and homelessness]" (22 p2). These findings from southern regions must be confirmed through northern research.

Based on findings from photovoice projects conducted in 2012 and 2013 in three communities in northeastern Ontario (31,32), this chapter strives to make visible the hidden homelessness of Indigenous Canadians living in rural northern Ontario, including a small town and two First Nation communities. It is intended to provide beginning insights into the linkages between hidden homelessness, substandard housing, and health for northern Indigenous residents, with some insights into the experiences of non-Indigenous people living in the small town of Cochrane.

Photovoice Projects on Homelessness in Three Northeastern Ontario Communities

The three communities chosen for the project included two northern Cree First Nation communities, one a remote James Bay coastal community and the other a rural northern inland community. The third, Cochrane, is a prosperous resource-based town located approximately one hour away from Timmins, a northern Ontario city. Its main population groups are anglophones and francophones of European origin, and Indigenous peoples, which makes it a bilingual and tri-cultural town. Cochrane is linked to James Bay by the Ontario Northland Railway and the Polar Bear Express train; it is often the first stop or even a destination for people migrating from James Bay communities. The three communities were selected because their differences allowed for the circumstances surrounding poor or inadequate housing to be compared across geographical and cultural bases. We did not identify the names of the First Nation communities to show respect for the communities and to ensure confidentiality for the participants. When reporting on results from interviews, however, the gender, age, and community type (Cochrane or a First Nation community) are noted, but all names are pseudonyms.

People living in substandard housing in one of the three communities who volunteered to participate were provided with cameras and invited to take photographs of their housing situations and living circumstances. Participants included 24 photographers, 17 from the two First Nation communities and seven from Cochrane. Twenty-two of 24 participants were Indigenous, with 21 identifying as Cree or Oji-Cree and one as Ojibway. The two non-Indigenous participants from Cochrane were anglophone men ages 47 and 85. Overall, half of the participants were men and half were women. The average age was 39.3 years, with a broad range from adolescence to 85 years. The participants collectively had 14 children, and some participants stated that their grandparents, aunts, or children in their extended families stayed with them.

In recorded interviews, the participants discussed the ideas behind their photographs and offered information they wanted to share; this allowed for comparison of the living and housing conditions of precariously housed people in Cree First Nation communities with those of people living with hidden homelessness in a town in the same general region – northeastern Ontario. The comparison makes this study unique. The project sought to understand whether variations in the context led to differences in the nature of difficult housing conditions or in the health impacts of living in challenging housing circumstances. The need for a comparative approach is increasingly necessary as the United Nations has described Canada's funding of First Nations housing as shamefully insufficient. Research that investigates this issue is required; the current project is a first step in providing photographic evidence about housing and living conditions.

Hidden from View: Homelessness in Three Northeastern Ontario Communities

It was really hard living in that house. But we had no choice, we had nowhere else to go, no other available housing anywhere. – Justine, First Nation, woman, age 56

Adequate housing is not just an important social determinant of health (33); it has been described as one of the most important: it creates a stable living environment, increases the opportunity for mental and physical health and well-being, and reduces the need for recourse to costly medical intervention (15,26).

The stories of the 24 photographers highlight the necessity of recognizing that accommodation with friends or family or substandard housing as the only option is a type of homelessness. The analysis of the photographs and their accompanying narratives uncovered eight central themes (Table 3.1) present in both Cochrane and the Cree communities. The following sections describe and illustrate each of these themes in the order shown in Table 3.1.

Couch Surfing or Sleeping Outdoors

Indigenous participants spoke about staying with family members or friends because of the lack of affordable housing in First Nations communities, and some participants spoke about extended family members who were staying with them. People in Cree communities have traditionally provided shelter to others in need, and interviews confirmed that the belief in providing this kind of support continues in the present, even though it often leads to overcrowding. A Cree participant in a First Nation took a photograph of a mattress on the floor that provided a temporary place to stay for a community member who did not have housing (see Figure 3.1).

Keeper, an Indigenous woman living in Cochrane, was familiar with Indigenous men who were living with absolute homelessness in outdoor locations in the town. She had spoken with some of them and described their circumstances:

> Here in Cochrane, there's a lot of Native men walking around; they don't have no home. And they're eating from the garbage, that's how bad it is. And they sleep in the bush with plastic tarps. I don't know why they don't let them in at the men's shelter. That's what it's for.

Members of our research team in Cochrane also observed the bush camps described by Keeper. The circumstances for Indigenous people are challenging when they remain outside the service system in northern towns, living in the bush with minimum shelter. Bush camps have been described as existing in other urban places in northern Ontario (9).

Table 3.1 Themes in photos and narratives about housing from Cochrane and Cree communities

Themes	Town of Cochrane	Cree First Nations
Couch surfing or sleeping outdoors	✓	✓
Unsanitary conditions: toilet, bath, mould, infestations	✓	✓
Lack of security: doors, windows, unsafe drinking water, wiring	✓	✓
Darkness, broken windows: dark, dingy, poor lighting, cold	✓	✓
Overcrowding: shared kitchen, bath, sleeping and living space	✓	✓
Loss of housing: eviction, fire, deterioration	✓	✓
Poor construction/maintenance: foundation, roofing	✓	✓
Health impacts: food insecurity; physical, mental, social	✓	✓

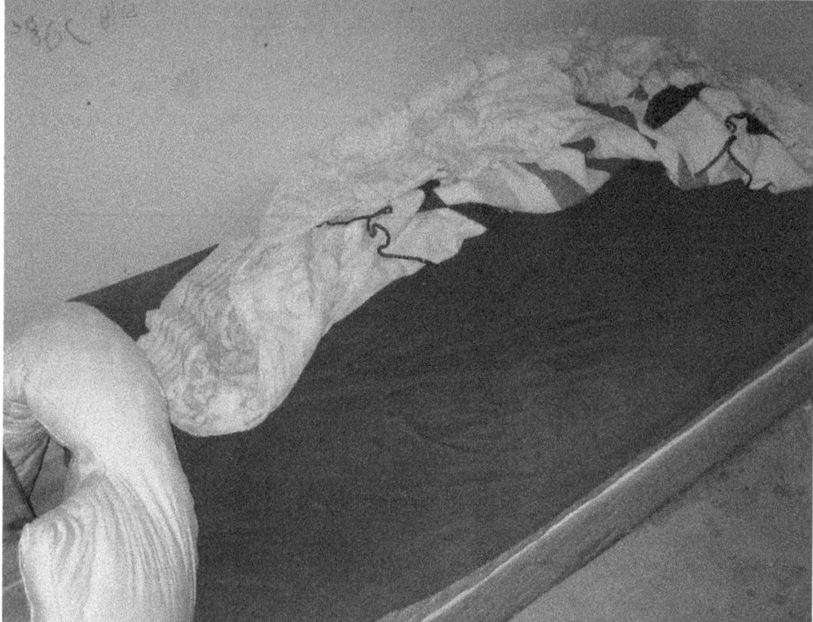

Figure 3.1 Couch surfing in a First Nation community: This mattress on the floor provided emergency shelter for a person who did not have housing.
Photo source: Carol Kauppi

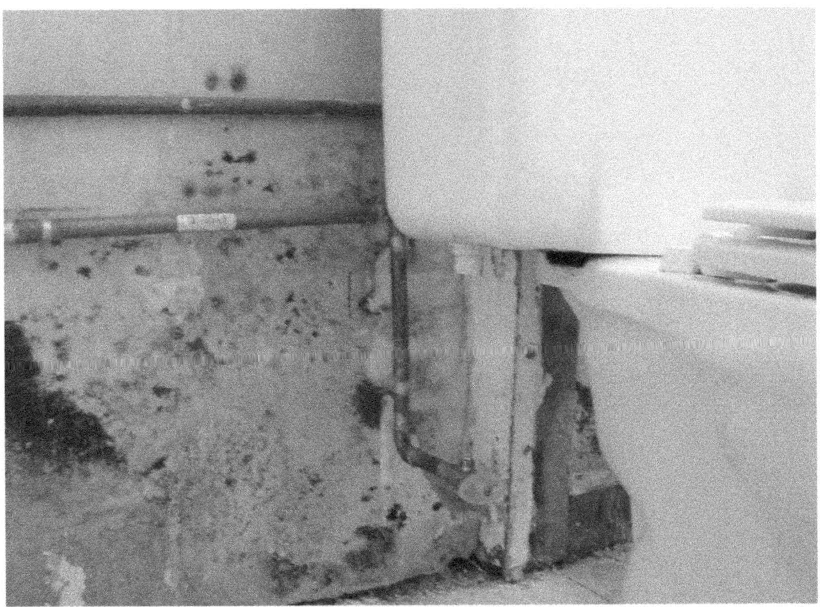

Figure 3.2 Moisture and extensive mould growth is shown on a wall and behind a toilet in a bathroom in a First Nation community.
Photo source: Carol Kauppi

Unsanitary Conditions

Participants in all three communities reported unsanitary housing conditions. A Cree participant in a First Nation community described a problem with the improper installation of bathroom fixtures such that water leakage creates conditions for the growth of mould:

> That's my washroom and I don't think it's been installed properly or something, like the tub, 'cause there's an open area or something. On the sides there's supposed to be glue or something. Yeah and then water goes through and makes all this mould. (Stevie, First Nation, adolescent girl, age 18)

In interviews, people have said that they try to clean away the mould but that it invariably reappears. An adolescent participant in a First Nation community was concerned about the health effects of breathing the damp, mouldy air in the home: "Water seeping through on the window – it's all mouldy and moist, really unhealthy to breathe in" (Robby, First Nation, adolescent boy, age 18). See Figure 3.2, which shows the moisture and mould on a bathroom wall.

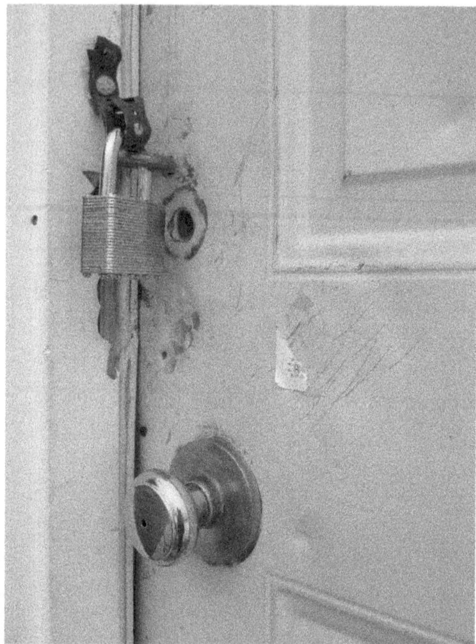

Figure 3.3 A padlock is rigged up to a front door to serve as an outside lock.
Photo source: Carol Kauppi

Lack of Security

"There's just no locks on the doors and we just tie them up with string – not good." – Noel, First Nation, man, age 41.

In Figures 3.3 and 3.4, a participant on a First Nation had found a way to lock the door securely, from the outside when leaving the house with a padlock, and from the inside when at home with a combination lock. The solution – using a combination lock on the inside – could pose a challenge in the event of an emergency, however, as opening a combination lock requires the person to know the combination and to manipulate the dial precisely.

People are fearful about their personal security given the condition of their doors and windows. This is a source of stress, which has a negative impact on health. Even with locks on their doors, participants reported that they were afraid that people would try to break in. The lack of security led many participants to supplement locking mechanisms by placing wooden bars or makeshift

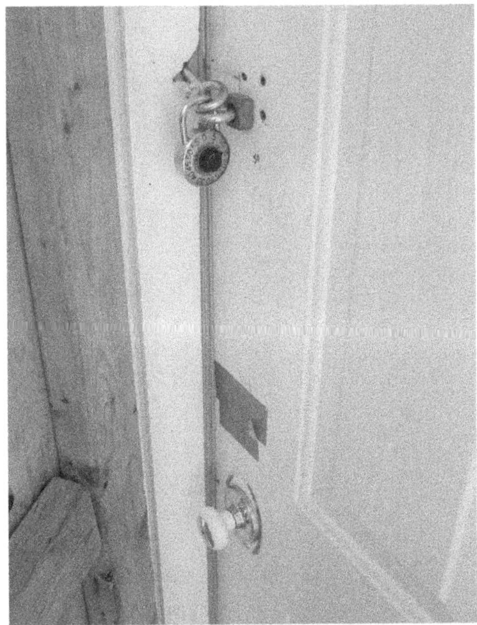

Figure 3.4 A combination lock is used on the front as an inside lock – a potentially deadly choice in an emergency.
Photo source: Carol Kauppi

locks across the door, by wedging the door firmly shut with improvised metal latches or a piece of wood, or by keeping large dogs as pets (see Figures 3.3, 3.4, and 3.5).

UNSAFE DRINKING WATER

Many First Nation participants took photographs of the containers they used to obtain potable water. This subtheme was not mentioned by participants in Cochrane. Figure 3.6 shows the water jug next to the makeshift security at the door. Gabe explained the ongoing problem with the water supply in the First Nation community:

> It's another issue about the water problem we have in our reserve. We are always spending money to go pick up fresh water, to get fresh water to drink and cook with. That takes a fair a bit of money out of our pocket to just to get to town. There is usually an advisory in our community saying that we can't drink the water and don't cook with it. (Gabe, First Nation, man, age 40)

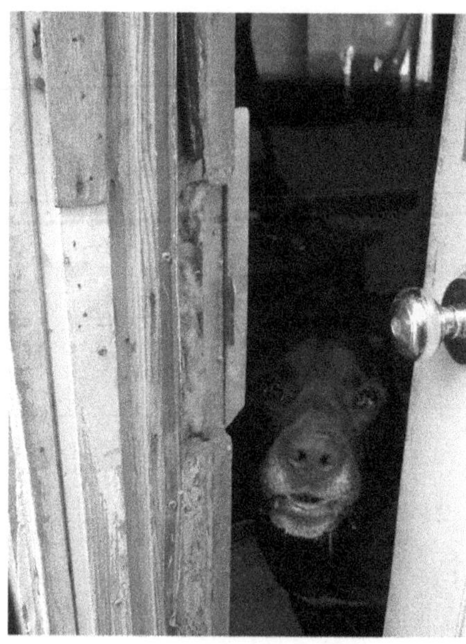

Figure 3.5 Keeping large dogs as pets helps some residents feel more secure when doors and windows are in disrepair.
Photo source: Carol Kauppi

Figure 3.7 also illustrates the problem with the water supply. The sink was being used for storage as there was no running water in the home.

WIRING

First Nation participants frequently photographed and discussed unsafe wiring; they showed the worst examples of improper electrical installations and spoke to concerns about water leaking through electrical fixtures when it rained. Figure 3.8 shows wiring that would not pass a safety inspection because of the exposed electrical boxes and wires. "I have a little niece that stays with us, she's like two … she might get like shocked or something" (Stevie, First Nation, adolescent girl, age 18).

Participants in First Nation communities also explained how the wiring had not been completed properly so that parts of the homes had no electrical outlets. This resulted in the overuse of extension cords, which can be a fire hazard.

Darkness

In general, the windows in rental accommodation in Cochrane and First Nation housing tended to be small. In addition, participants in all study communities spoke about living in dark, dingy housing, often a result of windows being broken and then covered with layers of plastic when replacement glass was not available or was unaffordable. Alternatively, it was a result of needing to cover up windows to keep the heat in, especially during the winter. As a consequence, their living accommodation receives less natural light at a time of the year with few hours of daylight because of the northern location of their communities.

Participants described the impacts. A lack of light can lead to depression and directly affect a person's mental health; it is also a physical hazard. Hallways are dark, and residents may be injured as they feel their way to a shared washroom; they may trip over something or fall down stairs. The photographs included many images in which windows and doors were covered in plastic. Figure 3.9 illustrates the dark interior in a photograph taken on a sunny day.

BROKEN WINDOWS

Participants in the First Nation communities photographed broken windows in their homes and discussed concerns about them (Figure 3.10). This subtheme was not evident among participants in Cochrane. Dene stated that the broken windows were drafty and cold in the winter. He mentioned that there was funding to repair some of the windows but not all. In addition to broken windows, participants in the other First Nation community in the study discussed problems with moisture, mildew, and mould that built up because of old windows in their home:

> Water seeping through on the window – it's all moldy and moist, really unhealthy to breathe in. Got some ice on the window. It's unsafe and it should be fixed. Shouldn't even have that in the first place. (Robby, First Nation, adolescent boy, age 18)

Overcrowding

Overcrowding was another common theme for all three communities. With many people living in a small house, every nook and cranny and all floor space was used (Figure 3.11). A participant from a First Nation community stated that all occupants of his home had to sleep in one room because of safety issues:

> They [band office] told me, like everything is all done, there is no problems. I don't think they are really qualified – the workers that did this. They're supposed to be certified people, and they tell the band office pretty much, "Okay, it's ready." So they moved us in here right away. It's pretty sad when you have to sleep everybody in the bedroom because of the stuff that hasn't properly been put together. It's unsafe. (Chase, First Nation, man, age 34)

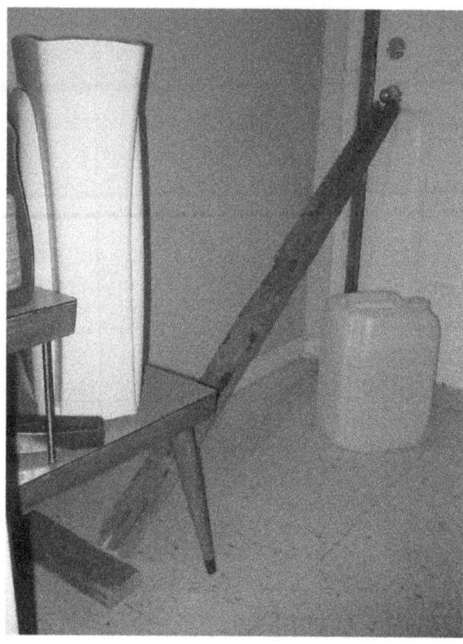

Figure 3.6 Because of water contamination, residents must bring in water in large, heavy jugs. Here, one is placed at the front door alongside a piece of wood wedged under the handle and braced against a piece of wood attached to the floor.
Photo source: Carol Kauppi

Other participants discussed similar problems from water leaking into various rooms of the house so that sleeping arrangements had to be altered. The issues with leaky roofs reduced the available space in homes where crowding was already an issue.

Participants also spoke of couch surfing – staying in other people's homes (refer back to Figure 3.1). We heard from many that Indigenous people who are vulnerably housed often have limited space but are generally willing to share it with family, friends, and even acquaintances.

Loss of Housing

Participants described the loss of housing in their interviews. A participant had received a notice of eviction and was facing the loss of her housing within days of the interview. The potential for a house fire was a concern expressed by Cree participants. The loss of housing is acutely felt given the shortage of affordable housing and the attendant difficulties in finding replacement shelter.

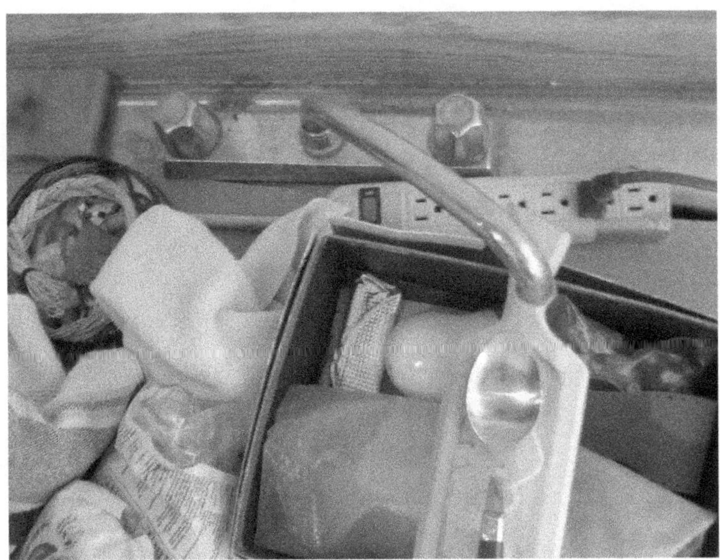

Figure 3.7 The lack of running water in many homes means the unused sinks double as storage space, something else lacking in crowded homes.
Photo source: Carol Kauppi

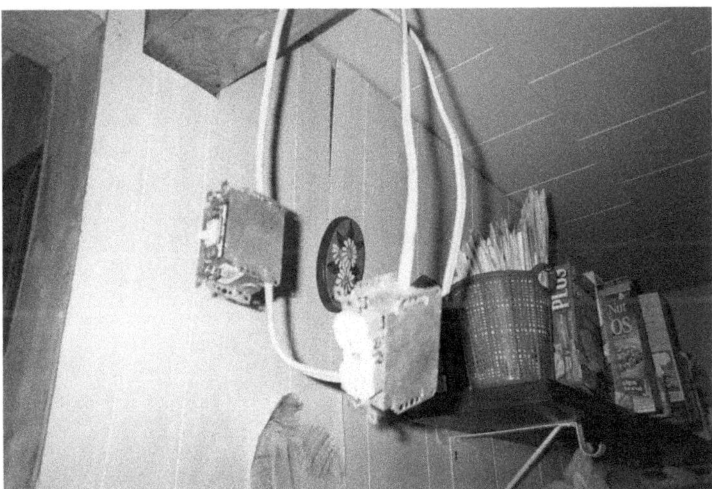

Figure 3.8 Unsafe wiring: Exposed wires and uncovered junction boxes are a common sight and create risks of fire and shock or electrocution.
Photo source: Carol Kauppi

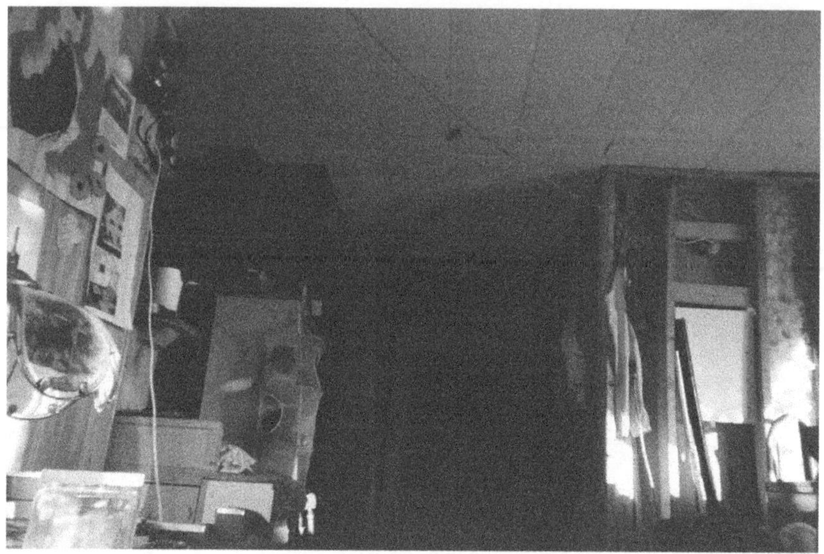

Figure 3.9 Small windows and windows covered with plastic or wood after being broken or to keep out the cold mean residents spend their time indoors in darkened rooms.
Photo source: Carol Kauppi

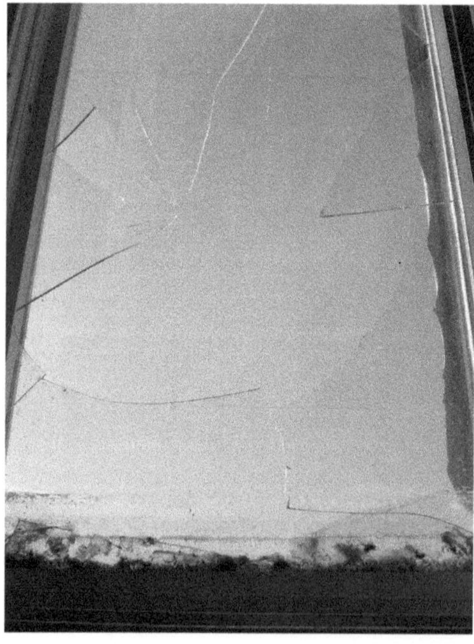

Figure 3.10 Broken windows left unrepaired are common in First Nation communities.
Photo source: Carol Kauppi

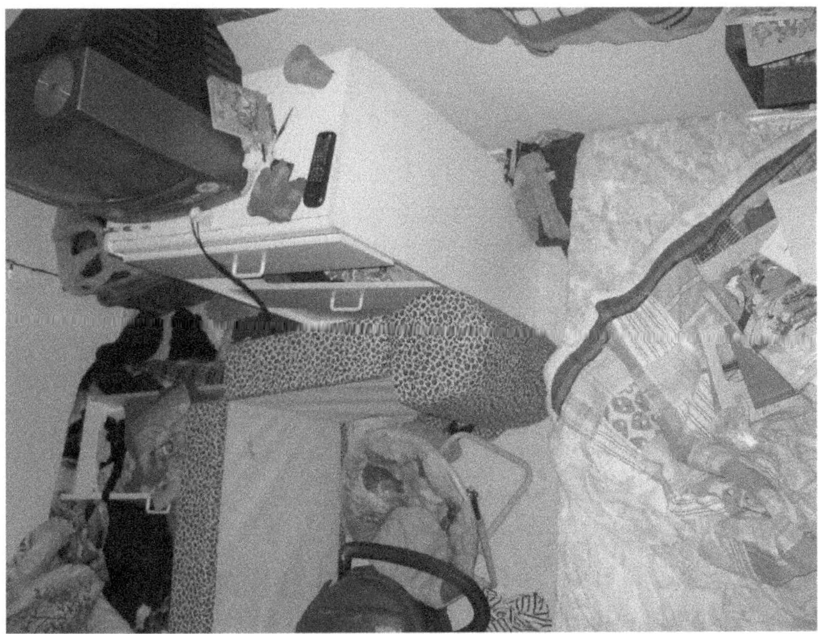

Figure 3.11 Every inch of space is filled to overflowing in a tiny bedroom. People are willing to endure severe overcrowding rather than turn away family or friends who need shelter.
Photo source: Carol Kauppi

First Nations participants reported that it is common to lose housing to arson (fire), flooding, and the gradual deterioration of housing stock because of age and poor construction. A Cree participant described how he had dealt with a potential threat of fire in his home:

> I'll point to something here, like, that might cause this house to get a fire. You see where the nail was there, do you see now? When I moved in, that nail was stuck into that wire, and I was scared to pull it but I just, I had a little stick I stand from over there and I just pulled it, so I don't want to get shock. (Noel, First Nation, man, age 41)

An Indigenous woman living in Cochrane had received an eviction notice because of complications with payment of her rent. She explained how problems with banking led to the circumstances involving the loss of her rent money:

> Just worried right now, I guess. Might be evicted on Monday. I had the rent money, but I gave it to my friend to hold on to. She has a safe over there. I got no bank account so I gave her 500 bucks to hold for me. And she got arrested. I won't be able to get it back. (Keeper, Cochrane, Indigenous woman, age 62)

Living on a limited income meant that Keeper did not have access to replacement funds to pay her rent; friends and family members could not provide financial support.

Poor Construction/Maintenance

Participants were worried about hazards in the home from shoddy construction and deteriorating conditions: "One nice step on one spot in this area, like it feels like my foot will go through" (Mari, First Nation, woman, age 41).

> You can tell that it's uneven, 'cause it shifts the house and sometimes the doors don't close properly. And that's [indicating part of the house], like half of it, where my house goes like this [shows with her hands how the house tilts at an angle]. (Stevie, First Nation, adolescent girl, age 18)

Tori explained that the discolouration of the insulation because of the roof leaking into all rooms of her trailer home was a concern, and it impacted her mental health (Figure 3.12):

> This is what the ceiling looks like. Not good. It's discouraging and depressing because it looks like crap. Almost ashamed to show my house, have company over. People see that when they first walk in my house, you know? The ceiling's had water damage before. The ceiling was leaking in every room. (Tori, Cochrane, Indigenous woman, age 34)

As an immediate response, people were dealing with water leaks by putting out pots or receptacles to catch the dripping water (Figure 3.13). However, some problems with the roof were so serious that temporary solutions became permanent. A Cree participant stated:

> That's the water seeping through the ceiling and going into the living room, we have to catch the water with bowls. That's a shelf just made for the bowls to sit there so we don't have to worry about it dripping everywhere – so it's easier for it to go on. It's been up there for a few years. I think since 2009. How do I feel? Feels gross that that's in the room. The water comes out brown, and sometimes it goes through the insulation. (Jani, First Nation, adolescent girl, age 17)

Coping with the leak in the roof and ceiling became part of their reality. A Cree participant spoke to the issue of the aging housing stock in the First Nation community:

> They renovated, they did the job, they fixed it up a little bit, in the afternoon they're gone and there's still houses like that. Yep, maybe say about twenty houses, yep,

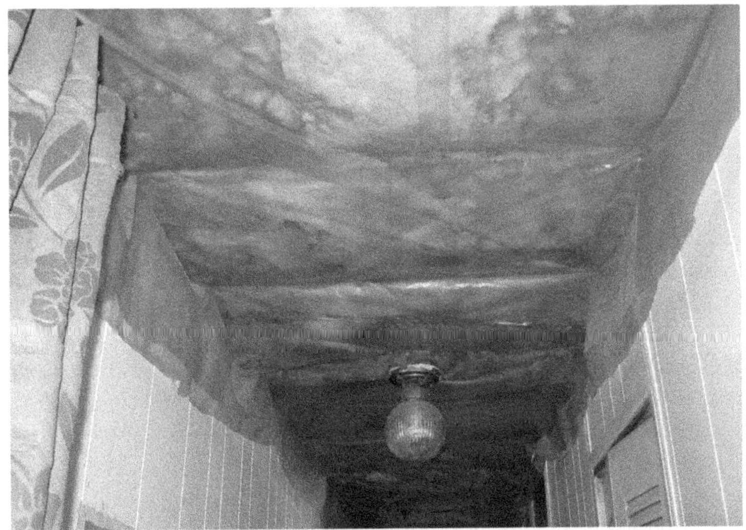

Figure 3.12 The ceiling in this home was removed because of water damage, but the mouldy insulation is clearly visible through the plastic tacked up in its place.
Photo source: Carol Kauppi

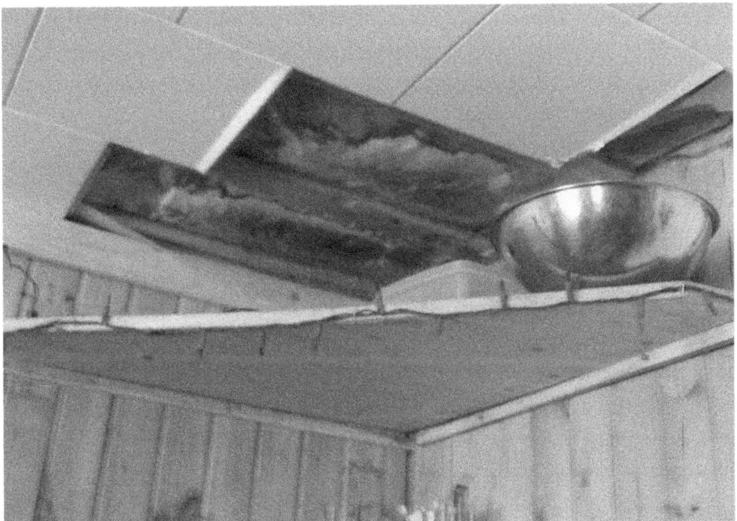

Figure 3.13 To deal with a perpetually leaky ceiling, one resident built a shelf under the missing ceiling tiles to hold the bowls and plastic containers that collect the water.
Photo source: Carol Kauppi

> and the worst ones, then after that they say they finished it but that's not true. There are houses still like that, old ones, yep, sad to see this. (Zack, First Nation, man, age 42)

A man in another First Nation community took photographs of many aspects of his housing, which was among the first homes constructed in his community. It had been deteriorating badly, and he stated that it was no longer on the list of homes that would be repaired. He was struggling to maintain the home so that he and his wife could live in it. Figures 5.14 and 5.15 show the roof and the foundation. He continually patched up the roof with tar to deal with leaks. He also identified problems with the structure of the home from its poor construction. His photograph of the foundation shows that the house was built on concrete blocks and lumber resting directly on the ground, without gravel for drainage.

An adolescent Cree participant referred to racism as an underlying factor in the poor housing in First Nation communities: "I feel like, just because I'm Native or something, we get, like, the lower class houses instead of like the higher stuff" (Stevie, First Nation, adolescent girl, age 18).

People have struggled to repair homes that should be removed from the housing stock. But as generally recognized, First Nation communities lack funds for both housing development and repair; thus, the shortage of adequate, affordable housing persists (2,34,35). The accommodations of low-income people were not well insulated and, consequently, were too warm or too cold. The homes also had inefficient and expensive forms of heating. As people who were on fixed or limited incomes, the participants were sometimes forced to choose between paying the bill for heat and paying the rent.

Health Impacts

Participants commented on the health effects of their housing for themselves and family members. Many spoke of negative impacts on their health such as coughs, numerous colds, runny noses, rashes, or general illness:

> Yeah, it was really bad, my kids were always coughing and like, rashes, I even had rash on my arm … [My three-year-old grandson] usually had colds like or sniffles all the time, runny nose, coughing, he was always sick, in that time when we were living there. (Rose, FN, woman, age 40)

> She [aunt who stays in the room] can get sick, and I used to stay in this room when I was young and I used to get sick all the time and it's hard for me to feel better fast. I think that I'm lucky I don't stay here anymore, but I am kind of worried for them because the house is falling apart. My grandmother tried but no one would do anything. (Jani, FN, adolescent boy, age 18)

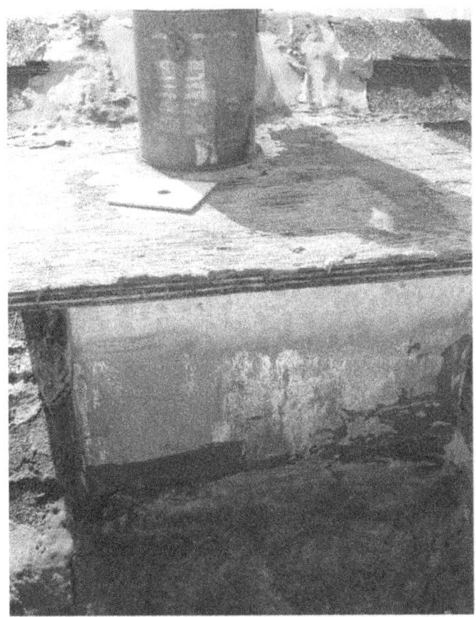

Figure 3.14 With hardly any shingles left on the roof of his house, one resident was forced to use plastic, wood, and tar to try to stop leaks.
Photo source: Carol Kauppi

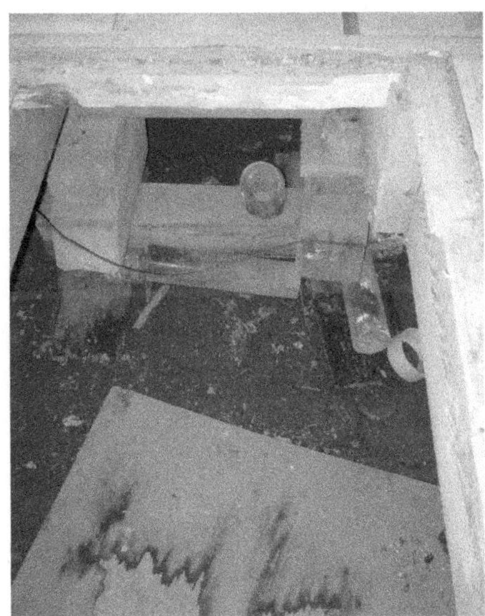

Figure 3.15 Substandard foundations mean no drainage, leaving homes vulnerable to seepage, frost heave, and rot. This home was built with concrete blocks and lumber sitting directly on the soil.
Photo source: Carol Kauppi

Dene, a Cree man, explained how broken windows, cold drafts, and illness were connected:

> As you can see, it's broken – the window – and didn't take much for it to break. You could feel drafts in the winter time, and, you know, you just worry about when's the next time it's gonna crack or shatter all of a sudden, especially when there's kids around. We get sick – so cold out – and the draft would come in and, you know, just get so cold sometimes that you catch a cold. (Dene, First Nation, man, age 26)

A participant in Cochrane explained that there were several ways in which her small apartment contributed to her health problems. Because of her disability, she used a walker and was in a wheelchair much of the time. However, her apartment was not accessible because of the concrete stairs without a ramp. Also, the concrete floor was cold and she stated: "So it really affects my, uh, osteoporosis and arthritis – I can feel it, eh, 'cause I get muscle spasms." Keeper also stated that she had asthma and that the mould in her apartment made her sick. A further problem was that she could not reach storage cupboards that were too high, given her disability. She relied on the help of people in her personal network to access items stored in these cupboards and to navigate in and out of her apartment. She felt frustrated and angry about the lack of attention on the part of the landlord to her request for modifications: "They ignore me and don't want to think about helping me." Keeper believed that she was experiencing discrimination. She stated that "those white neighbours" would not speak to her and that social assistance workers refused to give her access to particular benefits that she was entitled to receive. She stated: "It's sad, you know, how Natives are being treated bad. It's sad, yeah, it is [racism]" (Keeper, Cochrane, Indigenous woman, age 62).

FOOD INSECURITY

Food insecurity is linked to housing challenges as people must decide whether to spend their resources on shelter, food, or other basic necessities. A lack of food or food that is not nutritious is directly linked to health concerns. Some participants photographed food-related issues or spoke of the link between housing and food insecurity. Low income combined with the cost of housing and other expenses resulted in the need to make difficult decisions about whether to pay the rent or buy food:

> There's no housing in Cochrane, so to find an apartment, it's not feasible because it's not affordable anymore because of the Detour [mine]. As soon as Detour came in, the prices of houses has skyrocketed. It's ridiculous. You can't raise a family here. You're taking from your food and it's sad. It's sad when people have to struggle because of it. (Tori, Cochrane, Indigenous woman, age 34)

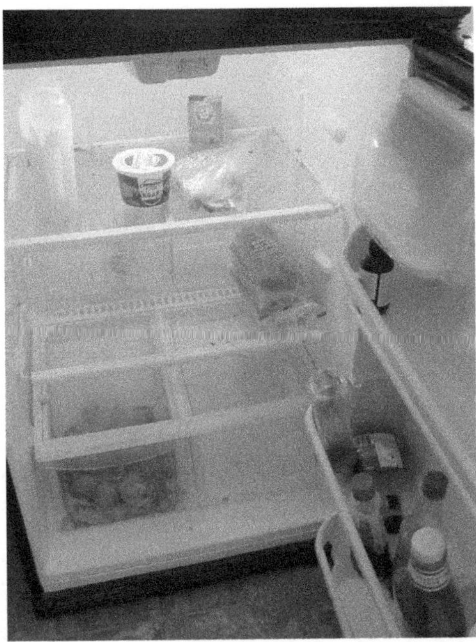

Figure 3.16 Fresh food in the rural and remote communities can be very expensive, leaving residents vulnerable to food insecurity. A nearly empty fridge with a loaf of bread, a container of margarine, some onions, one litre of milk, and some condiments has to keep this household going.
Photo source: Carol Kauppi

Cree participants took photographs of their refrigerators and cupboards (Figures 3.16 and 3.17), explaining that they wished they could keep them well stocked but were unable to because of competing expenses and the high cost of food.

MENTAL HEALTH IMPACTS: DEPRESSION, FRUSTRATION, ANGER, SHAME

Dene described how the lack of privacy affected his well-being. He was uncomfortable with the poor construction that had left the bathroom improperly completed – with no door – leading to feelings of depression:

> The bathtub, there's no doorway to this, so when you take showers and that, you gotta put a curtain up or something. It makes me feel a little depressed. It's not built properly, and, yeah, it's not your normal bathroom. When you're taking a shower, you think about someone's gonna walk in, you know, there's no door on it, no privacy really. That makes me feel kinda sad actually, you know, asking for renovations for so long. (Dene, First Nation, man, age 26)

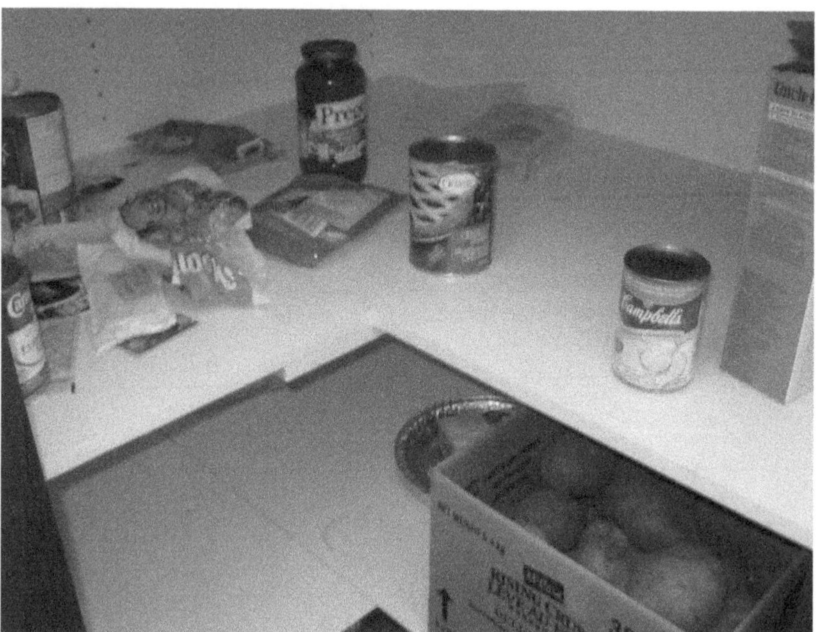

Figure 3.17 Processed food is also expensive in most communities. This kitchen cupboard has a handful of cans and packages, but the box of potatoes is the real staple.
Photo source: Carol Kauppi

Dene also explained that his bedroom did not have a door, that snow had come in from a broken window, and that people in his household felt very cold from the drafty conditions in the house. Other Indigenous participants stated that their housing conditions were linked to negative emotions, notably sadness, depression, frustration, and anger:

> There are many times when I get frustrated, you know, lay in bed and kind of seethe ... There are times when I get really frustrated, yeah and uh, yeah, I get frustrated ... I think that the housing is like ridiculous, it's ridiculous its way substandard ... But of course, we live in it. What I been told, it won't qualify for any of these upgrading programs. (Justine, First Nation, woman, age 56)

Participants living in First Nation communities felt sadness, frustration, and anger about their inability to make the substantial repairs to their homes and about the lack of action on the part of the band office to repair their homes. Such comments and reactions are consistent with testimony of witnesses to hearings of the Standing Senate Committee on Aboriginal Peoples (36) and the concerns of First Nation chiefs who acknowledged the inability to make repairs to housing because of insufficient government funding.

In Cochrane, both Indigenous and non-Indigenous participants spoke about the interconnected ways in which poverty and poor housing affected their physical or mental health. Skye, a 47-year-old anglophone man, expressed frustration about his living circumstances, which involved paying high rent and excessive heating bills on a limited income from the Ontario Disabilities Support Program. Because of shoddy construction, the heat loss meant that his heating bills were so high that he was forced to lower the heat and constantly felt chilly at home. He said that the cold often made him ill:

> Sick all the goddamn time, 'cause it was always so cold in here all the time, eh? And I had to bring the heat down cause there was no way I could afford it. You know, it would go so high there, if I left it up and kept it like 23, 24 all the time, in the winter time. Ugh, my bill would be up 500 dollars a month.

Because of a back injury, Skye needed regular medical care and believed that there was no one in the town who would help him, including government service providers. He said that he was "pissed off" with the power of the landlord to ignore his requests to correct the problems with his housing, and he was upset with the service system as a whole. He described his view of government supports:

> If the government could be one person, I'd love to have him in my back yard and beat him to death with a baseball bat, man, nice and slow. And watch every bit of it. You know, I'd enjoy every second of it. Oh yeah. (Skye, Cochrane, anglophone man, age 47)

Skye used words such as "frustrated," "pissed off," "drives me nuts," and "annoyed" to explain his emotional reactions to his living circumstances. However, his interview conveyed deep-seated feelings of rage over his helplessness to change his life circumstances.

Discussion

The photographs from two First Nation communities and the town of Cochrane, taken by Indigenous people along with two anglophone men, showed the same themes pertaining to housing issues and health. Our results are consistent with published literature (12,20,33,37). Housing hardship is not benign – it significantly affects physical and mental health.

Reach[3] reported on the physical and mental health issues experienced by people who do not have a healthy place to live (22). It stated that the most common physical health issues were chronic conditions, such as arthritis, hepatitis, asthma, high blood pressure, and chronic obstructive pulmonary disease. The most common mental health issues were depression and anxiety. Issues related to food insecurity were also cited, including insufficient food, poor-quality food, lack of nutritious food, and inability to follow a recommended special diet. Our participants in all three communities reported many of these same health-related challenges, with respiratory problems, depression, anxiety, and food insecurity being among the concerns most frequently expressed.

The high cost of heating and the absence of central heating and proper insulation, in combination with drafty windows and doors, led people with limited financial means to endure cold, damp conditions. Some participants resorted to using cooking stoves for heat, others lowered the inside temperature to save on heating costs, and many covered windows with blankets – particularly in the winter – creating dark and dank environments, all of which create ideal conditions for mould and mildew.

Dwellings with mould and mildew, poor ventilation, poor air quality, odours, allergens, and irritants affect the lung function of the inhabitants and cause respiratory infections and asthma, and spread tuberculosis – all of which participants mentioned – and are significant in the morbidity and mortality of precariously housed people (26,38,39). The poor air quality also affects the safety of the dwelling, which is often already compromised in other ways.

Unsafe housing structures such as steep stairs, a lack of railings, holes in the floors, and the absence of lighting can cause falls and physical injuries. Unsafe wiring, the use of back doorways for storage, and the absence of smoke alarms and emergency exits pose further risks to health and are hazards in the event of a fire. Some participants had rigged up methods of securing doors that would impede a quick exit to escape fire.

The worst examples of improper wiring – also a fire hazard – broken windows, and unsafe water were exclusively discussed by participants living in a First Nation community. That unsafe water was mentioned by a high number of participants living in First Nation communities should come as no surprise; more than half the water systems pose health risks according to the UN special rapporteur on the rights of Indigenous persons, James Anaya (40). The absence of functioning bathroom facilities and running water created challenges for personal hygiene, which is especially problematic for people with pre-existing physical conditions. The problems with water safety and sources raised issues not only about the physical and psychological health impacts but also about the burdens of having to haul water, bearing the costs associated with obtaining safe drinking water, and establishing additional housing on reserve, previously well documented (41,42).

While the traditional support mechanisms of opening one's home to those in need initially provides an informal type of social safety net, it also increases the likelihood of noise and overcrowding, associated with a lack of sleep and with stress, which can lead to both mental and physical health issues (38,39,43), including cardiovascular disease (44). In addition, overcrowding has been reported to be associated with food insecurity (42,45).

Food insecurity was discussed by participants in all three communities. It is widely recognized that food insecurity frequently occurs in households that are in core housing need in terms of adequacy, suitability, and affordability (42,46); northern and Indigenous communities experience especially high levels of food insecurity (45,47,48). First Nation participants in our study noted the high cost of food in their communities and, when the water supply was not safe, the exorbitant costs associated with obtaining safe water. Furthermore, First Nation and Inuit governments manage and maintain large portfolios for housing and infrastructure with limited resources; therefore, many have implemented maintenance fees or rents that apply to people occupying housing (36,49). Indigenous participants in our study commented on purchasing supplies to make repairs to their housing. Thus, while it may not be widely known, the housing costs in First Nation communities, combined with low income, contribute to housing hardship and food insecurity.

Participants recounted that poor housing conditions led to embarrassment, shame, sadness, depression, anger or rage, frustration, and loneliness, or even to attempted suicide. Living in substandard housing has negative effects on mental health, as well as on social supports and relationships, leading to social isolation and stress (42,23,24).

Conclusion

It has long been recognized that housing and living conditions in First Nations communities in Canada generally, and in northern First Nations communities specifically, are in a crisis. This situation has attracted international attention. Miloon Kothari (2), the UN special rapporteur on adequate housing, issued a report describing the situation as a national emergency. James Anaya (40), the UN special rapporteur on the rights of Indigenous peoples, noted the pressing need for additional housing and renovations to existing housing because of such issues as overcrowding, the spread of communicable diseases, and unhealthy living conditions. Anaya (40) stated that conditions linked to homelessness such as the lack of affordable housing are unacceptable in a country such as Canada, which has such great wealth. Like an echo to the statement of the UN special rapporteur, a Cree participant in one of our photovoice projects, the Poverty, Homelessness and Migration project (50) said: “So, it’s pretty sad, eh? In a country this rich, you know, this prosperous, to have people really living like that” (Wolfe, Sudbury, Indigenous man, age 45).

Through the act of taking a photograph, participants communicated their everyday realities. Many expressed the hope that greater familiarity among the Canadian public with these issues will lead to stronger pressure on those in power to bring about meaningful changes. The findings of this study reinforce understandings of the disadvantaged position of many northern Indigenous people whether they are residents of a First Nation community (i.e., "reserve") or urban Indigenous people. The results show that, overall, the same major themes were discussed by participants in all three communities. It is notable, though, that three subthemes were identified only by people in First Nations communities – unsafe drinking water, broken windows, and grossly substandard/dangerous electrical wiring – and that photographs from the First Nations communities showed conditions that appeared to be worse than those experienced by participants living in the urban context. That being said, this chapter delivers only a snapshot of findings and does not delve into every type of housing deficiency reported in participants photographs and narratives. A description of other findings from our photovoice projects have been published elsewhere (31,32).

Similar to the work of Reach[3] (22), our findings emphasize the need to recognize the health effects of housing hardship among people who have a roof over their heads. Much emphasis has been placed on forms of absolute, chronic, and episodic homelessness (51,52); it is vital to understand, however, that hidden homelessness often brings with it the same deleterious health outcomes. Substandard housing as an important social determinant of health needs to be more widely understood and acted upon. Poverty is linked to inadequate, substandard, and poor housing, which impacts health cumulatively over the life course and significantly contributes to morbidity and mortality (2,53). This has implications regarding advocacy for changes in housing policy.

Implications for Housing Policy

The federal government must address the crisis in housing in northern communities generally and in northern First Nations and Inuit communities specifically by providing sufficient funds to build the estimated 85,000 new units called for (54) and to make the repairs needed to an estimated 77,000 Indigenous people's homes across Canada (36). Without an appropriate response, a disproportionate number of northern Indigenous individuals and families will continue to face forms of hidden homelessness and the attendant health problems. Trends in census data show that, despite some improvements for Indigenous people living off reserve, there has been an increase in the number of Indigenous people in core housing need because of growth in the number of Indigenous households (55). The federal government's recent policy document entitled *Canada's National Housing Strategy* (5) provides funding for Indigenous and non-Indigenous Canadians to build a substantial number of new housing units and repair or retrofit existing units, outside First Nations communities, and provides housing subsidies and additional funding for homelessness and domestic violence. However, analyses of the new policy have raised concerns that it does not provide the level of financial investments that created Canada's social housing infrastructure in the post–World War II period. The National Housing Strategy has been described as a bold move (54), but one that is not likely to address the rising cost of housing unless all levels of government work together to ensure that low-income people can access decent affordable housing.

The Wellesley Institute (15) reviewed the published literature regarding evidence of the best housing strategies for improving health outcomes. It asserted that effective interventions "address indoor temperature control, the structural integrity and safety of buildings, access to water supply and control of chemical and biological hazards" (15 p5). Various levels of government must act in a coordinated manner to ensure that the required changes are made to develop and implement a national housing strategy that will respond to the needs of northern Indigenous people whether they live in urban settings or First Nation communities.

ACKNOWLEDGMENT

This research was supported by the Social Sciences and Humanities Research Council of Canada, the Ontario Arts Council, two First Nation communities in northeastern Ontario, and people in the town of Cochrane.

REFERENCES

1. Jones A, Jenkins K. Rethinking collaboration: working the Indigene-colonizer hyphen. In Denzin N, Lincoln YS, Tuhiwai Smith L, editors. Handbook of critical and indigenous methodologies. Thousand Oaks (CA): Sage Publications; 2008. p. 471–86.
2. Kothari M. Promotion and protection of all human rights, civil, political, economic, social and cultural rights, including the right to development. Report of the special rapporteur on adequate housing as a component of the right to an adequate standard of living, and on the right to non-discrimination in this context, Miloon Kothari, addendum. [Internet]. New York (NY): United Nations, Office of the High Commissioner for Human Rights; 2009 Feb 17 [cited 2017 Sep 1]. Available from: https://www2.ohchr.org/english/bodies/hrcouncil/docs/10session/A.HRC.10.7.Add.3.pdf
3. Kothari M. Affidavit, at para 66. Tanudjaja v Attorney General of Canada and Attorney General of Ontario (2011), ON SC File No. CV-10-403688.

4. Johal A. Housing crisis worse: Former UN special rapporteur Miloon Kothari revisits Vancouver. 2017 Dec 1 [cited 2019 Mar 28]. In: Policy Notes Blog [Internet]. Vancouver (BC): Canadian Centre for Policy Alternatives, BC Office. c2009 – . Available from: https://www.policynote.ca/housing-crisis-worse-former-un-special-rapporteur-miloon-kothari-revisits-vancouver/
5. Government of Canada. Canada's national housing strategy: a place to call home [Internet]. Ottawa (ON): Government of Canada; 2017 [cited 2020 Feb 5]. Available from: https://eppdscrmssa01.blob.core.windows.net/cmhcprodcontainer/sf/project/placetocallhome/pdfs/canada-national-housing-strategy.pdf
6. Falvo N. Ten things to know about Canada's newly-unveiled national housing strategy. 2017 Dec 18 [cited 2017 Dec 22]. In: Behind the Numbers Blog [Internet]. Ottawa (ON): Canadian Centre for Policy Alternatives. c2011 – . Available from: http://behindthenumbers.ca/2017/12/18/national-housing-strategy/
7. Pomeroy S. Making sense of the funding allocations in the National Housing Strategy [Internet]. Ottawa (ON): Centre for Urban Research and Education; 2017 [cited 2017 Aug 16]. Available from: https://carleton.ca/cure/wp-content/uploads/CURE-Brief-9-Assessing-the-Funding-in-the-National-Housing-Strategy.pdf
8. Schiff R, Turner A, Waegemakers Schiff J. Rural Indigenous homelessness in Canada. In: Peters E, Christianson J, editors. Indigenous homelessness. Perspectives from Canada, Australia, and New Zealand. Winnipeg (MB): University of Manitoba Press; 2018. Chapter 9.
9. Kauppi C, O'Grady B, Schiff R, Martin F, Ontario Municipal Social Services Association. Homelessness and hidden homelessness in rural and northern Ontario. Guelph (ON): Rural Ontario Institute; 2017.
10. Kauppi C, Pallard H, Hankard M, Faries E, Montgomery P. Homelessness in the Cochrane district: 2018 enumeration. Sudbury (ON): Centre for Research in Social Justice and Policy; 2019.
11. Kauppi C, Pallard H, Faries E. Homelessness in Cochrane, Ontario, final report. Sudbury (ON): Poverty, Homelessness and Migration, Centre for Research in Social Justice and Policy, Laurentian University; 2015 June.
12. Frankish C, Hwang S, Quantz, D. Homelessness and health in Canada: research lessons and priorities. Can J Public Health. 2005;96(Suppl 2):S23–9.
13. Gaetz S, Dej E, Richter T, Redman, M. The state of homelessness in Canada 2016 [Internet]. Toronto (ON): Canadian Observatory on Homelessness Press. 2016 [cited 2017 Aug 16]. Available from: http://www.homelesshub.ca/sites/default/files/SOHC2016.pdf
14. Hulchanski J. Homelessness in Canada: past, present, future. Keynote address at: Growing home: housing and homeless in Canada [Internet]. Calgary (AB): Canadian Policy Research Networks; 2009 Feb 18 [cited 2017 Aug 16]. Available from: http://tdrc.net/uploads/file/2009_hulchanski.pdf
15. Wellesley Institute. Housing and health: examining the links [Internet]. Toronto (ON): Wellesley Institute; 2012 [cited 2017 Aug 16]. Available from:

https://www.wellesleyinstitute.com/wp-content/uploads/2012/10/Housing-and-Health-Examining-the-Links.pdf
16. Wellesley Institute. Precarious housing in Canada 2010. Toronto (ON): Wellesley Institute; 2010.
17. Kohen D, Bougie E, Guèvremont A. Housing and health among Inuit children. Health Rep [Internet]. 2015 [cited 2017 Aug 16];26(11):21–7. Available from: http://www.statcan.gc.ca/pub/82-003-x/2015011/article/14223-eng.htm
18. Haley D, Parker K, Dauria E, Root C, Rodriguez L, Ruel E, Oakley D, Wang J, Jennings L, Soto-Torres l, Cooper H. Housing and health: exploring the complex intersections between housing environments and health behaviors among women living in poverty. In: O'Leary A, Frew P, editors. Poverty in the United States. New York (NY): Springer; 2017. p. 185–205.
19. Holton E, Gogosis E, Hwang S. Housing vulnerability and health: Canada's hidden emergency [Internet]. Toronto (ON): Research Alliance for Canadian Homelessness, Housing, and Health; 2010 [cited 2017 Aug 16]. Available from: https://www.homelesshub.ca/sites/default/files/attachments/HousingVulnerabilityHealth-REACH3-Nov2010_0.pdf
20. Webster P. Housing triggers health problems for Canada's First Nations. Lancet [Internet]. 2015 [cited 2017 Aug 16];385(9967):495–6. Available from: https://doi.org/10.1016/S0140-6736(15)60187-8
21. Whitzman C. At the intersection of invisibilities: Canadian women, homelessness and health outside the "big city." Gend Place Cult [Internet]. 2006 [cited 2017 Aug 16];13(4):383–99. Available from: https://doi.org/10.1080/09663690600808502
22. Reach[3]. Housing vulnerability and health: Canada's hidden emergency. Toronto (ON): Research Alliance for Canadian Homelessness, Housing, and Health; 2013.
23. Singh A, Daniel L, Baker E, Bentley R. Housing disadvantage and poor mental health: a systematic review. Am J Prev Med. 2019;57(2):262–72.
24. Magee C, Norena M, Hubley AM, Palepu A, Hwang SW, Nisenbaum R, Karim ME, Gadermann A. Longitudinal associations between perceived quality of living spaces and health-related quality of life among homeless and vulnerably housed individuals living in three Canadian cities. Int J Environ Res Public Health. 2019;16(23):4808.
25. Zhang L, Norena M, Gadermann A, Hubley A, Russell L, Aubry T, To MJ, Farrell S, Hwang S, Palepu A. Concurrent disorders and health care utilization among homeless and vulnerably housed persons in Canada. J Dual Diagn. 2018; 14(1):21–31.
26. Hernández D. Housing-based health interventions: harnessing the social utility of housing to promote health [Internet]. Am J Public Health. 2019 [cited 2020 Aug 26];109(S2):S135–S136. Available from: https://ajph.aphapublications.org/doi/pdfplus/10.2105/AJPH.2018.304914
27. Gultekin LE, Brush BL, Ginier E, Cordom A, Dowdell EB. Health risks and outcomes of homelessness in school-age children and youth: a scoping review of the literature. J Sch Nurs. 2020 Feb;36(1):10–18

28. Sandel M, Sheward R, de Cuba SE, Coleman S, Heeren T, Black MM, Casey PH, Chilton M, Cook J, Cutts DB, Rose-Jacobs R. Timing and duration of pre- and postnatal homelessness and the health of young children. Pediat. 2018;142(4):e20174254.
29. Christensen J. Indigenous housing and health in the Canadian north: revisiting cultural safety. Health Place. 2016;40:83–90.
30. Ontario Agency for Health Protection and Promotion (Public Health Ontario), Berenbaum E. Evidence brief: homelessness and health outcomes: what are the associations? Toronto (ON): Queen's Printer for Ontario; 2019.
31. Hein H, Kauppi C. Living on the outside: a photo exhibit using art in the struggle for social justice. Int J Soc Polit Commun Agendas Arts. 2014;8(3–4): 31–41.
32. Pallard H, Kauppi C, Hein J. Photovoice and homelessness in subarctic and urban communities. Int J Soc Polit Commun Agendas Arts. 2015;10(1):25–41.
33. MacKay K, Wellner J. Housing and health: OMA calls for urgent government action, housing-supportive policies to improve health outcomes of vulnerable populations. Ont Med Rev. 2013;80:10–2.
34. Walker R. Aboriginal self-determination and social housing in urban Canada: a story of convergence and divergence. Urban Stu. 2008;45(1):185–205.
35. Report of the special rapporteur on adequate housing as a component of the right to an adequate standard of living, and on the right to non-discrimination in this context [Internet]. New York (NY): United Nations; 2019 Jul 17 [cited 2020 Aug 26]. Available from: http://www.undocs.org/A/74/183
36. Standing Senate Committee on Aboriginal Peoples. Housing on First Nation reserves: challenges and successes [Internet]. Ottawa (ON): Senate Canada; 2015 Feb 8 [cited 2017 Aug 16]. Available from: https://sencanada.ca/content/sen/Committee/412/appa/rep/rep08feb15b-e.pdf
37. Shaw M. Housing and public health. Annu Rev Public Health. 2004;25:397–418.
38. Krieger J, Higgins D. Housing and health: time again for public health action. Am J Public Health. 2002;92(5):758–68.
39. Shannon H, Allen C, Dávila D, Fletcher-Wood L, Gupta S, Keck K, Lang S, Kahangire DA, World Health Organization. WHO housing and health guidelines: web annex A: report of the systematic review on the effect of household crowding on health. Geneva (CH): World Health Organization; 2018.
40. Anaya J. Statement upon conclusion of the visit to Canada by the United Nations special rapporteur on the rights of Indigenous Peoples [Internet]. New York (NY): United Nations, Office of the High Commissioner for Human Rights; 2013 Oct 15 [cited 2017 Aug 16]. Available from: https://www.ohchr.org/documents/issues/ipeoples/sr/a.hrc.27.52.add.2-missioncanada_auv.pdf
41. Standing Senate Committee on Aboriginal Peoples. On-reserve housing and infrastructure: recommendations for change. Senate 41st Parliament, 2nd Session [Internet]. Ottawa (ON): Senate Canada; 2015 Jun 12 [cited 2017 Aug 16]. Available

from: https://sencanada.ca/content/sen/Committee/412/appa/rep/rep12jun15-e.pdf

42. Reading CL, Wien F. Health inequalities and social determinants of Aboriginal peoples' health [Internet]. Prince George (BC): National Collaborating Centre for Aboriginal Health; 2009 [cited 2017 Aug 16]. Available from: http://www.ccnsa-nccah.ca/docs/determinants/RPT-HealthInequalities-Reading-Wien-EN.pdf
43. Coffey PM, Ralph AP, Krause VL. The role of social determinants of health in the risk and prevention of group A streptococcal infection, acute rheumatic fever and rheumatic heart disease: a systematic review. PLoS Negl Trop Dis. 2018 Jun 13;12(6):e0006577.
44. Hoevenaar-Blom M, Spijkerman A, Kromhout D, Verschuren W. Sufficient sleep duration contributes to lower cardiovascular disease risk in addition to four traditional lifestyle factors: the MORGEN study. Eur J Prev Cardiol. 2013;21(11):1367–75
45. De Shutter, O. Report of the special rapporteur on the right to food, Olivier De Schutter. New York (NY): United Nations General Assembly; 2012
46. Canada Mortgage and Housing Corporation. 2011 census/national housing survey housing series: issue 9 – the housing conditions of Canada's senior households. Ottawa (ON): Canada Mortgage and Housing Corporation; 2016.
47. Parker B, Burnett K, Hay T, Skinner K. The community food environment and food insecurity in Sioux Lookout, Ontario: understanding the relationships between food, health, and place. J Hunger Environ Nutr. 2019;14(6):762–79.
48. Tarasuk V, St-Germain AA, Mitchell A. Geographic and socio-demographic predictors of household food insecurity in Canada, 2011–12. BMC Public Health. 2019;19(1):12.
49. Standing Senate Committee on Aboriginal Peoples. We can do better: housing in Inuit Nunangat [Internet]. Ottawa (ON): Senate Canada; 2017 [cited 2018 Apr 2]. Available from: https://sencanada.ca/fr/comites/appa/42-1
50. Kauppi C, Pallard H, Faries E. Poverty, homelessness and migration In northeastern Ontario, Canada. OIDA Int J Sustain Dev [Internet]. 2015 [cited 2015 Apr 30];8(4):11–22. Available from https://ssrn.com/abstract=2612092
51. Ministry of Housing. Guidelines for service manager homeless enumeration [Internet]. Toronto (ON): Queen's Printer for Ontario; 2017 [cited 2018 Apr 2]. Available from: http://www.mah.gov.on.ca/AssetFactory.aspx?did=15968
52. Employment and Social Development Canada. Homelessness partnering strategy directives 2014–2019 [Internet]. Ottawa (ON): Government of Canada; 2016 [cited 2018 Apr 2]. Available from: https://www.unitedwaykfla.ca/wp-content/uploads/2016/10/HPS-Capital-Investments_2014-19-Directives.pdf
53. Shaw M. Housing and public health. Annu Rev Public Health. 2004;25:397–418.
54. Stuttor, G. Housing in the 2017 federal budget: the broad picture [Internet]. Toronto (ON): Wellesley Institute; 2017 [cited 2017 Aug 16]. Available from https://www.wellesleyinstitute.com/housing/housing-in-the-2017-federal-budget-the-broad-picture/

55. Canada Mortgage and Housing Corporation. 2011 census/national housing survey housing series: issue 10 – the housing conditions of off-reserve status Indian households [Internet]. Ottawa (ON): Canada Mortgage and Housing Corporation; 2016 Mar [cited 2017 Aug 16]. Available from: https://assets.cmhc-schl.gc.ca/sf/project/cmhc/pubsandreports/pdf/68547.pdf

4 Determinants of Infectious Diseases: Agent, Host, and Environmental Factors in Infectious Diseases

PAMELA ORR AND LINDA LARCOMBE

In Canada, provinces and territories vary in their collection, reporting, and publication of infectious disease data – which diseases are reportable, what data are collected and analysed (e.g., ethnicity), and what data are published. The lack of consistency in data collection, analysis, and availability is a barrier to a more complete understanding of infectious diseases in northern Canada. Other barriers include the multiplicity of jurisdictions (federal, provincial, territorial) involved, gaps in technical (including computer surveillance systems) and human resources, the concern about stigmatization and need for confidentiality, and unresolved issues regarding control and ownership of data.

Much of the information we have regarding infectious and other diseases in northern Canada comes from individual studies among selected regional groups. Such studies are driven by the availability of funds and the interests and priorities of granting agencies, researchers, and communities. They provide important information but are by their nature piecemeal and opportunistic. They do not paint a complete picture of health, illness, and the existing systems of care. It should also be noted that northern Canada is not homogeneous. Patterns of infectious diseases are explained by local social, economic, political, and biologic determinants, which vary across the North.

Infectious diseases may be viewed through the lens of the epidemiologic triangle of agent, host, and environment, recognizing that these are interactive and fluid components. The agent, or organism, that causes infection has characteristics that affect the transmission and severity of illness. The host, or person experiencing infection, has biologic and experiential characteristics that will affect that person's risk of, and immune response to, infection. The physical, socio-economic, and political environments affect the risk and experience of infection. As examples, the risk of gastric cancer is determined by a particular *Helicobacter pylori* (HP) genotype infecting a particular host (1–3). Vitamin D deficiency occurs in northern populations because of an environment of food insecurity, but the effect of a given level of vitamin D on an individual's resistance to infection is influenced by host genetics (4). Agent, host, and environment are frequently different in northern compared to southern Canada. An understanding of these factors, and their interplay, will allow for improved prevention and care for northern peoples.

Respiratory Diseases

The determinants of tuberculosis (TB) are prevalent in many regions of northern Canada. These include, but are not limited to, adverse environmental and host components of the epidemiologic triangle: crowded and poorly ventilated housing; comorbidities including diabetes, renal failure, substance abuse, and nutritional deficiencies; poverty; racism; social marginalization; and inadequate health systems. In 2017, the incidence of TB was 4.9 per 100,000 in Canada as a whole, while in Yukon, Northwest Territories, and Nunavut the incidence rates were 20.8, 6.7, and 265.8 per 100,000, respectively (5). From 2007 to 2008, the incidence of pulmonary TB was more than 300 per 100,000 person-years in 11 communities (10 First Nation and 1 Métis) north of the 53rd parallel in the Prairie provinces (6).

The epidemiology of TB in northern Canada is characterized by recurrent outbreaks with transmission of infection to large numbers of individuals across generations (7). The incidence of disease in children and young adults is high in some regions, including Nunavut and northern Manitoba and Saskatchewan, indicating ongoing transmission. Delays in diagnosis reflect failures at many levels (7–10).

Urgent action is required to ameliorate the social, economic, political, and environmental determinants of TB. TB prevention, diagnosis, and care programs in northern Canada also urgently need improvement (6–10). In the 1960s, an intensive mass TB campaign was instituted in northern Canada under the leadership of Dr. Stefan Grzybowski (7). The resultant 15 per cent annual decrease in TB incidence was greater than any previously recorded decline in the history of TB, and one that occurred despite the prevalence of significant adverse social determinants. From 2013 to 2015 a similar intensive door-to-door *Taima*, or Stop, TB campaign occurred on a small scale as part of a research study in Iqaluit, Nunavut (11). These projects demonstrate that significant gains in TB control require intensive resource allocation over many years (as long as it takes), integration into other health programs, and genuine partnership with the people served. Authoritarian approaches are not effective in tackling the complex issues involved in TB prevention and care (7,10,12).

Newer diagnostic technologies, such as interferon gamma release assays and rapid automated molecular DNA tests, are currently being studied in northern regions. An understanding of the genetic code (genotype) of a TB isolate (the agent) may aid epidemiologic understanding, but results are usually not available when decisions need to be made amid outbreaks. Successful TB programs assiduously identify, prioritize, and assess contacts with accuracy and speed to break the chain of transmission. The process must be thorough, trace upstream and downstream, and result in treatment completion for contacts with latent TB infection (LTBI), as well as those with active disease (7–10). Relationships of trust, respect, and understanding are required (12). The analysis of targets attached to performance measurements is also required, with dissemination of results (transparency) and public accountability (8).

While TB often dominates the discussion of respiratory disease in northern Canada, it is recognized that more common manifestations of lower respiratory tract infection (LRTI), including bronchitis, bronchiolitis, and pneumonia, are frequent causes of child and adult visits to health care centres. The determinants of LRTI include but are not limited to inadequate housing, poor sanitation, nutritional deficiencies, exposure to smoke, premature birth, genetic and epigenetic factors, and health system deficiencies.

A patient presents to a northern health centre with cough and wheezing. Is this an infectious or non-infectious process? If the history and clinical examination suggest infection, how do we know whether the causative agent is a virus or bacteria? In the absence of many diagnostic tools, overuse of antibacterial agents is hard to avoid. The potential consequences of undertreatment of bacterial infection in remote communities are substantial. Diagnostic and therapeutic algorithms are available, but most are developed in the context of southern populations and resources. Microbiologic testing of sputum, nasopharyngeal specimens, and blood is often not feasible given the cost, transport conditions, and turnaround time.

The need is urgent for research on the causes of LRTI in northern Canada and the development of effective preventive and therapeutic interventions. Empiric therapy is frequently given based on southern epidemiologic studies, but the types of organisms causing LRTI in northern Canada and their characteristics, such as antimicrobial susceptibility, may be different. For example, respiratory syncytial virus and adenoviruses are common causes of bronchiolitis, but what is the role, if any, of other organisms that we sometimes find in our investigations, such as *Simkania negevensis* and human metapneumovirus (13)?

Epidemic bronchiolitis occurs regularly in the spring in Nunavut, Northwest Territories, and the northern regions of many provinces. Morbidity and mortality vary from year to year but are higher for Indigenous than for non-Indigenous children. Noted morbidity includes prolonged mechanical ventilation, bronchiectasis, and Swyer-James syndrome. Palivizumab is not currently offered to Indigenous immune competent infants born at term in high-incidence communities in northern Canada (14). Studies suggest that it may be cost effective in this group depending on the severity of the seasonal outbreak (14).

The severity of seasonal influenza epidemics varies from year to year throughout Canada, but in northern and remote regions critical community services such as water delivery, sewage removal, airport maintenance, and health care services may be at risk if sufficient local persons are affected (15). During the first wave of the pH1N1 2009 (pandemic) influenza season, persons living in Nunavut and northern Manitoba communities were disproportionately among the critically ill (16). Risk markers included Indigenous ethnicity, predisposing comorbidities, time to treatment, rural residence, and income level. A severe inflammatory cytokine storm was observed in otherwise healthy young First Nations patients in intensive care units, pointing to the need to better understand the role of the host genetic determinants of immune response to influenza and other pathogens (16–18). We should not assume that preventive (particularly vaccines) and therapeutic interventions for influenza or other pathogens, which are developed for southern populations, will work for northern ones. The 2009 pandemic influenza, in particular, demonstrated that antibody response to the subunit influenza vaccine does not reflect the full story of immune protection; cellular immune response is critical (19).

Skin and Soft Tissue Infections (SSTIs), Invasive Bacterial Pathogens, and Otitis Media

Over the past 15 years, the incidence of skin and soft tissue infection from methicillin-resistant *Staphylococcus aureus* (MRSA) has increased in northern Canada, particularly in Nunavut, Northwest Territories, Labrador, and the northern regions of Saskatchewan, Manitoba, Ontario, and Alberta (20). An observed increase in complications from this agent, including bacteraemia, necrotizing pneumonia, and osteomyelitis, has also been reported. Those affected are predominantly young and healthy (21). Published reports have noted the predominance of community-associated MRSA clonal epidemic strains in northern regions of Saskatchewan, Manitoba, and Ontario, and the presence of virulence factors such as the Panton-Valentine leukocidin gene (20,21). Clinical suspicion of MRSA infection should be followed by testing and treatment protocols that account for local resistance patterns; effective antibiotics for resistant organisms must be available locally.

The determinants of northern SSTIs include environmental factors such as inadequate housing, water and sanitation systems, barriers to health, exposure to MRSA through the frequent travel of patients to large urban hospitals, and antibiotic overuse (20). Host comorbid conditions that affect the degree of sickness (morbidity) and risk of death (mortality) are prevalent in many northern communities; these include diabetes, obesity, and renal impairment. Collaborations such as the Northern Antibiotic Resistance Partnership provide research and education. Educational messages that relate to personal hygiene are likely to have limited efficacy if individuals are unable to change the unsanitary conditions in which they live. Systemic interventions are urgently needed.

The International Circumpolar Surveillance (ICS) project monitors invasive infections cause by bacterial organisms (*Streptococcus pneumoniae* (Sp), *Haemophilus influenzae* (Hi), *Neisseria meningitidis* (Nm), Group A *Streptococcus* (GAS), and Group B *Streptococcus*) in northern Canada (defined by the project as Yukon, Northwest Territories, Nunavut, Nunavik, and Labrador), Alaska (United States), Greenland, Norway, Sweden, Finland, and Russia (22). Between 2006 and 2013, the incidence of disease caused by each invasive organism (Sp, Hi, Nm, and GAS) was higher in the Canadian ICS regions than in Canada as a whole (22). The incidences of invasive Sp, Hi, and GAS disease were higher among Indigenous than among non-Indigenous persons. Reported incidences are likely underestimates as microbiologic cultures (taken before antibiotic administration) are not consistently collected in the North, and results, when available, may be compromised by transport conditions.

Invasive Sp serotypes differ in the northern ICS region compared to southern Canada. A large outbreak from a virulent clone of serotype 1 occurred in Nunavik in 2000, necessitating a massive vaccination campaign (23). More recently serotype 5 has been noted in northern Alberta and Saskatchewan (24). In children less than two years of age living in the northern ICS region of Canada, the average annual (2011–2015) incidence of invasive Sp was 141.1/100,000, which was 8.4 times the rate observed in the rest of Canada (25).

Past studies of various Sp polysaccharide and conjugate vaccines have raised concerns about their effectiveness among US Indigenous (including Navaho and Apache) populations, because of local differences in either epidemiology or immune response (26). Navaho and Apache peoples share common linguistic and ancestral origins with the Dene peoples of northern Canada. Therefore, as is the case with all vaccines developed and tested among mainstream North American populations, it is important to assess vaccine impact in northern Canada through careful active and passive surveillance. The 13-valent pneumococcal conjugate vaccine (PCV) was introduced into the paediatric vaccine schedule in 2010–2011 in most northern Canadian regions. It remains to be seen what effect this will have on the epidemiology of Sp. The 13-valent vaccine covers serotypes 1 and 5, but vigilance is required as new non-PCV-13 serotypes are emerging in Canada. In the case of Sp, and other invasive bacteria, emerging antimicrobial resistance is a concern, reinforcing the need in northern regions to take cultures in appropriate clinical settings, to support laboratory surveillance systems, and to stock health centres with a variety of potentially lifesaving antimicrobials (27).

The clinical presentation of invasive infections caused by Hi includes meningitis, pneumonia, bacteraemia, sepsis syndrome, bone and joint infection, SSTI, and epiglottitis. The incidence of invasive Hi disease decreased significantly in northern Canada after the introduction of the first serotype b (Hib) vaccine in 1986. However, serotype a (Hia) has emerged as a predominant strain in the Canadian ICS region (average annual incidence 5.3/100,000, 2000–2016) and in northwestern Ontario (average annual incidence 7/100,000, 2004–2008), with a higher incidence observed among Indigenous compared to non-Indigenous persons in those regions (28,29). Currently, there are no vaccines for Hi bacterial strains that are not serotype b, nor is there evidence that prophylaxis of contacts of these cases is efficacious.

Invasive Hi disease is associated with environmental and host determinants, which include poverty, crowded housing, inadequate water supply, exposure to indoor smoke, and lack of breastfeeding. A number of studies suggest that host genetic determinants also affect immune response to Hi and Sp natural infection and vaccination among some Indigenous Canadian (First Nations and Inuit) and US (Apache, Navajo, and native Alaskan) groups (26, 30). As was noted for influenza and pneumococcus, health interventions should be assessed in the specific locations and populations in which they are implemented. Northern health programs in Canada are often stretched for resources on all fronts. Partnerships with academic centres that have the wisdom, skills, and experience to successfully engage in northern community-based work, and which build local capacity, are often helpful. In terms of infectious disease prevention and care among Indigenous populations, the Center for American Indian Health (http://caih.jhu.edu) within the Johns Hopkins Bloomberg School of Public Health, serves as a model for epidemiologic and research partnerships.

Studies of Inuit and First Nations children living in northern Canada have reported an elevated (compared to non-Indigenous northern children and compared to southern children) incidence of acute (AOM) and prevalence of chronic (COM) infections of the middle ear (otitis media) (31). Determinants in this population include conditions in the social and physical environment (e.g., poverty, exposure to smoke), and host biologic factors; the latter include differences in the anatomy and function of the eustachian tube and immune factors influenced by breastfeeding and genetics (31,32). Studies of the microbiologic causes of AOM in northern Canada are lacking. In terms of prevention, it is unclear at present whether current Sp and Hi vaccines will result in decreased AOM and COM incidence in northern Canadian children. Guidelines on when to use antibiotics and which ones to use, if any, are urgently needed in northern Canada (33), and there is a need for research evaluation; those based on studies in southern populations may not be appropriate.

From 2006 to 2013, the average annual age-standardized incidence of invasive infection caused by the GAS bacteria in the ICS northern region of Canada was high (10.86/100,000) compared to Canada as a whole (4.20/100,000) (22). The incidence has been increasing since 1999 and is significantly higher among Indigenous than among non-Indigenous persons. Clinical presentations include pneumonia, empyema, bacteraemia, sepsis, necrotizing fasciitis, and bone and joint infection, among others.

The burden of illness from other conditions related to GAS infection, including pharyngitis, impetigo and other skin infections, glomerulonephritis, and acute rheumatic fever (ARF), has been noted in northern Canadian communities in which environmental determinants, particularly crowded and substandard housing, inadequate water and sewage systems, and inadequate health services, are prevalent. The average annual incidence of ARF is particularly high (21.3/100,000, 2013–2015) in northwestern Ontario, and delays in diagnosis, along with morbidity and mortality, are documented (34). Prevention and control measures for GAS include aggressive medical and social and environmental interventions. The former include development of locally appropriate algorithms for the diagnosis and treatment of pharyngitis, improved skills of primary health care providers, better surveillance (ARF is not currently a reportable disease), and systems that ensure adequate follow-up (34). Resistance to certain antibiotics, including macrolides and clindamycin, occurs in all regions of Canada; therefore, microbiologic culture and resistance testing have an important role in surveillance and care. The appropriate duration of follow-up penicillin prevention (prophylaxis) for those with cardiac involvement is unclear when patients remain in communities characterized by endemic and epidemic GAS.

The importance of surveillance for antimicrobial resistance (AMR) is also demonstrated in the context of upper and lower urinary tract infection (UTI). In a 2015 review of urine samples growing *Escherichia coli* (*E. coli*) bacteria from persons living in 19 northern Manitoba communities, 10.8 per cent produced an enzyme (extended spectrum beta-lactamase) that rendered the organism highly resistant to certain penicillin-type antibiotics, and 14 per cent were resistant to gentamicin, an antibiotic in another therapeutic class (35). This kind of regional data must be available to inform treatment decisions, which in the case of UTI are made before receiving microbiologic results, and to ensure that potentially lifesaving antimicrobials, such as those in the carbapenem class, are available in health centres.

Blood serology studies suggest that some northern trappers are exposed to the bacteria *Francisella tularensis*, but symptomatic illness is not common, possibly because the northern strain of this agent is less virulent. A case reported in Nunavut suggests a possible shift in the animal vectors that carry this organism related to environmental change (36).

Sexually Transmitted, Blood, and Body Fluid Infections

In 2015, the incidence of chlamydia was 11 times, 6 times, and 2 times higher in Nunavut, Northwest Territories, and Yukon, respectively, than the national average (37). For gonorrhea, the disparity in incidence was even higher in each territory. Sexually transmitted infection (STI) statistics are not published in a standardized fashion across provinces, but available data indicate an elevated incidence of gonorrhea and chlamydia in northern regions of British Columbia, Alberta, Saskatchewan, Manitoba, Ontario, and Quebec (Nunavik). Outbreaks of syphilis have occurred in Nunavut, Northwest Territories, northern Alberta, and Manitoba over the past five years. Data regarding HIV are problematic because of issues related to testing (such as accessibility and confidentiality) and reporting (such as migration and testing site). In 2015, HIV incidence was reported to be less than 3/100,000 in each territory (38). An elevated prevalence of HIV has been reported in northern communities in Saskatchewan (39). Reports have documented cases of another retrovirus, human T-cell lymphotropic virus (HTLV), among Inuit in Nunavut and First Nations in British Columbia (40).

Prevention of STIs requires overcoming barriers in the social and cultural environment to establish an open discourse about sex and sexuality. An increasing number of communication sites and methods focusing on sexual health, including websites, social media platforms, videos, theatre, and graphic novellas, have been developed for northern youth. Recent efforts to prevent and control STIs in the Northwest Territories and Nunavut have included community-based workshops (http://arcticfoxy.com) that foster sexual, emotional, mental, and spiritual health.

Secondary and tertiary STI prevention requires reaching out beyond health centres to identify, test, and treat asymptomatic and symptomatically infected persons. The challenges in northern communities include issues of confidentiality, stigma, fear, lack of point-of-care tests, and the limitation of tests that are sent to laboratories. STI programs will require new creative approaches that reach upstream to diagnose and treat the asymptomatically infected, and operate outside the health care box in terms of location and methods.

The prevalence of chronic hepatitis B infection among Canadian Inuit and Dene was approximately 2–5 per cent in the 1980s (41). The prevalence has fallen since the introduction of a vaccination program but remains high. The pattern of predominant genotypes in the Canadian Arctic (A, B6, D) is different from that seen in Alaska and Greenland, and within the Canadian North the pattern differs between western and eastern regions (41). These agent differences, along with possible host and/or environmental factors, may account for clinical differences: HBV sub-genotype B6 infection is associated with low risk for active liver disease and hepatocellular cancer.

Fewer data are available regarding hepatitis C in northern Canada. In a study of two Inuit communities, the prevalence of hepatitis C ranged from 1 to 18 per cent (42).

Gastrointestinal and Foodborne Infections

Data on the incidence of bacterial, viral, and parasitic gastrointestinal infection in northern Canada are not routinely available. Individual studies suggest that acute diarrheal illness is a common complaint in northern communities (43). The usually self-limited nature of the infections, and the barriers to obtaining and testing stool, promote an underestimation among patients and caregivers of associated morbidity. Research studies have identified bacterial (including *Salmonella*, *Shigella*, *Campylobacter*, *E. coli*), viral (enterovirus, norovirus, hepatitis A), and parasitic (*Giardia*, *Cryptosporidium*) pathogens as the cause of epidemic and endemic illness (43). Environmental determinants include prevalent deficiencies in water, sanitation, and housing infrastructure; climate change; and poverty.

Climate change, food insecurity, and shifts in cultural food practices have been implicated in northern foodborne illness. Outbreaks of botulism are seen when the traditional ways of fermenting whale and seal, which minimize the growth of anaerobic organisms, are not followed. Scarcity of country foods has forced an increased reliance on southern food, including meat, which may transmit bacterial infection if improperly handled or inadequately cooked (44). *Trichinella* infection is seen in the Arctic from consumption of infected marine animals and, less commonly, polar bear. It may present as diarrhea, with little or no myopathy. (45) Programs are available in Nunavut and Nunavik that allow hunters to submit meat for testing before consumption, but participation is low. *Brucella* and *Echinococcus* are endemic in northern caribou, and consumption of raw or undercooked meat is a risk factor for illness. Traditional knowledge indicates that hunters should inspect felled animals to ensure there are no signs of advanced *Brucella* infection, such as enlarged joints.

The seroprevalence of HP is high, compared to southern populations, in both Inuit and First Nations populations in northern Canada (1, 3). However, positive serology reflects past and present infection, not morbidity. Urea breath testing and stool antigen detection reflect current presence of the organism, but upper endoscopy with biopsy are required for more definitive diagnosis of potentially associated conditions, including gastritis, peptic ulcer, and gastric malignancy.

How do we diagnose and care for a patient who presents to a northern health centre with dyspepsia? Positive HP serology is of little help. Positive stool antigen shows infection but not disease. Endoscopy may diagnose disease but is not easily or widely available. Algorithmic treatment according to symptomatology and a combination of tests (if available) is used in many regions, but the efficacy and benefit of this approach is unclear, and the risks include antibiotic toxicity and promotion of resistance. HP infection is a risk factor for gastric cancer, but host susceptibility and strain genotype are key determinants. This may explain the perceived difference in the incidence of gastric cancer in Aklavik, Northwest Territories, compared to Manitoba, despite a high prevalence of HP infection in both regions (1–3).

Conclusion

A greater understanding of the interaction between host biology, agent characteristics, and environment will assist in the development of improved preventive (e.g., vaccine), diagnostic (e.g., for Hp induced gastritis), and therapeutic (e.g., use of antimicrobials) approaches to infectious diseases. Based on the issues discussed in this chapter, the following observations and suggestions may be considered:

1. In northern Canada, social, economic, political, and environmental factors are the primary determinants of the burden of infectious diseases and of disparities in relation to southern Canada. Interventions in these areas are a priority.
2. The social determinants are not an excuse for inadequate biomedical health programs. Interventions in the upstream determinants must be accompanied by improvements in the quality of local diagnostic, therapeutic, and rehabilitative health programs. Investment in human resources (e.g., the number and quality of local health workers) and in diagnostic and therapeutic approaches (e.g., antimicrobial stewardship) is recommended. Models of care from other circumpolar regions, such as the use of skilled community health aides in Alaska, are worthy of consideration (46).
3. Telling people what to do or not do is not a respectful or particularly effective approach in health care (STIs and LTBI being obvious examples). Effective health programs are designed and implemented in partnership with communities, are respectful of local knowledge and culture, and engage individuals, families, and communities in solutions.
4. Effective prevention and care programs need accurate data. The patterns and presentations of infectious diseases are different in the north than the south and change over time. We need to establish more prospective active surveillance networks.
5. Surveillance systems are not much good if there are no data to collect or if the data are not reliable. Improved diagnostic testing (including development and use of point-of-care tests) and increased availability, timeliness, and reliability of regional transport and diagnostic facilities are required.
6. Even with improved diagnostic systems, we will continue to rely on diagnostic and treatment algorithms for empiric approaches to illness in remote communities. We need research on the effectiveness of these algorithms in northern populations.

7. We must explore new technology and approaches, but not overlook or underestimate basic practices or methods (for instance, in TB programs) that have historically been proven to work.

REFERENCES

1. Bernstein C, McKeown I, Embil J, Blanchard J, Dawood M, Kabani A, Kliewer E, Smart G, Coghlan G, MacDonald S, Cook C, Orr P. Seroprevalence of *Helicobacter pylori*, incidence of gastric cancer, and peptic ulcer-associated hospitalization in a Canadian Indian population. Dig Dis Sci. 1999;44(4):668–74.
2. Kersulyte D, Bertoli MT, Tamma S, Keelan M, Munday R, Geary J, Veldhuyzen van Zanten S, Goodman KJ, Berg DE. Complete genome sequences of two *Helicobacter pylori* strains from a Canadian Arctic Aboriginal community. Genome Announc. 2015 Apr 16;3(2):e00209–15. doi: 10.1128/genomeA.00209-15
3. Cheung J, Goodman K J, Girgis S, Bailey R, Morse J, Fedorak RN, Geary J, Fagan-Garcia K, van Zanten SV; CANHelp Working Group. Disease manifestations of *Helicobacter pylori* infection in Arctic Canada: using epidemiology to address community concerns. BMJ Open. 2014 Jan 8;4(1):e003689. doi: 10.1136/bmjopen-2013-003689
4. Larcombe L, Orr P, Turner-Brannen E, Slivinski C, Nickerson P, Mookherjee N. Effect of vitamin D supplementation on mycobacterium tuberculosis-induced innate immune responses in a Canadian Dene First Nations cohort. PLoS One. 2012;7(7):e40692. doi: 10.1371/journal.pone.0040692
5. LaFreniere M, Hussain H, He N, McGuire M. Tuberculosis in Canada: 2017. Can Commun Dis Rep [Internet]. 2019 Feb [cited 2019 Feb 28];45(2/3):68–74. Available from: https://doi.org/10.14745/ccdr.v45i23a04
6. Long R, Hoeppner V, Orr P, Ainslie M, King M, Abonyi S, Mayan M, Kunimoto D, Langlois-Klassen D, Heffernan C, Lau A, Menzies D. Marked disparity in the epidemiology of tuberculosis among Aboriginal peoples on the Canadian prairies: the challenges and opportunities. Can Respir J. 2013 Jul–Aug;20(4):223–30.
7. Orr P. Tuberculosis in Nunavut: looking back, moving forward. CMAJ. 2013 Mar;185(4):287–8.
8. Basham CA, Elias B, Fanning A, Orr P. Performance measurement of a Canadian provincial tuberculosis programme: Manitoba, 2008–2012. Int J Tuberc Lung Dis. 2018 April;22(4):437–43.
9. Yuhui X. Investigation of tuberculosis outbreak in Nunavut, 2017. [SCRIBD Internet Site, uploaded by Nunatsiaq News]. [cited 2019 Feb 28]. Available from: https://drive.google.com/file/d/1M5il0FrsjEl0rswrLd6ux4znliIS8LrD/view
10. House of Commons Standing Committee on Health [Internet]. Ottawa (ON): Parliament of Canada. Evidence: Tuesday, April 20, 2010. Number 010, 3rd Session of the 40th Parliament; [cited 2019 Feb 28]. Available from: https://www.ourcommons.ca/DocumentViewer/en/40-3/HESA/meeting-10/evidence

11. Alvarez GG, VanDyk DD, Aaron SD, Cameron DW, Davies N, Stephen N, Mallick R, Momoli F, Moreau K, Obed N, Baikie M, Osborne G. Taima (stop) TB: the impact of a multifaceted TB awareness and door-to-door campaign in residential areas of high risk for TB in Iqaluit, Nunavut. PLoS One. 2014 July;9(7):e100975. doi: 10.1371/journal.pone.0100975
12. Orr P. Adherence to tuberculosis care in Canadian Aboriginal populations. Part 2: a comprehensive approach to fostering adherent behaviour. Int J Circumpolar Health. 2011 April;70(2):128–40.
13. Greenberg D, Banerji A, Friedman MG, Chiu C, Kahane S. High Rate of Simkania negevensis among Canadian Inuit Infants hospitalized with lower respiratory tract infections. Scand J Infect Dis. 2003 July;35(8):506–8.
14. Robinson JL, Le Saux N. Preventing hospitalizations for respiratory syncytial virus infection. Position statement: Canadian Pediatric Society, Infectious Diseases and Immunization Committee. Paediatr Child Health. 2015 Aug-Sept;20(6):321–6.
15. Van Caeseele P, Macaulay A, Orr P, Aoki F, Martin B. Rapid pharmacotherapeutic intervention for an influenza A outbreak in the Canadian Arctic: lessons from the Sanikiluaq experience. Int J Circumpolar Health. 2001 Nov;60(4):640–8.
16. Kumar A, Zarychanski R, Pinto R, Cook DJ, Marshall J, Lacroix J, Stelfox T, Bagshaw S, Choong K, Lamontagne F, Turgeon AF, Lapinsky S, Ahern SP, Smith O, Siddiqui F, Jouvet P, Khwaja K, McIntyre L, Menon K, Hutchison J, Hornstein D, Joffe A, Lauzier F, Singh J, Karachi T, Wiebe K, Olafson K, Ramsey C, Sharma S, Dodek P, Meade M, Hall R, Fowler RA; Canadian Critical Care Trials Group H1N1 Collaborative. Critically ill patients with 2009 influenza A(H1N1) infection in Canada. JAMA. 2009 Nov;302(17): 1872–9.
17. Keynan Y, Malik S, Fowke KR. The role of polymorphisms in host genes in determining the severity of respiratory illness caused by pandemic H1N1 influenza. Public Health Genomics. 2013 March; 16(1–2): 9–16.
18. Braun K, Larcombe L, Orr P, Nickerson P, Wolfe J, Sharma M. Killer immunoglobulin-like receptor (KIR) centromeric-AA haplotype is associated with ethnicity and tuberculosis disease in a Canadian First Nations cohort. PLoS One. 2013 July;8(7):e67842. doi: 10.1371/journal.pone.0067842
19. Rubinstein E, Predy G, Sauvé L, Hammond GW, Aoki F, Sikora C, Li Y, Law B, Halperin S, Scheifele D. The responses of Aboriginal Canadians to adjuvanted pandemic (H1N1) 2009 influenza vaccine. CMAJ. 2011 Sept 20;183(13):E1033–7. doi: 10.1503/cmaj.110196
20. Golding GR, Levett PN, McDonald RR, Irvine J, Nsungu M, Woods S, Horbal A, Siemens CG, Khan M, Ofner-Agostini M, Mulvey MR; Northern Antibiotic Resistance Partnership. A comparison of risk factors associated with community-associated methicillin-resistant and -susceptible *Staphylococcus aureus* infections in remote communities. Epidemiol Infect. 2010 May;138(5):730–7.

21. Kirlew M, Schroeter SRA, Makahnouk D, Hamilton M, Brunton N, Muileboom J, Schreiber Y, Saginur R, Kelly L. Invasive CA-MRSA in northwestern Ontario: a 2-year prospective study. Can J Rural Med. 2014 Summer;19(3):99–102.
22. Li YA, Martin I, Tsang R, Squires SG, Demczuk W, Desai S. Invasive bacterial diseases in North Canada, 2006–2013. Can Commun Dis Rep [Internet]. 2016 Apr 7 [cited 2019 Feb 28];42(4):74–82. Available from: https://doi.org/10.14745/ccdr.v42i04a01
23. Le Meur J-B, Lefebvre B, Proulx J-F, Dery S, Pepin J, De Wals. Impact of pneumococcal vaccines use on invasive pneumococcal disease in Nunavik (Quebec) from 1997 to 2010. Int J Circumpolar Health [Internet]. 2014 Jan [cited 2019 Feb 28];73:22691. Available from: https://doi.org/10.3402/ijch.v73.22691
24. Tyrrell GJ, Lovgren M, Ibrahim Q, Garg S, Chui L, Boone TJ, Mangan C, Patrick DM, Hoang L, Horsman GB, Van Caeseele P, Marrie TJ. Epidemic of invasive pneumococcal disease, Western Canada, 2005–2009. Emerg Infect Dis. 2012 May;18(5):733–40.
25. Huang G, Li AY, Martin I, Demczuk VBH, Tsang R. Epidemiology of invasive bacterial diseases among children under 2 years of age in northern Canada, 2011 to 2015 [abstract]. Presented at: 17th International Congress on Circumpolar Health [Internet]; 2018 Aug [cited 2019 Feb 29]; Copenhagen Denmark. Abstract no. 100. Available from: http://www.icch2018.com/wp-content/uploads/2018/08/AbstractList_Final_100818.pdf
26. Miernyk KM, Parkinson AJ, Rudolph KM, Petersen KM, Bulkow LR, Greenberg DP, Ward JI, Brenneman G, Reid R, Santosham M. Immunogenicity of a heptavalent pneumococcal conjugate vaccine in Apache and Navajo Indian, Alaska native, and non-native American children aged <2 years. Clin Infect Dis. 2000 Jul;31(1):34–41.
27. Helferty M, Rotondo JL, Martin I, Desai S. The epidemiology of invasive pneumococcal disease in the Canadian North from 1999 to 2010. Int J Circumpolar Health [Internet]. 2013 Aug 5 [cited 2019 Feb 29];72. Available from: https//doi.org/10.3402/ijch.v72i0.21606
28. Kelly L, Tsang R, Morgan A, Jamieson FB, Ulanova M. Invasive disease caused by Haemophilus influenza type A in Northern Ontario First nations Communities. J Medical Microbiology. 2011;60:384–90.
29. Bruce M, Zulz T, Johnson K, Hurlburt D, Rudolph K, Debyle C, Tsang R. The epidemiology of Haemophilus influenza serotype a disease in the North American Arctic, 2000–2016 [abstract]. Presented at: 17th International Congress on Circumpolar Health [Internet]; 2018 Aug [cited 2019 Feb 29]; Copenhagen Denmark. Abstract no. 263. Available from: http://www.icch2018.com/wp-content/uploads/2018/08/AbstractList_Final_100818.pdf
30. Guenter D, Siber G, Law B, Moffatt M. Antibody to *H. influenza* type B capsular polysaccharide in maternal and cord sera from Inuit, Native Indian and Caucasian subjects in the Northwest Territories and Manitoba. Arctic Med Res. 1991;Suppl: 344–5.

31. Bowd A. Otitis media: health and social consequences for Aboriginal youth in Canada's North. Int J Circumpolar Health. 2005 Feb;64(1):5–15.
32. Bluestone CD, Klein JO. Otitis media in infants and children. 2nd ed. Toronto (ON): WB Saunders; 1995.
33. Martin BD, Macdonald SM. The management of ear disease: guidelines for Aboriginal health care programs. Int J Circumpolar Health. 1998;57(Suppl 1):268–75.
34. Gordon J, Kirlew M, Schreiber Y, Saginur R, Bocking N, Blakelock B, Haavaldsrud M, Kennedy C, Farrell T, Douglas L, Kelly L. Acute rheumatic fever in First Nations communities in northwestern Ontario: social determinants of health "bite the heart." Can Fam Physician. 2015 Oct;61(10):881–6.
35. Bogaty C, Kassam S, Walkty A, Orr P. Frequency of extended-spectrum beta-lactamase-producing *Escherichia coli* urinary isolates from nursing stations in northern Manitoba, Canada [abstract]. Presented at: Association of Medical Microbiology and Infectious Diseases annual conference [Internet]; 2018 May 3 [cited 2019 Feb 28]; Vancouver (BC) Canada. Abstract PT15. Available from: http://www.ammi.ca/AnnualConference/2018/Abstracts/%202018%20JAMMI%20Abstracts.pdf
36. Silverman M, Law B, Carson J. A case of insect borne tularemia above the tree line. Arctic Med Res. 1991;Suppl:377–9
37. Public Health Agency of Canada. Report on sexually transmitted infections in Canada: 2012 [Internet]. Ottawa (ON): Centre for Communicable Diseases and Infection Control, Infectious Disease Prevention and Control Branch, Public Health Agency of Canada; 2015 [cited 2019 Feb 28]. Available from: http://www.catie.ca/ga-pdf.php?file=sites/default/files/Report-on-STIs-in-Canada-2012.pdf
38. Public Health Agency of Canada [Internet]. Ottawa (ON): Government of Canada. HIV in Canada: surveillance summary tables, 2014–2015; [modified 2016 Nov 30; cited 2019 Feb 28]. Available from: http://www.canada.ca/en/public-health/services/publications/diseases-conditions/hiv-in-canada-surveillance-summary-tables-2014-2015.html
39. Population Health Branch, Ministry of Health (SK). Saskatchewan HIV prevention and control report 2017. Saskatoon (SK): Government of Saskatchewan; 2018 [cited 2019 Feb 28]. Available from: http://publications.gov.sk.ca/documents/13/108029-2017-Saskatchewan-HIV-Prevention-and-Control-Report.pdf
40. Andonov A, Coulthart MB, Perez-Losada M, Crandall KA, Posada D, Padmore R, Giulivi A, Oger JJ, Peters AA, Dekaban GA. Insights into origins of human t-cell lymphotropic virus type 1 based on new strains from Aboriginal people of Canada. Infect Genet Evol. 2012 Dec;12(8):1822–30.
41. Osiowy C, Simons BC, Rempek JD. Distribution of viral hepatitis in indigenous populations of North America and the circumpolar Arctic. Antivir Ther. 2013 Jun;18(3 Pt B):467–73. doi: 10.3851/IMP2597

42. Rempel JD, Uhanova J. Hepatitis C in American Indian/Alaskan Native and Aboriginal Peoples of North America. Viruses. 2012 Dec;4(12):3912–31.
43. Harper SL, Edge VL, Ford J, Thomas MK, Pearl D, Shirley J, IHACC, RICG, McEwen SA. Healthcare use for acute gastrointestinal illness in two Inuit communities: Rigolet and Iqaluit, Canada. Int J Circumpolar Health. 2015; 21;74 (1):26290. doi: 10.3402/ijch.v74.26290
44. Orr P, Lorencz B, Brown R, Kielly R, Tan B, Holton D, Clugstone H, Lugtig L, Pim C, Macdonald S, Hammond G, Moffatt M, Spika J, Manuel D, Winther W, Milley D, Lior H, Sinuff N. An outbreak of diarrhea due to verotoxin-producing Escherichia coli in the Canadian Northwest Territories. Scand J Infect Dis. 1994 Dec;26(6):675–84.
45. Proulx J-F, MacLean JD, Gyorkos TW, Leclair D, Richter A-K, Serhir B, Forbes L, Gajadhar AA. Novel prevention program for trichinellosis in Inuit communities. Clin Infect Dis. 2002 Jun;34(11):1508–14.
46. Golnick C, Asay E, Provost E, Van Liere D, Bosshart C, Rounds-Riley J, Cueva K, Hennessy TW. Innovative primary care delivery in rural Alaska: a review of patient encounters seen by community health aides. Int J Circumpolar Health. 2012 Jun 29;71:18543. doi: 10.3402/ijch.v71i0.18543

5 Women's Health: What Does It Mean to "Be Well"? A Qualitative Case Study to Explore Inuit Women's Conceptions of Wellness

GWEN HEALEY AKEAROK, LYNN M. MEADOWS, THERESA KOONOO, AND KATHY MICHAEL

Introduction

Women's health and well-being in northern Canada has been the subject of some study, primarily focusing on topics related to childbirth, midwifery, and the impact of colonial policies and sedentarization of northern Indigenous communities (1–4). It is well known in Canada that Nunavummiut (people of Nunavut) face a number of barriers when it comes to achieving and maintaining good health: poor access to services (5); understaffed health centres (6); a transient workforce of health professionals (6,7) (see also Møller, chapter 8, and Pong, chapter 7, both this volume); serious issues related to mental wellness, addiction (8,9) (see also Mushquash, Drawson, and Toombs, chapter 15; and Tan, chapter 13, both this volume), historical trauma, and acculturation (10–14); a high prevalence of communicable diseases, such as tuberculosis (TB) (15,16) (see also Orr and Larcombe, chapter 4, this volume); and geographically and politically isolated communities (17–19). There are also tremendous strengths in communities to address local health concerns, such as a willingness to work together, strong social support, Inuit ways of knowing and living that foster healthy lifestyles and activity, the continuation of the sharing of Inuit knowledge in new and innovative ways, and strong cultural pride (20–24) (see also Crawford, Waddell, and Lund, chapter 17, this volume).

Greater disparities in health status exist between men and women in Inuit communities than in the general population (25). Serious health issues that affect Inuit women include high rates of sexually transmitted infections (26), high levels of smoking (24), and food insecurity (23). Mental health and wellness play a significant role in the overall health of women. *Mental health, wellness*, and *well-being* are terms that are often used interchangeably to describe psychological health, the perception of health, an overall sense of health, and an overall satisfaction with our health (27). In Nunavut, challenges to mental health and wellness have been described as one of the most prevalent and concerning health issues (28–30). Past epidemiological research has documented high rates of depression (9,31–33), violence (34,35), and deaths by suicide (33,36,37) in our communities. It is important to hear and understand the voices of our community members on the topic of mental health and wellness to build on our strengths and move forward in supporting each other on a journey to wellness. In this chapter, we share the perspectives of a group of Inuit women to shed light on some of the health and social challenges that affect individual, family, and community wellness.

There is a paucity of literature that shares the voices of women and their insights into the strengths, protective mechanisms, experiences, and contexts they feel impact wellness. The research discussed in this chapter was carried out a decade ago and since then, little other research has been published on this topic outside policy documents, but, more importantly, very little has changed in women's health since that time. A new literature search was conducted for this chapter, and the contents of the original paper were reviewed again by the authors. The information was found to still be relevant today because women still hold the same perspective and challenges persist, such as obstetric evaluation (38,39), the lack of culturally appropriate health care options (12), and the need for care provided in local language (40). More recent literature published in other areas, such as suicide and the lives and concerns of Inuit women, are considered in the discussion section. This chapter presents and discusses the determinants of health and wellness as identified by a group of Inuit women in Nunavut.

Historical Context – Colonization and Wellness

During the 1920s, 1930s, and 1940s, TB and influenza repeatedly ravaged Inuit populations (15,41,42), and many of the same illnesses continue to present in high numbers in northern communities today (26). The process of relocation off the land and into communities initially began as a response by Inuit to the presence of fur traders, explorers, and missionaries; however, it took new form with the systematic efforts of the government in the 1950s to "resettle" Canada's North. Inuit were relocated to southern Canada to cut relief costs and for them to receive medical care, in particular for TB; to remote High Arctic regions to maintain sovereignty and support the economic initiatives of the Hudson's Bay Company; and off the land and into settlements to facilitate the provision of supplies, education, and medical care (3,43,44). The significant and life-altering movement of Inuit to either southern, High Arctic, or community-based locations had an impact on the transmission of Inuit knowledge and language, and Inuit ways of teaching and learning, and on the mental health and wellness of community members.

In 1951, the first government-regulated residential school for Inuit was opened in Chesterfield Inlet (45). Exposure to residential schools for Inuit in the eastern Arctic occurred in recent history – in the living memory of our Elders and community members – resulting in extreme culture shock and abrupt alteration of Inuit life and pathways to well-being. Some communities have experienced up to three generations of Inuit children being sent away from their families to attend day schools in the larger communities (45,46). Many of the students who attended residential school in Nunavut, similar to Indigenous people elsewhere, experienced mental, verbal, physical, and emotional abuse in these institutions (13,45–47). These students are the parents, grandparents, uncles, and aunts of today.

Contemporary Context – Wellness in Today's Communities

Communities in Nunavut are now permanent settlements ranging between 110 and 7000 in population. The size and location of a community play significant roles in wellness among members, with some perceiving less control and greater influence on behaviour from other sources or individuals, depending on whether the community is a regional transportation centre, whether the population is more or less transient, or whether there is access to alcohol (48). Influences from media, television, and the education system (49,50); residential schooling (45,46); medical evacuation for birthing and treatment of communicable diseases, such as TB; and settlement in permanent communities have contributed to significant acculturative stress and mental health and wellness issues (42,43,51–53) for Inuit women, families, and communities today.

Canada's chief public health officer from 2014 to 2016, Dr. Gregory Taylor, stated in a report that "family violence is an important public health issue. Its impacts on health go beyond direct physical injury, are widespread and long-lasting and can be severe, particularly for mental health. Even less severe forms of family violence can affect health" (35 p3). In Nunavut, the Crime Severity Index, the measure of the seriousness of a crime, is four times the level in Canada as a whole (54). In the Inuit Health Survey, 52 per cent of women and 46 per cent of men reported having experienced at least one form of physical violence as an adult (24). Thirty-one per cent of respondents experienced severe physical abuse as children, and 38 per cent reported that as adults they have sometimes or often experienced verbal abuse. A survey conducted by Pauktuutit Inuit Women of Canada on shelter service needs in Inuit Nunangat stated that 27 per cent of those seeking shelter are turned away because of a lack of space (55). Although it is a very complex issue, the stress of rapid social change, colonization, trauma, and the inadequacy of programs and services in communities have been identified as barriers to meaningfully addressing interpersonal violence (55–58).

Suicide is also a serious concern that affects many Inuit communities in Nunavut; it has received much media attention in recent years from both the research community and the media. Kral and Minore (59) conducted a study in which 90 Inuit – an equal number of men and women – were interviewed about suicide and wellness in Igloolik, Nunavut, and Qikiqtarjuaq, Nunavut. Having someone to talk with, having connections to family, having connections to the land, and being familiar with other forms of *Inuit Qaujimajatuqangit* (Inuit knowledge) were identified as important factors in wellness, happiness, health, and healing. Those themes remain prevalent today (9,30). In research studies conducted in recent years, suicide was identified with being disconnected from family and with the breakup of romantic relationships, substance and cannabis use, depression, and personality disorders (60–62). Mancini Billson and Mancini (63) and Pauktuutit Inuit Women's Association (45,64) have identified childhood sexual abuse as a factor in suicide attempts among Inuit women and as a serious concern in northern communities in Canada, particularly in the context of residential schooling and its intergenerational effects.

Alcohol and substance abuse and exposure to violent situations endanger both the health and the safety of Inuit women and their families in Nunavut. Suicide continues to be a concern among community members and organizations in Nunavut, and new initiatives are being implemented to address this (31,37,65,66).

Case Study: A Qualitative Exploration of Inuit Women's Conceptions of Wellness

We conducted an exploratory qualitative case study to investigate a research question that was raised by several women in the community: What does it mean to "be well" and how do we support women to achieve well-being? The study used an Inuit research framework, which privileged Inuit research and knowledge production constructs: *Unikkaaqatigiiniq* (storytelling), *Inuuqatigiittiarniq* (respect for all people), *Pittiarniq* (to be good or kind), *Piliriqatigiiniq* (working together for the common good), and *Iqqaumaqatigiinniq* (thinking deeply in ways that lead to understanding or innovation) (20).

The approach included an iterative process for recruitment, sampling, data collection, and analysis. Individual face-to-face interviews were conducted to gather data from a sample of Inuit women living in Iqaluit, Nunavut, between August 2005 and January 2006. As stated earlier in this chapter, although this research was carried out more than a decade ago, little other research has been published on this topic since this study was conducted.

Purposive sampling strategies (67) allowed for a sample of women that included a wide range of characteristics, such as age, family status, and educational background, that were representative of the variables of interest in the population (68). Participants were recruited until the data reached saturation or until new interviews no longer contributed to the themes identified in analysis

(67,68). With participant permission, interviews were audio recorded with a digital recorder and transcribed verbatim. Interviews ranged between 30 and 90 minutes and took place at a location chosen by the participant. Interviews were conducted by the researcher using a semi-structured, eight-question guide. Participants were asked to comment on the contexts and issues that affected their health (e.g., broad determinants of health). In particular, the participants were asked to comment on how these issues contributed to their well-being and impacted their daily lives. Data were coded with QSR*N6 software and analysed by the researcher using a process of immersion and crystallization (69). Issues of rigour were addressed using established qualitative techniques, which included a thorough review of the literature (67,70), bracketing (a process of critical self-reflection to acknowledge and "bracket" preconceptions about the research topic) and researcher reflexivity (68), debriefing with colleagues and co-researchers (20), and member checking by verifying data and analyses with participants (68,71,72).

Locating the Researcher Position

Gwen Healey Akearok: My engagement in this research emerged from a lifelong pursuit to understand and build on the aspects of my community that contribute to wellness. I was born and raised in Iqaluit, Nunavut. My ancestry is not Inuit. I was raised to know, respect, and live by Inuit values as a member of the community – a community that did not point out to me in any way that I was not Inuit. I did not grow up feeling that I was different. My husband and my children are Inuit. Inuit ways of knowing and understanding are embedded in my world view. I love my community and where I come from. I feel privileged to have been taught and mentored by Elders of my community, including Aalasi Joamie, Martha Tikivik, and the late Andrew Tagak, Sr. My research position was to meaningfully engage in what other scholars outline as methodologies that weave ethical approaches, participatory research, self-reflexivity, and community research practices and world views, with particular emphasis on addressing inequity in our communities.

Theresa Koonoo: Originally from Pond Inlet, Nunavut, Theresa is now the territorial coordinator for community health representatives in Nunavut. At the time of the original study, Theresa provided advice, insight, and guiding questions, and reviewed the study findings again in preparation of this manuscript.

Kathy Michael: The late Kathy Michael was from Iqaluit, Nunavut. She was the community health representative when the research was carried out and contributed to the study as a research assistant, helped to shape questions, and shared advice and direction. Her contribution is acknowledged posthumously with the permission of her daughter.

Lynn M. Meadows: I am a southern researcher from Calgary and provided a supportive role in the research. I was privileged to support Gwen's MSc research, sharing perspectives, knowledge, and experience to better understand the health of Inuit women. Additionally, I worked with Gwen and another southern college on a funded grant to explore Inuit women's bone health from 2005 to 2007. During my career, I have striven to make visible women's experiences and voices related to their health and well-being. I have had the honour of doing research through three visits to Iqaluit between 2005 and 2018. Inuit women have helped me gain insight into their lives and culture when I have worked directly with them through research.

In addition to being granted the approval of the University of Calgary's Conjoint Health Research Ethics Board, this research project was licensed by the Nunavut Research Institute and guided by the *Ethical Principles for the Conduct of Research in the North*, published by the Association of Canadian Universities for Northern Studies (73). Above all, participants were treated with respect, appreciation, and dignity.

Similar to participatory action research, an Inuit research framework stresses the relationship between researcher and community, the direct benefit to the community of the potential outcome of the research, and the community's involvement as beneficial in and of itself (74). Participants in this study individually member checked the research findings in one-on-one discussions and were provided opportunities to incorporate the results into their work or their community involvement, or to share information with family or friends.

Results: Women's Perspectives on Wellness

Eight self-identified Inuit women between 27 and 51 years of age participated in this study and provided data through nine in-depth interviews in Iqaluit, Nunavut. One participant requested a second interview the following day after thinking about the questions more deeply. Mental health and well-being were discussed by participants in terms of a transition from traditional to southern values and ways of living, the changing gender roles in families and in the workforce, and any issues of identity related to the feeling that they are torn between two cultures. Women discussed mental health and well-being in terms of (1) culture and identity; (2) self-esteem and self-confidence; (3) relationships with family, partners, and the community; and (4) alcohol and substance abuse.

Culture, Knowledge, and Identity

Culture was discussed by the participants in terms of shared practices and beliefs and the use of common Inuktut language. Personal identity was tied to articulations of culture for women in this study. Women felt they were caught between wanting to respect Inuit traditions and ways of living and living in a rapidly changing world where formal education, gainful employment, and growing communities have altered the way of life for Nunavummiut. Participants felt that young Inuit women were facing internal struggles to forge the pathways forward while remaining true to the many cultures, Inuit and non-Inuit, that are converging in Nunavut.

> Knowing your culture, it'll affect your health mentally and knowing who you are and if you know who you are, then … you'll have more confidence in yourself … I know with me I went [away for high school] … which I'm happy about but … I had a lot of struggles in finding out who I am … I'd say I'm an Inuk but I'm living in a qallunaat [white person] world. Where does that leave me? Am I betraying my Inuk culture or what am I doing? I had a lot of personal struggles and finding out who I really am. – Participant #2

In some cases, this tension came from, for example, having one parent who is Inuk[1] and the other non-Inuk. For others, it originated from education and travel experiences in the south or the growing population of non-Inuit in the territory. Young women in the study felt that their identity as Inuit would be defined by others based on their ability to speak Inuktitut. The young women themselves also correlated their language abilities with the extent to which they felt they were Inuit, which challenged their sense of identity.

> When I was at school, I felt like I had to find myself and kind of accept who I am … there's a lot of Western influence … when I came back [from boarding school] I knew how to speak Inuktitut but … it wasn't really good. I felt kind of stupid for not being able to speak Inuktitut – kind of shy. I [was discouraged] and didn't want to [try to] speak Inuktitut anymore … I think [what I felt is experienced] by a lot of people. Younger people … they don't really know their language … Because they're Inuk but [people say you're not] if you can't speak the language and then that's when I started questioning … then what am I, you know? I'm supposed to be Inuk and I can't speak my language fully. I kind of got lost. It was not fair … I'm supposed to be Inuk, I should know how to do this kind of thing and it still affects me now. – Participant #7

Overall, women talked about the general move away from Inuit cultural practices as a type of grief, a grief resulting from the experience of culture loss, and that this grief can cause significant problems related to identity, social inclusion, wellness, and suicide. They discussed the Inuit knowledge and practices that they treasured and that gave them strength, such as stories of childrearing, midwifery, harvesting and preparing food, and sewing.

> And when my [children] come in, they eat fish or take out some clams or whatever I have available. I pick them myself in the bay. – Participant #3

> It's like it makes me [think] sometimes … What's their life like compared to the way we are now? My Anaana (mother) says they were taught respect. They were taught how to live out on the land. They were taught how to make clothing out of animal hides and things like that … I think one of the problems we have now is multicultural [values] mingling together … I think that one of the reasons why there is more family violence … unhealthy relationship is that you are told [to behave a certain way] by your parents. But then you are told by the government you need good education and you have to do things a different way … like so right now it's two [messages] at the same time … The woman does not have enough education, can't work … I think that's what's causing a lot of frustration in life right now. If I didn't get an education like I did, I think I'd be in the gap. I'd be right where I cannot go forward or backwards to fix it 'cause there's a barrier there. – Participant #5

Women described owning and sharing of this knowledge as contributing to positive well-being. They highlighted the importance that knowing or learning Inuktitut (or the more localized Inuktut) has for them; the importance of valuing opportunities to spend time with and learn from Elders; and the importance of practising skills, such as sewing or harvesting, with more knowledgeable role models. These activities created important opportunities for learning and sharing Inuit knowledge, fostering healthy relationships with community members, and keeping a positive outlook on life. This, in turn, fostered community wellness.

> I believe with anything, if we dwell on the positive side of things even though you're passing by some negative stuff, when you look at the positive side of things it makes it that much easier for you to deal with … It energizes you more. I find that when I start to look at things in such a dreary way, in a negative way, it weighs me down. It really weighs me down and it takes away lots of energy … And I think keeping a positive attitude towards those things helps to alleviate it much quicker and easier. Although it may not be alleviated totally, it makes it easier. – Participant #6

Self-Esteem and Self-Confidence

Participants were concerned that among Inuit women, low levels of self-esteem and confidence were developed early in childhood (e.g., already present at elementary school levels) and continued throughout their lives. They identified this as a problem affecting women's well-being. However, they were unable to articulate why they felt low levels of self-esteem develop and exist. Women were concerned with what they described as a general lack of parenting skill among parents in the community. Younger participants, in particular, discussed wellness and self-esteem in terms of what one participant called living a "dramatic lifestyle" – characterized by a combination of drinking, partying, drug use, and high-risk sexual activity in the community.

> Understanding how people conduct themselves in their relationships with whomever, I think is a really big determinant of how you expect your life will be ... If you have a constant presence of unhealthy relationships ... that unhealthiness that comes with living an unnecessarily dramatic lifestyle ... if you live in that kind of constant uncertainty and drama, I think that really takes a toll on you ... These are the things that you have to challenge and you have to work through yourself ... I think that's the hardest thing about being healthy is that you have to make the commitment to yourself to work through those problems ... I think once you have figured out how to take care of yourself that way, that's when you're really, really healthy. – Participant #1

Participants felt that this "dramatic" lifestyle could put women at risk for sexually transmitted infections and unwanted pregnancies and expose them to situations where they might consume alcohol during pregnancy, be sexually assaulted, or be vulnerable to situations of violence. In addition, the "drama" described by women also referred to community gossip. Community gossip, they felt, resulted from or led to gossip about an individual's choices and risky lifestyle and only contributed negatively to the self-esteem of women.

Women described harvesting; sharing food; having positive relationships with family and friends; pursuing different forms of education, such as school or learning from Elders; and exploring creative and artistic pursuits as being positive contributors to self-esteem.

Relationships

Women spoke about relationships and their effect on wellness in terms of family dynamics; personal and intimate relationships with partners; and relationships within the community.

Family: Participants felt that Inuit women often have sole responsibility for children in separated relationships, even in partnered relationships, and identified that responsibility as a source of both mental and financial strain. Mothers in the study had both biological and adopted children and spoke to "worrying" about their children, their health, their education, their exposure to sexually transmitted infections as teenagers, and their choices in relationships. They noted that stress had a considerable impact on the wellness of both women and men. When asked about the origin of stressors, women reported that it was largely based in family dynamics and relationships. Women discussed family relationships in terms of multiple generations, including their own parents, siblings, and children. These relationships were described as valuable but also challenging to manage and as both a source of stress in their lives and a source of support. Women perceived poor relationships among parents and children to generally be attributable to poor communication skills, a lack of knowledge about parenting, or a lack of understanding of traditional values related to childrearing.

Inuit values that women noted included celebrating the strengths and abilities of children, acknowledging the naming relationships, helping and learning from Elders, and making positive contributions to family and community. The interviewed women's perspectives illustrated the complex relationships between parents, children, extended family, and community, and highlighted the need to support positive Inuit values and practices both now and for the future.

> I think that's a big part of the health issues, managing family dynamics … I think it's also a good way to [move towards a] healthier life, stronger living. Family relationships, with partners, with children. Childrearing practices, having good communication with the family network. [Sharing] the values of our traditional Inuit childrearing practices and family beliefs in general. They're not lost; you cannot lose what you still have. They're not being learned. They're not being shared. And they need to be shared more. And we need to hear the values, … from our traditional background. Because they are so very important. And very important to be passed on. We come from an oral history and how we know about our culture and so on is through oral storytelling, being passed on from generation to generation. It was very easy to do that when your families lived together in one dwelling, but that is not the situation anymore. And there's nothing wrong with that; it's just the fact that we need to continue the sharing of information in a different medium now I think. Ah, we have lived, passed on that information orally, now we need to look at more effective ways because we're not living with our parents and grandparents anymore in a close-knit way. Then, we should rely more on perhaps different medium like reading material and books and videos and all kinds of radios and all kinds of other medium that is more effective in a way that we're living in our [current] society. –Participant #4

Partners: Women highlighted the particularly demanding role of intimate partner relationships in their lives and in the lives of their friends and family in the community. Participants felt many Inuit women experience violence and anger in intimate relationships. When women spoke of domestic violence it was primarily in terms of how male partners needed help. Several participants noted that Inuit men were coping with their own personal trauma and pain and felt these underlying issues needed to be addressed. Women also described situations where women acquaintances were reluctant to leave a violent relationship because they did not have their own money and could not afford to take their children and leave. If they did leave, they and their children potentially had to rely on friends or family members for a period, becoming part of the "hidden homeless"[2] in Nunavut. Several of the participants in the older age group (over 40 years of age) highlighted the importance of communication with partners, indicating that poor communication in partnerships came from either not knowing its value or needing guidance in effective communication. In addition, effects of rapid cultural change were highlighted as influencing personal, familial, and community relationships. One participant stated,

> Lack of communication, lack of trust and [the effect of] two cultures mingling together are the three factors I could think of for [contributing to] unhealthy relationships … There's lack of communication between Elders and the younger generation and when we listen to our parents talking about how it was back then, I say "wow" … Communication is important … Like communicate … it gives us a healthier home environment, family environment and I feel that communication [and storytelling] … is the major medications for your life. – Participant #5

Community: The importance of having strong relationships within the community to share experiences and impart health knowledge was clearly articulated. However, the women described some aspects of community relationships as negative. For example, women spoke of how the community views a person, how they felt judged by community members regarding their life decisions, or how family members may band together against an individual or another family over a personal issue.

Substance Use and Coping

Use of substances, such as alcohol, was often brought into the conversation indirectly through issues dealing with sexual abuse or the supports that are needed to cope with emotionally difficult times. A few women had participated in addictions recovery programs and had sought counselling to address the anger and hurt they carried as a result of experiencing childhood sexual abuse.

> I was majorly stressed I think between 15 and 21. Um, I was learning to live away from home and learning to be on my own and figuring out how you live on your own. Once I got used to that it, it's pretty easy. I learned then it takes a long time to recover, to get healthy again when you have been sexually abused or raped. The last five years I have been accepting and moving on and being healthy about it. I went to a post-traumatic recovery for 10 weeks and also went to a detox rehab to deal with all these issues. Even after I left I went on, went to [continue] counselling for that … I recommend it to women, or even men, that have been abused to take that move. Because I always used to think I would be able to heal by myself … but I was wrong. It takes a lot of work to get over that. Because in smaller communities, family is involved. Your abuser is part of the family. So for us women, for any women,

> it's slowly getting better where sexual abuse used to be just swept under our carpet, and if you voiced about it you were considered a "shit disturber." So you always had to watch yourself, because you're the one, even though you're the victim, they would turn on you and say, "You're wrecking the family … Just sweep this under the carpet." And, your abuser; they don't even bother with that person regardless of how much damage they have done. So, that's the unhealthy part. I do recommend very much [for women and men] to seek help. – Participant #8

Participants described sexual abuse as a terrible and widespread issue that they felt affected both men and women in many communities in Nunavut, and that they felt was often ignored. Additionally, participants linked sexual abuse and its repercussions (for both victim and aggressor) to ongoing trauma, domestic violence, and substance use by participants. One participant described losing many years of her life to alcoholism in her attempt to cope with years of sexual abuse as an adolescent. She felt that this issue was not uncommon and described situations of other women known to her who use alcohol to cope with their own personal history of abuse. Women also identified coping mechanisms that contributed to a positive sense of wellness, such as pursuing counselling and addictions treatment, spending time with children and grandchildren, harvesting and sharing food, helping with community sport events, joining a sewing club, and spending time on the land. Referring again to strengths and positive protective practices, one participant described the role of spirituality and spiritual guidance in maintaining motivation and finding contentment when faced with extraordinary hardship. In her description of spirituality, she included Inuit shamanism, organized religion, and therapeutic relationship with the land.

> I find if you practice some sort of spiritual activity like you know being religious and stuff, it kind of empowers you to continue on and give you hope. It is there for you when you're at your weakest because who else are you going to turn to if you've tried all kinds of other stuff that's possible. I find it's very important to have a kind of spiritual guidance or belief or something, practise spirituality because … I may not need it all the time now, but come down the road, I need something to fall back on just having support … kinda give you strength and kinda motivates you to keep on going … And that's how I see spirituality being important in any woman. Once they are spiritually content, then they're more content with themselves you know. It helps when you're at your weakest or … even when you're at your happiest … it helps. – Participant #4

Discussion: What We Learned about Inuit Women's Conceptualizations of Wellness

Understanding wellness in communities and for populations requires an acknowledgement that it is multifaceted, complex, and experienced in the day-to-day context of people's lives. What has been made more explicit through this study is the important role of Inuit culture and knowledge for Inuit women and the strengths that they draw from both each other and this knowledge. The women in this study provided rich examples of how an amorphous concept such as culture is experienced in people's day-to-day lives as social beings. As articulated earlier, to address health concerns, it is important to work together as a community to build upon strengths, such as social and familial supports; to use Inuit ways of being and living that support health and well-being; to continue sharing of Inuit knowledge in new and innovative ways; and to maintain strong cultural pride.

Previous and recent research on Canadian Inuit women's health has primarily focused on specific issues, such as nutrition and contaminants, alcohol and substance use, or pregnancy and childbirth (24,33,34,38,75–78). A review of published research in this field revealed no published literature that shared women's perceptions of wellness (79). The wellness issues Inuit women from Nunavut discussed in this study included Inuit culture, knowledge, and identity; self-esteem and self-confidence; substance abuse and coping; and relationships. Through sharing their experiences and the stories of women in their community, they provided a window through which to begin to understand the interplay of historical events, location, culture, community, and self that determines health and well-being in our region. The women's accounts illustrate that wellness determines the nature of how we interact with our families, friends, and the world around us and the constraints and supports, both personal and communal, that affect it. It is over time and in this complex context that these factors play very strongly into our overall health and well-being.

This study has highlighted the importance of several key issues in Inuit women's health, including the role of Inuit culture and identity, the development of self-esteem for young women, and the mental and emotional strains women experience through family and personal relationships. Participants also reinforced the reality that women's health is only one part of community health and that efforts must be made to approach health holistically and inclusively in Nunavut communities. It is apparent from the women's stories that early childhood experiences and other determinants of health across the lifespan accumulate in women's lives. This is an essential contribution to the public health and community health discourse. As articulated earlier, to address health concerns, it is important to work together as a community to build upon strengths, such as social and familial supports; to use Inuit pathways to wellness that support health and well-being; to continue sharing of Inuit knowledge in new and innovative ways; and to maintain strong cultural pride. It is also important to stress the role Inuit language plays in women's health, lending an urgency to supporting people's well-being through their mother tongue.

Conclusion

Knowledge generated from this study can make positive contributions to evidence-based policy and decision making in Nunavut, as well as contribute to the territorial initiatives underway to develop strategies for mental health and wellness promotion and suicide prevention. Furthermore, the findings may be useful in other northern and circumpolar jurisdictions. This study, conducted more than 10 years ago, was the catalyst for an expanded program of research exploring the perspectives of parents and youth on a multitude of issues, including health communication in families, ways to support adolescent well-being, and the importance of storytelling as a methodology in health research in northern communities (22,80–83). Further community-driven research addressing local health needs is required to improve the health of Nunavut communities. Future research should investigate the concerns raised by women in this study, including perceptions of wellness, men's and women's experiences with sexual abuse and domestic violence, and Inuit women's views of self-esteem and self-confidence and the protective factors that contribute to positive mental health. Drawing upon existing community strengths and resources and building capacity to conduct research in the North is the key to addressing a number of health concerns in the North now and over the coming years.

NOTES

Author contributions: conceptualization, GHA, LM; methodology, GHA, LM, TK, KM; data curation, GHA, TK; writing – original draft preparation, GHA; writing – review and editing, GHA, LM, TK.

1 *Inuit* is the Inuktitut word for "people." *Inuk* is the singular form, meaning "person."

2 The *hidden homeless* is a term used in Nunavut to describe single-parent families, primarily single moms, who have no permanent residence. They "couch surf" from relative to relative, taking shelter with whomever will help them. They are considered to be "hidden" because they do not live on the streets but are cared for by their friends and family, as is typical in northern communities.

REFERENCES

1. Moffitt P, Vollman AR. Photovoice: picturing the health of Aboriginal women in a remote northern community. Can J Nurs Res. 2004;36(4):189–201.
2. Moffitt PM. Colonialization: a health determinant for pregnant Dogrib women. J Transcult Nurs. 2004;15(4):323–30.

3. Indigenous and Northern Affairs Canada. Health and healing. Ottawa (ON): Government of Canada; 1996.
4. Jasen P. Race, culture and the colonization of childbirth in northern Canada. Soc Hist Med. 1997;10(3):385.
5. Qaujigiartiit Health Research Centre. Needs assessment of mental health services for children and youth in Nunavut. Iqaluit (NU): Qaujigiartiit Health Research Centre; 2010.
6. Office of the Auditor General of Canada. Health care services—Nunavut. Ottawa (ON): Office of the Auditor General of Canada; 2017.
7. Cherba M, Healey G. Impact of health care provider turnover on health outcomes: a scoping review. Iqaluit (NU): Qaujigiartiit Health Research Centre; 2017.
8. Kral MJ, Idlout L, Minore JB, Dyck RJ, Kirmayer LJ. Unikkaartuit: meanings of well-being, happiness, health, and community change among Inuit in Canada. Am J Community Psychol. 2011;48:426–38.
9. Redvers J, Bjerregaard P, Eriksen H, Fanian S, Healey GK, Hiratsuka V, Jong M, Larsen CV, Linton J, Pollock N, Silviken A, Stoor P, Chatwood S. A scoping review of Indigenous suicide prevention in circumpolar regions. Int J Circumpolar Health. 2015 Mar 4;74:27509.
10. Healey G. (Re)settlement, displacement, and family separation: contributors to health inequity in Nunavut. Northern Rev. 2016;42:1–22.
11. Healey GK, Meadows LM. Tradition and culture: an important determinant of Inuit women's health. J Aborig Health. 2008;4(1):25–33.
12. Nunavut Tunngavik Inc. Annual report on the state of Inuit culture and society: Nunavut's health system. Iqaluit (NU): Nunavut Tunngavik Inc.; 2008.
13. Qikiqtani Inuit Association. Qikiqtani Truth Commission final report: achieving Saimaqatigiingniq. Iqaluit (NU): Inhabit Media; 2012.
14. Nunavut Tunngavik Inc. Annual report on the state of Inuit culture and society: Inuit children and youth. Iqaluit (NU): Nunavut Tunngavik Inc.; 2011.
15. Sandiford Grygier P. A long way from home: the tuberculosis epidemic among the Inuit. Montreal (PQ): McGill-Queen's University Press; 1994.
16. Orr P. Tuberculosis in Nunavut: looking back, moving forward. CMAJ. 2013;185(4): 185–6.
17. Legare A. Inuit identity and regionalization in the Canadian central and eastern Arctic: a survey of writings about Nunavut. Polar Geogr. 2004; 31(3–4):99–118.
18. Loukacheva N. The Arctic promise: legal and political autonomy of Greenland and Nunavut. Toronto (ON): University of Toronto Press; 2007.
19. Nunavut Bureau of Statistics. Nunavut quick facts. Panniqtuuq (NU): Government of Nunavut; 2016.
20. Healey G, Tagak Sr. A. Piliriqatigiinniq "working in a collaborative way for the common good": a perspective on the space where health research methodology and Inuit epistemology come together. Int J Crit Indig Stud. 2014;7(1):1–8.

21. Annahatak B. Quality education for Inuit today? Cultural strengths, new things, and working out the unknowns: a story by an Inuk. Peabody J Educ. 1994;69(2):12–18.
22. Healey G, Noah J, Mearns C. The eight ujarait (rocks) model: supporting Inuit adolescent mental health with an intervention model based on Inuit ways on knowing. Int J Indig Health. 2016;11(1):92–110.
23. Egeland G, Faraj N, Osborne G. Cultural, socioeconomic, and health indicators among Inuit preschoolers: Nunavut Inuit child health survey, 2007–2008. Rural Remote Health. 2010;10(1365).
24. Galloway T, Saudny H. Nunavut community and personal wellness, Inuit health survey (2007–2008). Montreal (QC). Centre for Indigenous Nutrition and the Environment, McGill University; 2012.
25. Morgan C. The Arctic: gender issues [Internet]. Ottawa (ON): Library of Parliament, Social Affairs Division (CA); 2008 [cited 2021 Feb 4]. Publication No.: PRB08-09E. Available from: http://publications.gc.ca/collections/collection_2010/bdp-lop/prb/prb0809-eng.pdf
26. Nunavut Department of Health. Reportable communicable diseases in Nunavut, 2007 to 2014. Iqaluit (NU): Government of Nunavut; 2016.
27. World Health Organization. Mental health: a state of well-being. Geneva (CH): World Health Organization; 2017.
28. Eggertson L. Nunavut suicides a "public health emergency." CMAJ. 2015;187(16):E462.
29. Inuit Tapiriit Kanatami. National Inuit suicide prevention strategy. Ottawa (ON): Inuit Tapiriit Kanatami; 2016.
30. Nunavut Tunngavik Inc. Recommendations for federal actions to address suicide prevention in Nunavut as submitted to the Parliamentary Standing Committee on Indigenous and Northern Affairs. Ottawa (ON): Government of Canada; 2016.
31. Government of Nunavut, Nunavut Tunngavik Inc., Embrace Life Council, Royal Canadian Mounted Police. Nunavut suicide prevention strategy [Internet]. Iqaluit (NU): Government of Nunuvut; 2010 Oct 26 [cited 2021 Feb 4]. Available from: https://www.tunngavik.com/wp-content/uploads/2010/10/2010-10-26-nunavut-suicide-prevention-strategy-english.pdf
32. Statistics Canada. Suicides and suicide rate, by sex and by age group (both sexes). Ottawa (ON): Statistics Canada; 2012.
33. Chachamovich E, Haggarty J, Cargo M, Hicks J, Kirmayer LJ, Tureck G. A psychological autopsy study of suicide among Inuit in Nunavut: methodological and ethical considerations, feasibility and acceptability. Int J Circumpolar Health. 2013;72:1–10.
34. Schmidt R, Hrenchuk C, Bopp J, Poole N. Trajectories of women's homelessness in Canada's 3 northern territories. Int J Circumpolar Health. 2015;74(1):29778–9.
35. Taylor G. The chief public health officer's report on the state of public health in Canada 2016 – a focus on family violence in Canada [Internet]. Ottawa (ON):

Government of Canada; 2016. Publication No.: 160152. Available from https://www.canada.ca/content/dam/canada/public-health/migration/publications/department-ministere/state-public-health-family-violence-2016-etat-sante-publique-violence-familiale/alt/pdf-eng.pdf

36. Tester FJ, McNicoll P. Isumagijaksaq: mindful of the state: social constructions of Inuit suicide. Soc Sci Med. 2004;58:2625–36.
37. Government of Nunavut, Nunavut Tunngavik Incorporated, Royal Canadian Mounted Police V-Division, Embrace Life Council. Resiliency within: an action plan for suicide prevention in Nunavut 2016/2017 [Internet]. Iqaluit (NU): Government of Nunavut; 2016 [cited 2021 Feb 4]. Available from: https://www.tunngavik.com/files/2017/07/Resiliency-Within-_ENG.pdf
38. Lauson S, McIntosh S, Obed N, Healey G, Asuri S, Osborne G, Arbour L. The development of a comprehensive maternal-child health information system for Nunavut – Nutaqqavut (our children). Int J Circumpolar Health. 2011;70(4): 363–72.
39. Department of Health and Social Services. Nunavut maternal and newborn health care strategy, 2009–2014. Iqaluit (NU): Government of Nunavut; 2009.
40. Office of the Languages Commissioner of Nunavut. "If you cannot communicate with your patient, your patient is not safe": final report of the Office of the Languages Commissioner – Qikiqtani General Hospital. Iqaluit (NU): Legislative Assembly of Nunavut; 2015.
41. Inuit Tapiriit Kanatami. 5000 Year heritage. Ottawa (ON): Inuit Tapiriit Kanatami; 2005.
42. Waldram JB, Herring A, Young TK. Aboriginal health in Canada: historical, cultural, and epidemiological perspectives. Toronto (ON): University of Toronto Press; 2007.
43. Kirmayer LJ, Brass GM, Tait CL. The mental health of aboriginal peoples: Transformations of identity and community. Can J Psychiatry. 2000;45:607–16.
44. Tester FJ, Kulchyski, P. Tammarniit (mistakes): Inuit relocation in the eastern Arctic, 1939–63. Vancouver (BC): UBC Press; 1994.
45. Pauktuutit Inuit Women's Association of Canada. Sivumuapallianiq: national Inuit residential schools healing strategy – the journey forward. Ottawa (ON): Pauktuutit Inuit Women's Association of Canada; 2007.
46. King D. A brief report of the federal government of Canada's residential school system for Inuit. Ottawa (ON): Aboriginal Healing Foundation; 2006.
47. Chrisjohn R, Young, S. The circle game: shadow and substance in the residential school experience in Canada. A report to the Royal Commission on Aboriginal Peoples. Penticton (BC): Theytus Books; 1995.
48. Archibald L. Teenage pregnancy in Inuit communities: issues and perspectives. A report prepared for the Pauktuutit Inuit Women's Association. Ottawa (ON): Pauktuutit Inuit Women's Association; 2004.
49. Condon RG. Inuit youth: growth and change in the Canadian Arctic. London (GB): Rutgers University Press; 1987.

50. Condon RG. The rise of adolescence: social change and life stage dilemmas in the central Canadian Arctic. Hum Organ. 1990;49:266–79.
51. Kirmayer LJ, Valaskis GG. Healing traditions: The mental health of Aboriginal peoples in Canada. Vancouver (BC): UBC Press; 2009.
52. Wolsko C, Lardon C, Mohatt GV, Orr E. Stress, coping and well-being among the Yup'ik of the Yukon-Kuskokwim Delta: the role of enculturation and acculturation. Int J Circumpolar Health. 2007;66(1):51–62.
53. Curtis T, Kvernmo S, Bjerregaard P. Changing living conditions, life style and health. Int J Circumpolar Health. 2005;64(5):442–51.
54. Statistics Canada. Police-reported Crime Severity Index and crime rate, by province and territory, 2018. Ottawa (ON): Government of Canada; 2018.
55. Pauktuutit Inuit Women of Canada. Study of gender-based violence and shelter service needs across Inuit Nunangat. Ottawa (ON): Pauktuutit Inuit Women of Canada; 2019.
56. Bjerregaard P, Young TK, Dewailly E, Ebbesson SO. Indigenous health in the Arctic: an overview of the circumpolar Inuit population. Scand J Public Health. 2004;32:390–5.
57. Ilagiitsiarniq family violence prevention framework for action. Iqaluit (NU): Legislative Assembly of Nunavut; 2013.
58. Arnakak J. Indigenous knowledge and its role in the healing of deep-rooted conflicts. Paper presented at: Mimesis, creativity and reconciliation. Annual Conference of Colloquium on Violence and Religion; 2006 May 31–Jun 4; St. Paul University, Ottawa, Canada.
59. Kral MJ, Minore JB. Arctic narratives: Participatory action research on suicide and wellness among the Inuit. Paper presented at: Biennial Conference of the Society for Community and Action; 1999 Jun; New Haven, CT, United States. As cited in Tester FJ, McNicoll P. Isumagijaksaq: mindful of the state: social constructions of Inuit suicide. Soc Sci Med. 2004;58:2625–36.
60. Beaudoin V, Seguin M, Chawky N, Affleck W, Chachamovich E, Turecki, G. Protective factors in the Inuit population of Nunavut: a comparative study of people who died by suicide, people who attempted suicide, and people who never attempted suicide. Int J Environ Res and Public Health. 2018;15:144.
61. Chachamovich E, Kirmayer LJ, Haggarty J, Cargo M, McCormick R, Turecki G. Suicide among Inuit: Results from a large, epidemiologically representative follow-back study in Nunavut. Can J Psychiatry. 2015;60(6):268–75.
62. Morris M, Crooks C. Structural and cultural factors in suicide prevention: the contrast between mainstream and Inuit approaches to understanding and preventing suicide. J of Soc Work Pract. 2015;29(3):321–38.
63. Mancini Billson J, Mancini K. Inuit women: Their powerful spirit in a century of change. Lanham (MD): Roweman and Littlefield; 2007.
64. Pauktuutit Inuit Women's Association. There is a need, so we help: services for Inuit survivors of child sexual abuse. Ottawa (ON): Pauktuutit Inuit Women's Association; 2003.

65. Anang P, Naujaat Elder EH, Gordon E, Gottlieb N, Bronson M. Building on strengths in Naujaat: the process of engaging Inuit youth in suicide prevention. Int J Circumpolar Health. 2019;78(2):1508321.
66. Lys C. Exploring coping strategies and mental health support systems among female youth in the Northwest Territories using body mapping. Int J Circumpolar Health. 2018;77(1):1466604.
67. Morse JM, Swanson J, Kuzel AJ. The nature of qualitative evidence. Thousand Oaks (CA): Sage Publications; 2001.
68. Creswell JW. Qualitative inquiry and research design. 3rd ed. Thousand Oaks (CA): Sage Publications; 2013.
69. Borkan J. Immersion/crystallization. In: Crabtree B, Miller W, editors. Doing qualitative research. 2nd ed. Thousand Oaks (CA): Sage Publications; 1999. p. 179–94.
70. Morse JM, Barrett M, Mayan M, Olson K, Spiers J. Verification strategies for establishing reliability and validity in qualitative research. Br Med J. 2002;1(2):13–22.
71. Creswell JW. Research design: quantitative, qualitative, and mixed methods approaches. Thousand Oaks (CA): Sage Publications; 2003.
72. Meadows LM, Verdi AJ, Crabtree B. Keeping up appearances: using qualitative research to enhance knowledge of dental practice. J Dent Educ. 2003;67(9):981–90.
73. Association of Canadian Universities for Northern Studies. Ethical principles for conduct of research in the North. Ottawa (ON): Association of Canadian Universities for Northern Studies; 2003.
74. Macaulay AC, Commanda LE, Freeman WL, Gibson N, McCabe ML, Robbins CM, Twohig PL. Participatory research maximizes community and lay involvement. Br Med J. 1999;319:774–8.
75. Kilabuk E, Momoli F, Mallick R, Van Dyk D, Pease C, Zwerling A, Potvin SE, Alvarez GG. Social determinants of health among residential areas with a high tuberculosis incidence in a remote Inuit community. J Epidemiology Community Health. 2019 May;73(5):401–6.
76. Corosky GJ, Blystad A. Staying healthy "under the sheets": Inuit youth experiences of access to sexual and reproductive health and rights in Arviat, Nunavut, Canada. Int J Circumpolar Health. 2016;75(1), Article 31812.
77. Beaumier M, Ford J. Food insecurity among Inuit women exacerbated by socio-economic stresses and climate change. Can J Public Health. 2010;101(3):196–201.
78. Nelson C, Lawford K, Otterman V, Darling E. Mental health indicators among pregnant Aboriginal women in Canada: results from the maternity experiences survey. Health Promot Chronic Dis Prev Can. 2018;38(7–8):269–76.
79. Young TK. Review of research on Aboriginal populations in Canada: relevance to their health needs. Br Med J. 2003;327:419–22.
80. Healey GK. Applying Indigenous analytical approaches to find answers to a public health question: a reflection on ᐅᓂᒃᑲᖅᑕᑎᒋᐃᓐᓂᖅ Unikkaqatigiiniq (storytelling) and ᓴᓇᓂᖅ Sananiq (crafting). In: Humble AM, Radina ME,

editors. How qualitative data analysis happens: moving beyond "themes emerged." New York (NY): Taylor & Francis; 2018.

81. Healey GK. Exploring the development of a health care model based on Inuit wellness concepts as part of self-determination and improving wellness in Northern communities. In: Piggot T, Arya N, editors. Under-served: health determinants of Indigenous, inner-city and migrant populations in Canada. Toronto (ON): Canadian Scholar Press; 2018.
82. Healey G. Youth perspectives on sexually transmitted infections and sexual health in Northern Canada and implications for public health practice. Int J Circumpolar Health. 2016;75(1):30706.
83. Healey G. Inuit parent perspectives on sexual health communication with adolescent children in Nunavut: "It's kinda hard for me to try to find the words." Int J Circumpolar Health. 2014;73(1).

6 Assessing the Health Impacts of a Mine: Attending to the Prevailing Epistemology and Erasure of Indigenous Peoples' Well-Being

JEN JONES AND LESLEY JOHNSTON

Introduction

Making sense of both the positive and the negative ways in which health and mining intersect in northern Canadian Indigenous communities is an involved undertaking. This task is particularly important since the techniques used to assess the health impacts of extractive industries on proximate Indigenous populations continue to be contested. As extractive industries develop in northern Canada, opportunities have emerged for Indigenous governments to secure access to community and individual economic wealth in the form of employment, payments, and preferential treatment for community businesses, often through commonly termed impact and benefit agreements (IBAs)(1). These agreements, part of the larger governance of the extractive industries, facilitate direct negotiation between mine developers and Indigenous governments with little state interference (1,2). Yet these economic benefits have not necessarily translated into better health status for Indigenous communities (1,3). The development of extractive industries and subsequent new earnings for northern communities often result in problematic issues, such as family stress, substance abuse, crime, mental health impacts, physical injury, changes to nutrition, and increased instances of chronic disease (3–8). These issues compound existing health disparities experienced by northern Indigenous communities (9–12).

The persistence of health inequities in the face of economic stimulus has made northern Canadian jurisdictions noteworthy sites for examination of the efficacy of governance efforts to mitigate impacts to health and well-being. Alongside the settlement of land claims, self-government agreements, and advancements in the governance of extractive industries for better engagement with Indigenous communities, novel mechanisms to assess and account for health impacts of extractive industries have been developed. Tools such as health impact assessments (HIAs), used in conjunction with IBAs and environmental assessments, have received increased attention for their abilities to attend to health and social issues related to extractive industries.

HIAs have moved assessment processes beyond the quantitative appraisal of health risks associated with the contamination of air, water, and soil to a more holistic understanding of impacts, aiming to identify, evaluate, and mitigate the many pathways through which extractive industries affect health (13). Using the social determinants of health (SDoH) in the analysis of impacts of extractive industries can, and has, led to further understanding of the underlying social inequities that help to determine health disparities. Moreover, the application of SDoH in governance mechanisms offers an opportunity to critically analyse the challenges specific to Indigenous communities proximate to extractive industries (14–17).

Though governments (Indigenous and non-Indigenous) are increasingly requesting that assessments include greater consideration of health impacts, supplementary health assessment mechanisms, such as HIAs, are voluntary rather than being a legal requirement for the environmental assessment. As such, the implementation of the resulting health action plan is not legally required (18–20). As an output primarily of industry to be included in the IBA, HIAs have been accused of adopting actions that better suit the needs of industry than those of community, calling into question the neutrality of assessments (21–23). Further, despite the application of SDoH, efforts to assess health impacts often fail to adequately predict, respond to, and mitigate the ways in which Indigenous health and well-being are affected by mining (24,25). This failure, in addition to the questionable objectivity of the tools, may lie in the reductionist approach inherent to health assessment mechanisms. These mechanisms are challenged to capture and address a fundamental experience shared across all proposed resource projects in northern Canada. This foundational experience is the effects of settler colonialism on the health and well-being of Indigenous people. Persisting legacies of environmental dispossession, loss of language and culture, ongoing trauma (experienced both directly and via intergenerational transmission), and structural and political inequities continue to shape Indigenous people's well-being and perpetuate health disparities (10,12,26).

In this chapter, we explore the limitations of the assessment of impacts on health and suggest that to critically analyse the potential impacts of a mine on the health and well-being of northern Indigenous populations, extractive industries must be understood to affect not only land and health but land and health as understood within the context of the political and structural forces of settler colonialism. Critical to this analysis is understanding that settler colonialism is the domination and control over a people and land, secured through social and political relations and structures committed to maintaining power imbalance (27) – an essential consideration when reviewing existing assessment mechanisms.

Yet how do we tangibly and effectively relate these complex and nuanced experiences, particularly in the context of ongoing legacies of settler contact and settler colonialism? In so doing, how do we circumvent further essentializing Indigenous communities as homogenous or pathologizing communities as ill (28)? How can we recognize the agency of northern Indigenous communities and the efforts and successes they have had in asserting their rights? Further, we are two non-Indigenous researchers writing on Indigenous issues. We are both settler Canadians; one of us (Jones) works and lives in northern Canada, and the other (Johnston) lives in southern Canada and has experience working in mining issues in the Global South. Naming ourselves as settler Canadians is to recognize our positionality and situate ourselves away from the unmarked and unnamed status that comes with being researchers of settler descent (29,30). In naming our non-Indigeneity, we hope that the information shared here is understood to be filtered through our lens and experiences as settler Canadians researching Indigenous issues.

Wrestling with these questions and experiences, the lead author called up a community member she knew from conducting research in Yukon. After explaining the need to write about the SDoH and their limited ability to address fully the complex intersection of extractive industries, Indigenous people's health, and the persistent impacts of settler colonialism, the community member said: "Use my story." The community contact then proceeded to speak of mining – weaving past, present, and future.

The story told was not dissimilar to other stories heard during interviews with Yukon First Nations' people, and we share it in this chapter to illustrate why we need to transform the way in which we address and mitigate negative health impacts. The stories of disquiet and expectation that result from proposed extractive industry proximate to Indigenous communities or territory in northern Canada are complex. They are tied to a history of settler contact and political and structural inequities, and are often informed by a world view different from one that informs existing governance mechanisms. Despite modern-day treaties, such as self-government and land claim agreements, that would seem to indicate a new era of relationships between Indigenous peoples and Canada, and efforts to understand complex histories, the development of novel mechanisms to assess health and well-being continue to make invisible northern Indigenous peoples' experiences with extractive industries. Framed differently, mechanisms used to address, assess, and mitigate impacts to health and well-being apply an epistemology and ontology that do not necessarily reflect Indigenous world views. This is a form of settler colonialism. The reliance on a perceived apolitical approach, and without consideration of the world view informing the decisions, can result in community concerns seldom being wholly reflected in assessments, even with the application of the SDoH.

Like the genesis of this chapter, it is the community's story that drives the following background information and analysis. The narrative becomes a method of illustrating the ways in which ongoing legacies of settler contact and settler colonialism, changes to land, and opportunity for economic wealth intersect and ultimately impact health and well-being. It helps elucidate what is often missing in an assessment of impacts on health. To assist with understanding the limitations of assessment mechanisms and their inability to respond wholly to Indigenous communities' concerns and expectations, we begin this chapter with a history of mining exploration in the North, with a specific focus on Yukon. This history is situated within a context of settler contact and Indigenous resistance and successes and, as we explain, is important context to understanding the current intersection of health and extractive industries. We then draw attention to the contributions and limitations of normative health frameworks used to assess the health impacts of mining or other extractive industries. It is only then that we introduce the community narrative as a way of illustrating the challenges and limitation of SDoH as used in existing health assessment mechanisms to respond to Indigenous communities' concerns regarding extractive industries. We hope that you, as a reader, will gain an appreciation for the differing world views and experiences of settler contact, contested treaties, and other ongoing legacies of settler colonialism that are foundational to understanding and addressing the health and well-being of northern Indigenous populations.

Mining in Northern Canada

Understanding the impacts of mining on Indigenous people's health in northern Canada requires consideration of the history of mining that is inextricably connected to the history of settler contact and Indigenous resistance and resilience (27). The North is diverse in both its people and its landscape. In this chapter, we focus primarily on events in Yukon, Canada's most westward northern territory. The first settlers in the region were Russians who had travelled over mountains from the west coast and traded with coastal First Nations, before moving into interior Yukon and bringing new wares from afar. Fur traders making their way from eastern Canada soon followed, introducing sugar and tobacco. It was, however, the rush for gold and subsequent development of mining that most profoundly impacted northern Indigenous populations (31). During the Klondike Gold Rush of 1890, northern Yukon became home to over 40,000 non-Indigenous prospectors who had made their way through territory that had previously experienced little incursion by non-Indigenous populations (32).

As the gold rush ended, hard-rock mining found a foothold in parts of what is now known as central Yukon. Mining for copper, silver, zinc, and nickel led to the development of towns. By World War II, mining towns in central

Yukon were hubs for miners and industries (33). With these mines and mine towns came roads, opening up land and water previously only accessed by the local First Nations people, making way for other extractive resource initiatives, including oil and gas.

By this time, the North was seen by the south as the land of opportunity (34). Wealth awaited those who dared venture into these perceived wilds. The discourse of *terra nullius*, the colonial doctrine premised on the belief that undeveloped land or land without a sovereign or governing power is "no one's land" and therefore open for settlement, was employed by Canada and resulted in the displacement of Indigenous peoples from their land (34,35). By the mid-twentieth century, the once nomadic northern Indigenous peoples of Yukon moved into settler settlements (36).

The experience of dispossession, including the separation from the therapeutic qualities of land – which meant a loss of the ways in which land has benefit for physical, mental, emotional, and spiritual health (37) – was met with resistance from northern Indigenous peoples. In neighbouring Northwest Territories, the *1970 Mackenzie Valley Pipe Line Report* (commonly referred to as the Berger Inquiry) lobbied for a 10-year moratorium to be placed on resource development in the North to allow for Indigenous rights and governance to be addressed. Indigenous peoples in Yukon were concurrently campaigning for recognition that the North was their homeland, not the hinterland it was commonly purported to be (34). In 1973 the Yukon First Nations presented to then prime minister Pierre Trudeau a document outlining a list of grievances and an approach for the settlement of land claims. The historic document, *Together Today for Our Children Tomorrow* (31), laid the foundation for present-day land claims in Yukon and resulted in a novel environmental assessment mechanism and the devolution of administrative authority of lands and resources to the First Nations in the form of self-governing First Nations.

These milestones have yet to result in forms of resource governance that respond fully to Indigenous peoples' relationship with land or that addresses the colonial relationship between Canada and northern Indigenous peoples. Indeed, the settlements of modern-day treaties were motivated by access to land and the natural resources they represent, similar to the Royal Proclamation of 1763 signed over 250 years ago (38). Historic treaties were signed by Indigenous peoples in Canada in good faith – with the understanding of pre-existing sovereignty – to ensure good relations (38,39). However, despite modern-day treaties negotiated in the language of self-determination, the ontologically distinct positioning of the signing parties has led to different understandings and expectations by the powers invested in the process (40).

As argued by some, the settlement of land claims and the establishment of self-government is a cumbersome and rigid process – and an extension of colonial control (36,38,41). Indeed, the western-Eurocentric concept of rights and property (crucial to the discourse of treaties, self-government, and land claims) are themselves contested terms (42). Both terms suggest ownership, a concept not recognized in an Indigenous relationship with land. This tension has real implications. For example, one outcome of the Yukon land claims was the development of the Yukon Environmental and Socio-economic Assessment Act, which was "established, in part, to protect, promote and where possible enhance the *well-being* [italics added] and traditional economies of Yukon First Nations persons and their special relationship with the land" (43). Although this recognizes First Nations peoples' special relationship with land and well-being, the use of a settler-centric world view continues to dominate. First Nation governments are expected to negotiate mitigations and benefits of extractive industries using terms and concepts that neglect their approach to land and its relationship to health and well-being.

Assessing Health and Population Health

Over the past few decades, the ways in which health is defined and addressed has begun to change. In part this is a result of the ascendance of population health and SDoH frameworks that have broadened our scope of understanding health beyond the individually oriented, biomedically focused methodologies previously used in health analysis (44). These new approaches for addressing health and health disparities have done much for our understanding of the interactions between social and political determinants and their role in modifying health outcomes (16,17).

Population health is an approach that looks beyond sick or at-risk individuals to the factors that contribute to the health of society as a whole (45). Though criticized for undervaluing the role of social structures and overvaluing positivist approaches, it aims to incorporate factors ranging from the biological to the social and has succeeded in broadening our understanding of health. The SDoH, developed through the World Health Organization's commission of the same name and as embodied in the 1986 Ottawa Charter, have done much for our understanding of the interactions between determinants and their role in modifying health outcomes. The approach reveals that it is not just the presence of health-supporting resources being made available to the population as a whole that matters; rather, it is the *distribution* of these resources within the population that determine health and well-being (12,46). This distinction has been useful in making connections between political decision making, policy creation, and health outcomes.

Despite contributions made through the use of the SDoH and population health frameworks, tensions continue to exist among scholars as to the effectiveness of these tools (47–50). Some scholars contend that insufficient attention has been paid to how societal structures, including power, mediate the ways in which these social determinants shape a population's health. Although the use of qualitative research methods and the application of community participatory research principles are more evident in health research today, there is still a staunch reliance on population health data, including census data, vital statistics, disease surveillance or registries, and national health surveys that neglect the social, political, and geographic structures that underlie this evidence (51).

Understanding and defining the factors that determine health impacts is complex. When we begin to consider these within the context of large-scale industrial practices like mining, the task becomes even more challenging. Mining directly impacts health outcomes through occupational exposures and injuries; it also indirectly impacts health determinants, such as migration and housing, nutrition, and social cohesion – and more. Any project that affects the determinants of health has the potential to cause both positive and negative change in a population. It is widely acknowledged that extractive industries have the ability to fundamentally transform a region's environmental, social, cultural, and health makeup – not always for the better (5,7,8,52–55).

Even with the most straightforward projects, the assessment mechanisms used in mining are challenged to predict and fully capture the multiple and overlapping health impacts of projects. HIAs, a relatively recent addition to the assessment suite, negotiate the limitations of environmental assessment mechanisms that traditionally rely on quantitative measurements of risk (1). HIAs attempt to analyse the impacts of extractive industries by examining multiple pathways in which no one determinant is independent of another (56). Therefore, HIAs are promoted as a mechanism that seeks to identify health consequences of a project, policy, or program by examining the broader determinants of health (20,56,57). However, in practice, HIAs are challenged to recognize, let alone respond to, nuanced and complex health concerns. It may be argued that this is, in part, a result of the lack of agreement or understanding that still exists in the literature to explain the ways in which social, economic, and political structures govern the determinants of health – or even what constitutes a determinant (58–60). Given these limits to understanding, it is no wonder that the mechanism struggles to encapsulate health impacts. More pragmatically, the completion of a comprehensive HIA requires multiple types of data – both qualitative and quantitative – to create a profound understanding of potential project impacts. For voluntary, industry-led processes this requirement poses significant resourcing challenges. Consequently, HIAs generally continue to rely on population health data and health risk assessment measures that focus on air emissions and contamination of water or soil – with limited consideration of how multiple effects and existing health status interact with one another (61,62). Furthermore, it is industry and banks that often develop supporting documents for the implementation of mechanisms such as HIAs, with a one-size-fits-all mandate (63–65). Because of that universal approach, effective identification of community-specific impacts, benefits, and mitigation requirements is problematic. For Indigenous communities, generic efforts imposed to mitigate negative impacts and maximize benefits from potential economic stimulus often fail, as industry may overlook what really matters. Industry, seeking social licence and ongoing support from the communities in which the project is based, may find this backing compromised when promised benefits fail to materialize (3,66).

Further, the criticisms levelled against population health and SDoH frameworks apply to HIAs. The use of normative health frameworks that categorize impacts into health effect categories, such as exposure to potential hazardous materials; infectious disease; injury; stress and mental well-being; and food, nutrition, and subsistence activity to name a few, fail to capture the context in which these impacts exist (14,67). Unsurprisingly, the erasure of context, or more specifically the erasure of the relationships between settler society and experiences specific to Indigenous communities – namely, the processes of settler colonialism – limit the effectiveness of HIAs and other hegemonic mechanisms.

Conceptualizing Indigenous Health

Fully grasping the conditions and processes that determine health outcomes within the context of a mine is already a challenge, yet a further dynamic is at play – the need to comprehend and appropriately incorporate Indigenous health concepts that differ fundamentally from Eurocentric biomedical concepts enshrined in frameworks like population health or even those of the SDoH.

Indigenous health and well-being is conceived more broadly than that typified by a biomedical definition of health (9,26,68). Often described in an Indigenous conceptualization of health and well-being is the interconnection between "physical, mental, emotional and spiritual [domains of] health as well as a healthy lifestyle, cultural continuity with the past and future opportunities and a healthy connection to culture, family and community" (51 p73). The introduction of biomedical approaches initiated the move away from holistic health conceptualizations, which is often cited as being fundamentally dissimilar to an Indigenous understanding of wellness (9,35).

It is recognized – though rarely applied to policy matters and programming – that Indigenous well-being, for many Indigenous peoples, is ontologically distinctive. Through an Indigenous world view, the unique relationship Indigenous peoples have with the land and the environment should not be overlooked or perceived as merely a discrete determinant that informs health. The fundamental importance of the relationship with the land and Indigenous ways of knowing differ profoundly from conventionally applied Western-capitalist-biomedical ontological positioning and ways of knowing or explaining health and well-being (69). Land is not separate or an inanimate object; rather, land figures centrally in Indigenous understandings of well-being (35,70). In these conceptualizations, land is noted for providing traditional medicines and being a source of cultural and spiritual well-being (70,71). This relationship between land and well-being is not easily understood, let alone explained, through conventionally applied, Western biomedical definitions and concepts of health.

The application of normative or biomedical health frameworks, terms, and concepts in mechanisms governing extractive industries, including HIAs, force Indigenous peoples' experiences and concerns into health categories that are not representative of their way of interacting with the world and their well-being within it. Along with the erasure of an Indigenous world view, the health impacts of dispossession and loss of language and culture have been overlooked in these frameworks.

Recognizing this criticism, critical health scholarship has made efforts to reflect an Indigenous ontology in the SDoH. Scholarship has revealed how poverty, stress, trauma (both directly experienced and via intergenerational transmission), cultural erosion, and environmental dispossession contribute to health disparities as experienced by Indigenous populations (1,10,35). These distal determinants further an understanding of the nuanced role of the legacies of colonization and continued settler colonialism in shaping Indigenous people's well-being and perpetuating existing health disparities (10,12). Indeed, colonialism is identified as perhaps the most important determinant of health (72). Research has revealed how the forced removal of Indigenous children, their placement in residential schools, and the relocation or forced resettlement of once nomadic communities have contributed to higher rates of cardiovascular disease, diabetes, injury, and increasingly high levels of obesity (9,10). Further work has sought to conceptualize how traumatic events of the past, including experiences of the Indian residential school system affect individual health today. Some researchers, such as Reading and Wien (12), and de Leeuw, Lindsay, and Greenwood (72), among others, have sought to address these concerns by proposing a specific set of Indigenous determinants of health. This is not easy work, challenged as it is by the spectre of biological reductionism (73). Understanding the pathway between experiences of dispossession and other assimilation policies and historical trauma is its own fundamentally distinct process that has profound effects on health, and while these impacts are often exacerbated by mining development, they are not addressed in extractive industries' assessment of health impacts. Though the impacts are known to be unrelenting, trauma is often placed in the past, and mechanisms like HIA thus fail to capture and address structural and politically informed issues (74).

How this relates to understanding the impacts of a mine on the health of northern Indigenous populations may be a stretch for some. Yet in speaking with citizens of northern communities who have experienced mining in the past or are preparing for new mines in the near future, the link between legacies of settler contact, dispossession, and residential school and mine experiences – past, present, or future – is all too evident. As demonstrated in the following narrative, this reality confounds the practice of assessing health impacts of extractive industries.

Sharing a Story

We have shared the history of mining and self-governance in the North, the advances and continued limitations in population health and SDoH frameworks, and a brief overview of conceptualizations of health. These are a precursor to the narrative that follows. We have used a narrative to give you insight into the history of a people and their resilience in the face of settler colonialism and to help you better understand why the context and these experiences are fundamental to the ways in which health is conceived and must be considered when conducting HIAs on extractive industries and beyond. We also hope that the following story will demonstrate how community narratives eclipse common categories used in the governance of extractive industries to explain impacts on health – even with the application of population health and SDoH frameworks.

To be clear, the following narrative is not one person's story; it a composite of narratives gathered through research conducted with citizens of a Yukon First Nation. Through the narrative, we aim to illustrate the complexity of Indigenous health and the ways in which settler colonialism persists, or is reproduced, through the assessment procedures and governance processes that are ostensibly intended to mitigate the impacts of the contemporary extractive industries on Indigenous peoples' health. The composite first person narrative is derived from 42 interviews with Yukon First Nation citizens and draws from narrative interpretive methods (75). The pronoun *I* is used not to imply a simple retelling of one person's story but rather to reflect the common themes arising from the interviews. Not all the themes documented in the original research are addressed in this composite. The question driving the following narrative, and asked of all community members involved in the research project, was "What are your health concerns and expectations with mining in the area?"

A Community Contribution

My father worked in the coal mine; my brother and my uncle work in a mine now. That coal mine provided jobs for the men and access to goods that we needed. Other family members had good jobs as well. But with jobs came access to more money and then more access to alcohol. This had an impact on us kids. Also, people got sick or became hurt. Accidents on the site happened. The Elders who worked in those mines, they got sick, really sick. We still get sick from those mines; the water, the air, the land has changed.

Our people were healthier living on the land. We didn't have diabetes. When I was little, I walked a long way. I hunted rabbit and picked berries with grandmother, but it's not like that anymore. Things have changed. I still like to go out and set nets. I feel better on the land. I feel peace of mind. Being on the land helps citizens cope with the trauma of residential school. I didn't go to those schools, but a lot of our community members did. There are mothers who came back from those schools who had a hard time raising their kids. Being on the land helps them.

There are stories from our Elders that are attached to places. What happens when those places are disturbed or changed? It has happened in the past where mining came in and destroyed our sacred areas. I don't trust they won't do this again. Will this new mine be like the others? Those other mines affected the water; not even our moose are safe because of the mine.

Mines bring roads and bring more people. It cuts us off from our land. I also worry about the drugs and alcohol that come with new workers. It's not safe for young girls; I worry about them too. We can't protect everyone, and lots can happen at once and we are a small community. Our community workers are already busy; how can we do more with the same number of support staff when there will be more people in our community?

I want more economic opportunity in our town. We need to find jobs for our people. But there are risks. What do you think will happen to us when those mines shut down? We live here, the mine owners don't. We have knowledge, but no one listens to our First Nation governments; our First Nation governments are walked over and disregarded. You know, we have been tricked and altered into not being. I didn't know my culture or my language. I still don't. My kids and grandkids don't. How will a mine help with that?

Conclusion

We have presented this chapter by setting the context and the scholarly foundation and then sharing a community narrative. The choice to present the issue of mining and Indigenous health in this format was made to demonstrate the experience of attempting to apply health assessment mechanisms in northern Canadian jurisdictions in which the health of Indigenous citizens is considered. Made evident, we hope, is a tension between what is shared in the community narrative and what assessment mechanisms are able to grasp, and the reasons for their limitations. One of the obvious challenges is how to "fit" a community narrative into any one health category, such as injury, family stress, substance abuse, crime, or mental health, and how, when one attempts to force a fit, these mechanisms contribute to erasing the underlying narrative of experiences of removal from land, assimilation, and structural and political inequities backed by policies of settler colonialism.

To conclude this chapter, we draw attention to items discussed earlier in the chapter and how they may be differently understood or considered given the sharing of the community narrative, as well as questions they pose for moving forward. Notable in the narrative is the interweaving of historic experiences with mining past and present, distrust of the government and its processes, and reference to the impacts of assimilation and colonial policies that have stripped Indigenous peoples of their language and culture.

The reliance of assessment mechanisms on contemporary settler and biomedical methods has resulted in accusations of essentializing Indigeneity, suppressing Indigenous world views, and erasing Indigenous experiences of settler contact and settler colonialism (69,76,77). So, while the assessment of health impacts that result from extractive industrial development are required under modern-day treaties – written with the language of self-determination or recognition – these mechanisms, and even treaties themselves, rely on contemporary Western and settler colonial concepts and fail to recognize and accept ontological pluralism. Although scholarship on HIA attempts to recognize different approaches to health and persisting social and political inequities, little is presented on how mechanisms can address in practice this awareness, other than to suggest "fitting in Indigenous issues" or offering training to communities to lessen dependence on non-Indigenous negotiators, thereby lessening the chance that community issues are taken out of context (62,78).

Just as relevant and important is the reliance of these mechanisms on population health and its use of large data modelling and categorized health effects. Even with the application of the SDoH, assessment mechanisms are hard-pressed to incorporate the ways in which societal structures and values shape the lives of Indigenous peoples (47,50). This problem exists even in an era when Indigenous scholars and communities have called upon health researchers to scrutinize assumptions; recognize the complex historical, political, and social contexts that shape Indigenous health; and, more recently, be deliberate in reversing the impacts of colonization (79).

Finally, we conclude that mechanisms used to assess impacts resulting from, or to negotiate the benefits of, extractive industries proximate to Indigenous communities are similarly challenged by the use of concepts and terms that perpetuate power imbalances (41). Arguably, the persistent use of mechanisms that fail to address the underlying political and structural disparities and Indigenous peoples' relationship with land may indeed be perpetuating settler colonialism.

If we understand settler colonialism to be a process grounded in a quest for resources, as well as through cultural and structural dominance achieved by the enforcement of specific beliefs, values, and principles (80), then the reliance on existing health assessment mechanisms that erase the experiences of

Indigenous peoples by using contemporary or normative concepts and terms may indeed be persisting colonialism. This is a strong assertion yet an important consideration as we hope and intend to transform the way in which we address and mitigate negative health impacts of extractive industries on Indigenous populations. Given what has been presented as background and in the community narrative, do we not need to recognize and find ways to integrate Indigenous ontologies and conceptions of health, as well as experiences of settler colonialism, in efforts aimed at mitigating the impacts of the extractive industries? Left unchecked, would this not result in assessment mechanisms that continue to ignore their contribution to structural and politically informed health disparities? Alternatively, can a change in approach lead to better policies and practices? The final considerations we leave with you.

REFERENCES

1. Jones J, Bradshaw B. Addressing historical impacts through impact and benefit agreements and health impact assessment: why it matters for Indigenous well-being. Northern Rev. 2015;41:81–109.
2. Galbraith L, Bradshaw B, Rutherford MB. Towards a new supraregulatory approach to environmental assessment in northern Canada. Impact Assess Proj Apprais. 2007;25(1):27–41.
3. Cameron E, Levitan T. Impact and benefit agreements and the neoliberalization of resource governance and indigenous-state relations in northern Canada. Stud Polit Econ. 2014;93(1):25–52.
4. Shandro JA, Veiga MM, Shoveller J, Scoble M, Koehoorn M. Perspectives on community health issues and the mining boom – bust cycle. Resour Policy. 2011;36(2):178–86.
5. Lenné MG, Salmon PM, Liu CC, Trotter M. A systems approach to accident causation in mining: an application of the HFACS method. Accid Anal Prev. 2012;48:111–17.
6. Masuda JR, Zupancic T, Poland B, Cole DC. Environmental health and vulnerable populations in Canada: mapping an integrated equity-focused research agenda. Can Geogr. 2008;52(4):427–50.
7. Yu L, Wang Y-b, Xin G, Su Y-b, Gang W. Risk assessment of heavy metals in soils and vegetables around non-ferrous metals mining and smelting sites, Baiyin, China. J Environ Sci (China). 2006;18(6):1124–34.
8. Friesen MC, Demers PA, Spinelli JJ, Eisen EA, Lorenzi MF, Le ND. Chronic and acute effects of coal tar pitch exposure and cardiopulmonary mortality among aluminum smelter workers. Am J Epidemiol. 2010;172(7):790–9.
9. Adelson N. The embodiment of inequity: health disparities in Aboriginal Canada. Can J Public Health. 2005;96(Suppl 2):S45–S61.

10. Czyzewski K. Colonialism as a broader social determinant of health. Int Indig Policy J. 2011;2(1):5.
11. Gracey M, King M. Indigenous health part 1: determinants and disease patterns. Lancet. 2009;374(9683):65–75.
12. Reading CL, Wien F. Health inequalities and the social determinants of Aboriginal peoples' health. Prince George (BC): National Collaborating Centre for Aboriginal Health; 2013.
13. Banken R. From concept to practice: including the social determinants of health in environmental assessments. Can J Public Health. 1999;90:S27.
14. Brisbois BW, Reschny J, Fyfe TM, Harder HG, Parkes MW, Allison S, Buse, CG, Fumerton, R, Oke, B. Mapping research on resource extraction and health: a scoping review. Extr Ind Soc. 2018;6(1):250–9
15. Mactaggart F, McDermott L, Tynan A, Gericke C. Examining health and well-being outcomes associated with mining activity in rural communities of high-income countries: a systematic review. Aust J Rural Health. 2016 Aug;24(4):230–7.
16. Schrecker T, Birn A-E, Aguilera M. How extractive industries affect health: political economy underpinnings and pathways. Health Place. 2018;52:135–47.
17. Jacka JK. The anthropology of mining: the social and environmental impacts of resource extraction in the mineral age. Annu Rev Anthropol. 2018;47:61–77.
18. Byambaa T, Wagler M, Janes CR. Bringing health impact assessment to the Mongolian resource sector: a story of successful diffusion. Impact Assess Proj Apprais. 2014;32(3):241–5.
19. Byambaa T, Janes C, Davison C. Challenges of building health impact assessment capacity in developing countries: a review. J Glob Health. 2012;2(2):5–8.
20. Harris-Roxas B, Viliani F, Bond A, Cave B, Divall M, Furu P, Harris, P, Soeberg, M, Wernham, A, Winkler, M. Health impact assessment: the state of the art. Impact Assess Proj Apprais. 2012;30(1):43–52.
21. O'Faircheallaigh C. Making social impact assessment count: a negotiation-based approach for Indigenous peoples. Soc Nat Resour. 1999;12(1):63–80.
22. Banerjee SB. Corporate social responsibility: the good, the bad and the ugly. Crit Sociol. 2008;34(1):51–79.
23. Esau G, Malone M. CSR in natural resources: rhetoric and reality. J Glob Responsib. 2013;4(2):168–87.
24. Kwiatkowski RE. Indigenous community based participatory research and health impact assessment: a Canadian example. Environ Impact Assess Rev. 2011;31(4):445–50.
25. Jones J, Nix NA, Snyder EH. Local perspectives of the ability of HIA stakeholder engagement to capture and reflect factors that impact Alaska Native health. Int J Circumpolar Health. 2014;73:24411.
26. Richmond CAM, Ross NA. The determinants of First Nation and Inuit health: a critical population health approach. Health Place. 2009;15(2):403–11.

27. Alfred T, Corntassel J. Being Indigenous: resurgences against contemporary colonialism. Gov Oppos. 2005;40(4):597–614.
28. Tuck E. Suspending damage: a letter to communities. Harv Educ Rev. 2009;79(3):409–28.
29. de Leeuw S, Hunt S. Unsettling decolonizing geographies. Geogr Compass. 2018;12(7):e12376.
30. Anthony-Stevens V. Cultivating alliances: reflections on the role of non-indigenous collaborators in indigenous educational sovereignty. J Am Indian Educ. 2017;56(1):81–104.
31. Yukon Indian People. Together today for our children tomorrow: a statement of grievances and an approach to settlement by the Yukon Indian People. Bampton (ON): Charters Publishing Company Limited; 1973.
32. Neufeld D. Our land is our voice: First Nation heritage-making in the Tr'ondëk/Klondike. Int J Heritage Stud. 2016;22(7):568–81.
33. Keeling A, Sandlos J, editors. Mining and communities in northern Canada: history, politics, and memory. Calgary (AB): University of Calgary Press; 2015.
34. Christensen J, Grant M. How political change paved the way for Indigenous knowledge: the Mackenzie Valley Resource Management Act. Arctic. 2007;60(2):115–23.
35. Tobias JK, Richmond CA. "That land means everything to us as Anishinaabe …": Environmental dispossession and resilience on the north shore of Lake Superior. Health Place. 2014;29:26–33.
36. Nadasdy P. Boundaries among kin: sovereignty, the modern treaty process, and the rise of ethno-territorial nationalism among Yukon First Nations. Comp Stud Soc Hist. 2012;54(03):499–532.
37. Wilson K. Therapeutic landscapes and First Nations peoples: an exploration of culture, health and place. Health Place. 2003;9(2):83–93.
38. Alcantara C. To treaty or not to treaty? Aboriginal peoples and comprehensive land claims negotiations in Canada. Publius: J Fed. 2008;38(2):343–69.
39. Youngblood Henderson J. Treaty governance. In: Belanger YD, editor. Aboriginal self-government in Canada: current trends and issues. Saskatoon (SK): Purich Publishing Ltd.; 2008. p. 20–38.
40. Irlbacher-Fox S. Finding dahshaa: self-government, social suffering and, Aboriginal policy in Canada. Cambridge University Press; 2009.
41. O'Faircheallaigh C. International recognition of indigenous rights, indigenous control of development and domestic political mobilisation. Aust J Polit Sci. 2012;47(4):531–45.
42. Franks C. Rights and self-government for Canada's Aboriginal peoples. In: Cook C, Lindau, JD, editors. Aboriginal rights and self-government the Canadian and Mexican experience in North American perspective. Montreal (QC): McGill-Queen's University Press; 2000, p. 101–34.

43. Yukon Environmental and Socio-economic Assessment Board [Internet]. Whitehorse (YK): Yukon Environmental and Socio-economic Assessment Board; 2021. Purpose of YESAA [cited 2016 Jul 31]. Available from: https://www.yesab.ca/the-assessment-process/purpose-of-yesaa/
44. Raphael D. Social determinants of health: Canadian perspectives. Toronto (ON): Canadian Scholars' Press; 2009.
45. Young TK. Population health: concepts and methods: Oxford (GB): Oxford University Press; 2004.
46. Waldram JB, Young TK, Herring A. Aboriginal health in Canada: historical, cultural, and epidemiological perspectives. Toronto (ON): University of Toronto Press; 2006.
47. Coburn D, Denny K, Mykhalovskiy E, McDonough P, Robertson A, Love R. Population health in Canada: a brief critique. Am J Public Health. 2003;93(3):392–6.
48. Braveman P. Health disparities and health equity: concepts and measurement. Annu Rev Public Health. 2006;27:167–94.
49. Navarro V. What we mean by social determinants of health. Int J Health Serv. 2009;39(3):423–41.
50. Raphael D, Bryant T. The limitations of population health as a model for a new public health. Health promotion international. 2002;17(2):189–99.
51. Smylie J, Firestone M. Back to the basics: identifying and addressing underlying challenges in achieving high quality and relevant health statistics for Indigenous populations in Canada. Stat J IAOS. 2015;31(1):67–87.
52. Hendryx M, Wolfe L, Luo J, Webb B. Self-reported cancer rates in two rural areas of West Virginia with and without mountaintop coal mining. J Community Health. 2012;37(2):320–7.
53. Goessling KP. Mining induced displacement and mental health: a call for action. Int J Adv Couns. 2010;32(3):153–64.
54. Jobin W. Health and equity impacts of a large oil project in Africa. Bull World Health Organ. 2003;81(6):420–6.
55. World Health Organization. Managing the public health impacts of natural resources extraction activities. A framework for national and local health authorities [Internet]. Geneva (CH): World Health Organization; 2010 Nov 17, discussion draft [cited 2016 Sep 28]. Available from: https://commdev.org/pdf/publications/WHO-Managing-the-public-health-impacts.pdf
56. Winkler MS, Krieger GR, Divall MJ, Cissé G, Wielga M, Singer BH, Tanner M, Utzinger J. Untapped potential of health impact assessment. Bull World Health Organ. 2013 Apr 1;91(4):298–305.
57. Bhatia R, Wernham A. Integrating human health into environmental impact assessment: an unrealized opportunity for environmental health and justice. Cirn Saude Colet. 2009;14(4):1159–75.
58. Native Women's Association of Canada. Social determinants of health and Canada's Aboriginal women: NWAC's submission to the World Health

Organization's Commission on the Social Determinants of Health. Navan (ON): Native Women's Association of Canada; 2007.

59. Raphael D. A discourse analysis of the social determinants of health. Crit Public Health. 2011;21(2):221–36.
60. Krieger N. Proximal, distal, and the politics of causation: what's level got to do with it? Am J public health. 2008;98(2):221.
61. Morgan RK. Health and impact assessment: are we seeing closer integration? Environ Impact Assess Rev. 2011;31(4):404–11.
62. Noble B, Bronson J. Practitioner survey of the state of health integration in environmental assessment: the case of northern Canada. Environ Impact Assess Rev. 2006;26(4):410–24.
63. International Council on Mining and Metals. Good practice guidance on health impact assessment. London (GB): International Council on Mining and Metals; 2010.
64. International Finance Corporation, World Bank Group. Introduction to health impact assessment. Washington (DC): International Finance Corporation; 2009.
65. Equator Principles Association [Internet]. Eastbourne (GB): Equator Principles Association. The equator principles; 2011 [cited 2016 Sep 28]. Available from: https://www.equator-principles.com/
66. Knotsch C, Warda J. Impact benefit agreements: a tool for healthy Inuit communities. Ottawa (ON): National Aboriginal Health Organization; 2009.
67. Butler P. Colonial extractions: race and Canadian mining in contemporary Africa. Toronto (ON): University of Toronto Press; 2015.
68. de Leeuw S, Maurice S, Holyk T, Greenwood M, Adam W. With reserves: colonial geographies and First Nations health. Ann Assoc Am Geogr. 2012;102(5):904–11.
69. Castellano MB. Ethics of Aboriginal research. Int J Indig Health. 2004;1(1):98.
70. Cunsolo Willox A, Harper SL, Ford JD, Landman K, Houle K, Edge VL, Rigolet Inuit Community Government. "From this place and of this place:" climate change, sense of place, and health in Nunatsiavut, Canada. Soc Sci Med. 2012;75(3):538–47.
71. Kral M, Idlout L, Minore J, Dyck R, Kirmayer L. Unikkaartuit: meanings of well-being, unhappiness, health, and community change among Inuit in Nunavut, Canada. Am J Community Psychol. 2011;48(3–4):426–38.
72. de Leeuw S, Lindsay NM, Greenwood M. Introduction: rethinkging determinants of Indigenous peoples' health in Canada. In: Greenwood M, De Leeuw S, Reading C, editors. Determinants of Indigenous peoples' health. Toronto (ON): Canadian Scholars' Press; 2015.
73. Bombay A, Matheson K, Anisman H. The intergenerational effects of Indian residential schools: Implications for the concept of historical trauma. Transcult Psychiatry. 2014;51(3):320–38.
74. Kirmayer L, Gone J, Moses J. Rethinking historical trauma. Transcult Psychiatry. 2014;51(3):299–319.

75. Wertz MS, Nosek M, McNiesh S, Marlow E. The composite first person narrative: texture, structure, and meaning in writing phenomenological descriptions. Int J Qual Stud Health Well-being. 2011;6(2).
76. Agrawal A. Dismantling the divide between Indigenous and scientific knowledge. Dev Change. 1995;26(3):413–39.
77. Cochran PA, Marshall CA, Garcia-Downing C, Kendall E, Cook D, McCubbin L, Gover RM. Indigenous ways of knowing: Implications for participatory research and community. Am J Public Health. 2008;98(1):22.
78. Kwiatkowski RE, Tikhonov C, Peace DM, Bourassa C. Canadian Indigenous engagement and capacity building in health impact assessment. Impact Assess Proj Apprais. 2009;27(1):57–67.
79. Truth and Reconciliation Commission of Canada. Honouring the truth, reconciling for the future: summary of the final report of the Truth and Reconciliation Commission of Canada. Winnipeg (MB): Truth and Reconciliation Commission of Canada; 2015.
80. Harris C. How did colonialism dispossess? Comments from an edge of empire. Ann Assoc Am Geogr. 2004;94(1):165–82.

SECTION II

Health Care in Northern Canada

HELLE MØLLER

As the federal legislation for publicly funded health care, the Canada Health Act (CHA) "establishes criteria and conditions related to insured health services and extended health care services that the provinces and territories must fulfil to receive the full federal cash contribution under the Canada Health Transfer (CHT)" (1 p6). In the CHA annual report, the minister of health has reiterated that the objectives of the CHA are to ensure that "all Canadians have equitable access to health care services based on their need and not on their ability, or willingness, to pay" (1 p6). Part of the CHA reads, "The primary objective of Canadian health care policy is to protect, promote and restore the physical and mental well-being of residents of Canada and to facilitate reasonable access to health services without financial or other barriers" (1 p6). It is important to note that "reasonable access" to health services' is interpreted

> using the "where and as available" principle. Thus, residents of a province or territory are entitled to have access on uniform terms and conditions to insured health care services at the setting "where" the services are provided and "as" the services are available in that setting." For example, if a hospital in one region of a province was providing highly specialised services, that would not mean that all hospitals in the province would be required to provide the same service. Rather, it means that all residents of the province should have access to the service wherever it is being offered, on the same basis. (1 p10).

Most communities in northern Canada have less easy access to health care services when compared to the south (2–5). Several factors contribute to shaping this reality, including geographical, infrastructural, financial, and political ones, and the impacts of climate change that compound all other factors. The cost of delivering services is rising in Canada as a whole, rendering the sustainability of the health care systems (particularly in the North) a key concern (5–7).

Access to hospitals, health centres, and other facilities that provide care, services, and programs that restore, support, and maintain health and well-being is, in many northern communities, not equivalent to access in southern Canada (8–10). Residents of rural and remote communities located at a distance from larger population centres often need to travel to larger northern centres or southern Canada for services. This is particularly so for residents of many northern and remote Indigenous communities to which access is possible only by plane, boat, or winter roads. The need to leave your family and support system when you, your children, or close relations have health concerns or health care needs (beyond what can be addressed in your home community), can cause financial, emotional, and social strain for the individual, the family, and the wider community (9–12). For residents of remote communities, these impacts are often compounded by services being disjointed, that is, not coordinated between the care providers in a home community and those in the urban centre. For residents in some remote communities, the hospital in the nearest urban centre does not provide all the services needed. Rather, residents are directed to larger hospitals even further away, and residents with specialty needs, such as the elderly, disabled, or chronically ill, often require several different access points (13). These various access points generally do not share records or have easy lines of communication as they may be situated in different provinces or territories and/or be located at different jurisdictional levels (federal, provincial, territorial, or Indigenous government). Such conditions render the health and social systems in northern Canada fragmented and uncoordinated, contributing to symptoms and issues being addressed in silos rather than holistically, leading to increased suffering, distress, prolonged health risks, and ill health (5,14,15).

In addition to specialized health facilities, services, and programs being scarce, staffing the facilities and programs that do exist in northern communities, whether hospitals or health centres, has proved difficult. Recruiting and retaining health professionals has historically been very challenging in northern communities (16–18). In some areas of the North, health professionals are generally hired from southern Canada. Although southern professionals provide the best care they can, southern health professionals often do not speak the mother tongue of the community members they serve, which can result in miscommunication of key information, create frustration and distress for both health care users and health care providers, exacerbate suffering, and prolong ill health for northern residents (17,18).

A key response to recruitment and retention challenges has often been to promote educating local residents to become health care providers (16–18). Promoting education for "home-grown" health care providers proves difficult when access to education and levels of educational attainment are significantly lower in northern than in southern Canada. For example, in 2016, of Inuit ages 25–64 living in Inuit Nunangat, 44.4 per cent had a postsecondary qualification, and of these, 14.3 per cent had a university degree. In comparison, 64.8 per cent of Canada's population overall ages 25–64 had a postsecondary qualification, and of these, 28.5 per cent had a university degree (19; see also Walton, chapter 1, this volume). Many factors contribute to low educational levels, including that schools were, and to a large degree continue to be, developed and controlled by southern institutions, with the language of instruction and educational culture being dissimilar to – rather than drawing from or sensitive to – northern Indigenous languages and cultures (17,18,20,21; see also Walton, chapter 1, this volume).

Still, improving educational preparedness for training and actual training of health care providers with a focus on the North does occur locally. Preparing for training happens through particular programs, for example, those offered at Thompson Rivers University in Kamloops, British Columbia (Aboriginal pathways to health careers (22)) and Lakehead University (Native Nurses Entry Program (23)). Training of northern (and Indigenous) providers also happens through the nursing program in Iqaluit that has run since late 1990 (17,20); the midwifery program in Cambridge Bay, Nunavut, that started in 2010 (24); and the Northern Ontario Medical School in Thunder Bay, Ontario (25, see also Pong, chapter 7, this volume). There are also great examples of local groups and initiatives that have succeeded in securing government funding to offer particular services for Indigenous people – for example, midwifery clinics and programs across Ontario (26,27) and in Nunavut (28); doula programs for First Nations mothers, as discussed by Cidro and Sinclair, chapter 9, this volume; and community therapy assistant programs in Nunavut (29), northern BC, northern Quebec, and northern Ontario (30).

In addition to promoting the education of local or home-grown health professionals, telehealth has been introduced in many communities (31). In rural and northern Ontario, for example, the Ontario Telemedicine Network has provided virtual health care services across the province since 2006, allowing rural and remote residents access to specialized care that was otherwise not available to them (32). This has decreased the need to travel and improved health care access for hundreds of thousands of residents (32). Despite these efforts, health care providers are still in high demand and it remains a challenge to recruit and retain them in northern Canada – particularly in the more remote communities (33–38).

In this section, health care access and delivery in northern Canada is described from a variety of viewpoints, starting with issues related to the shortage of health care professionals, with particular attention to physicians and nurses. The section begins with chapter 7 by Raymond Pong, which examines the strategies that have been and are used to recruit medical doctors to northern and remote areas historically and presently. Pong describes the severity of need experienced in northern Ontario and how an intensified focus on education of medical doctors in northern districts, including training students in remote and northern communities, may be a big part of the solution to addressing the physician shortage. The chapter draws specifically on Pong's experience with training Northern Ontario Medical School students in remote districts and the positive outcomes of this approach. Pong highlights the gape in specialized care and providers felt across remote and northern communities. This does not mean that specialists can or necessarily should be available in all communities; it does mean, however, that it is necessary to work towards innovative solutions that enable northern and remote residents access to the specialist care they need, when they need it, without any additional financial burden, wait time, or undue social disruption. Simultaneously, it is of utmost importance that we support the health and well-being of northern and remote residents by addressing the social determinants of health and focusing on health promotion and illness prevention, as discussed in chapter 8, this volume. Such a focus would have the added benefit of decreasing the need for specialist care.

Helle Møller, who has also educated health care professionals (nurses and medical interpreters) in northern communities (Nunavut and Greenland), picks up the topic of the shortage of health care professionals. In chapter 8, Møller starts with a historical review of nursing in northern Canada, concentrating on the presence, roles, and working conditions of nurses in the North after the end of World War II, when many of the nurses working in the Canadian North were British nurse-midwives who often collaborated with local, traditionally educated midwives. Møller continues with an appraisal of nursing in northern Canada as it looks today and how nurses' roles have evolved (both narrowing and expanding) before and after the introduction of nurse practitioners. The chapter then moves to a more focused discussion of the contemporary nursing shortage and some of the recruitment and retention strategies that have been used. It uses Nunavut as a case study – the need is felt most strongly in this territory (as revealed through current data on nursing shortages), and nurses are often the health professionals most present. The chapter ends with a discussion of what has been done and needs to be done to ensure that communities in northern Canada can attract, recruit, and retain the nurses they need. The solutions, the author contends, lie not only in attempting to attract and retain (or educate locally) but also in improving the social determinant conditions in remote communities since they are key for education and retention.

Following the discussions of critical health human resources shortages in the North, this section moves on to look at health care for a few specific populations that demand special consideration; in particular, we consider health care for pregnant women, Elders, and persons living with mental health challenges. In chapter 9, Cidro and Sinclair discuss the historical and current challenges maternal health care faces in the Canadian north, particularly for Indigenous women. The authors highlight how the Westernization and medicalization of birth have resulted in significant social and cultural disruptions and discontinuation of Indigneous traditional midwifery and traditional doula care. The evacuation policy that forces all Indigenous women to be transferred out of their home community weeks before their due date to give birth at tertiary care centres has been and continues to be particularly disruptive. As a response to this and with the ultimate goal of returning birth to communities, the authors started their ongoing research on the roles that doulas can have in supporting First Nations women and families during the perinatal period, focusing on three Cree communities located in northern Manitoba: Pimicikamak Cree Nation (Cross Lake), Nisichawayasihk Cree Nation (Nelson House), and Misipawistik Cree Nation (Grand Rapids First Nation). Both authors note that as Indigenous researchers working with Indigenous peoples, they look first at community priorities, and then start with spirit, bind people together with friendship, and focus on relationships. They acknowledge that to overcome the challenges that many Indigenous people face, there is a need to go back to the beginning, and the beginning is birth. As the authors maintain in their closing paragraph, "Training Indigenous doulas in First Nations is a first step in revitalizing Indigenous birth knowledge and creating a path to returning birth to communities."

In chapter 10, Beatty and McKay deal with a topic that has been significant in Canada for decades and continues to be an issue today: the presence, or absence, of specific health support for Elders in many northern communities. The authors explore the distribution of, access to, and delivery of long-term-care services in the North specifically in relation to Indigenous Elders (seniors). The chapter describes the general organization and delivery of formal continuing care services across the North and the difficulty caused by services being a patchwork of federal and territorial responsibility and funding. The authors describe this patchwork system as being far from able to provide the long-term care and support needed. They portray the shortcomings of existing care and services in the North generally and describe the findings from a case study that illuminate perspectives and common concerns among First Nation family care providers in northeastern Saskatchewan. Important recommendations from the authors include the necessity of enhancing homecare programs in northern communities to allow Elders to age in place and of building First Nation long-term-care facilities on reserve to allow Elders who require a higher level of care to stay in known environmental, cultural, and linguistic surroundings, close to family and friends.

Access to appropriate, timely, and culturally safe care is also very difficult for those living with mental health challenges in northern communities. Chapter 11 by Azaad Kassam highlights how the history and legacy of colonization have resulted in significant concerns related to addiction, depression, abuse, and suicide. Kassam draws on his own experience as a northern mental health care professional, particularly in northeastern Ontario and northern Quebec, and eloquently reinforces a common thread in all the chapters of this section: to address inequity (including in mental health and addictions prevention and care) northern communities must be provided with adequate support and self-determination to lead and develop their own approaches to healing and prevention, including reappropriation and renewal of traditional cultural values. Solutions to these challenges are further discussed through an Indigenous lens, in chapter 15 by Mushquash, Drawson, and Toombs in Section III.

Climate change is acutely felt in northern Canada, and research has been emerging especially in the last decade that describes not just the physical and mental health impacts of climate change. The magnitude and early impacts of climate change in the North are having a significant impact on social and ecological determinants of health for northern communities. Another concerning impact of climate change is the disruption of health services in the North, which is the focus of chapter 12 by Cunsolo, MacLeod, Shiwak, Wood, the Inuit Mental Health and Climate Change Adaptation Team, and Harper. The authors highlight how climate change compounds the health impacts experienced within the already-present health disparities stemming from the legacies of colonization, forced acculturation, and systematic marginalization – contexts that have contributed to lower life expectancy, higher prevalence of chronic disease, higher incidence rates of infectious disease, and higher rates of substance usage, suicide, and addiction than the Canadian average. A case study from Nunatsiavut, Labrador, contextualizes the effects of climate change through the perspectives of northern residents. It highlights the important role that health care providers have in responding to climate-related health impacts. The authors conclude with suggestions for a move towards adaptive systems, strategies that can mobilize northern health care providers and communities and move them towards resilient health care systems.

This section concludes with a critical issue in the North that has been described as a crisis in many northern communities: suicide. This issue is also discussed by Kassam, but its significance – and an assets-based focus on solutions and prevention strategies – warrants a dedicated chapter. In addition to mental health care and support being limited, Josephine Tan explains in chapter 13 that a local perspective and approach that builds on local strengths is needed to address the underlying factors leading to suicide ideation, attempts, and completed suicides in Inuit communities. Further, Tan observes that limited financial, health, and social support make it more challenging to develop and offer traditional suicide prevention initiatives, and that federal government support is crucial. The territorial and federal governments have both pledged financial support to address this important issue. In 2017, the Nunavut government pledged $4.5 million to support mental health in the territory; in the same year the federal government pledged $70 million to help address mental health issues and suicide by Indigenous people in Canada.

In sum, this section provides the reader with a review of some of the challenges that exists to providing the quality and quantity of care needed in northern and remote communities and highlights the need for educating professionals close to home. It also highlights the need to address determinants, focus on innovative solutions that suit the needs of northern and remote residents, and enhance intersectoral and interprofessional collaboration to improve health and well-being and decrease the need for care, specialized and otherwise.

REFERENCES

1. Health Canada. Canada Health Act: Annual report 2018–2019 – public administration, comprehensiveness, universality, portability, accessibility [Internet]. Ottawa (ON): Government of Canada; 2020 [cited 2020 May 15]. Available from: http://www.canada.ca/content/dam/hc-sc/documents/services/publications/health-system-services/canada-health-act-annual-report-2018-2019/pub1-eng.pdf
2. Young TK, Chatwood S, Ng C, Young RW, Marchildon, GP. The north is not all the same: comparing health system performance in 18 northern regions of Canada. Int J Circumpolar Health. 2019 Dec;78(1):1697474. doi: 10.1080/22423982.2019.1697474
3. Health Quality Ontario. Northern Ontario health equity strategy [Internet]. Toronto (ON): Health Quality Ontario; 2018 [cited 2020 Jan 20]. Available from: http://www.hqontario.ca/Portals/0/documents/health-quality/health-equity-strategy-report-en.pdf
4. Ferguson M. Spring 2015 report of the Auditor General of Canada – Report 4: access to health services for remote First Nations communities [Internet]. Ottawa (ON): Auditor General of Canada; 2015 Jun 1 [cited 2020 Jan 10]. Available from: http://www.oag-bvg.gc.ca/internet/English/parl_oag_201504_04_e_40350.html
5. Ferguson M. Report of the Auditor General of Canada to the Legislative Assembly of Nunavut – 2017: Health care services – Nunavut [Internet]. Ottawa (ON): Auditor General of Canada; 2017 Mar 7 [cited 2020 Jan 10]. Available from: http://www.oag-bvg.gc.ca/internet/English/nun_201703_e_41998.html
6. Government of Northwest Territories. Caring for our people: strategy plan for the NWT Health and Social Services System, 2017 to 2020 [Internet]. Yellowknife (NT): Government of Northwest Territories; 2017 [cited 2020 Jan 10]. Available from: https://www.hss.gov.nt.ca/sites/hss/files/resources/caring-our-people-strategic-plan-2017-2020.pdf
7. Canadian Institute for Health Information. National health expenditure trends, 1975 to 2019. Ottawa (ON): Canadian Institute for Health Information; 2019.

8. The National. Canada's struggle to provide healthcare to Northern communities. CBC Online [Internet]. 2018 Mar 5 [cited 2020 Jan 10]. Available from: http://www.cbc.ca/news/thenational/canada-s-struggle-to-provide-health-care-to-northern-communities-1.4563721
9. Bourassa C. Addressing the duality of access to healthcare for Indigenous communities: racism and geographical barriers to safe care. Healthc Pap. 2018;17(3):6–10. doi: 10.12927/hcpap.2018.25507
10. Huot S, Ho H, Ko A, Lam S, Tactay P, MacLachlan J, Raanaas RK. Identifying barriers to healthcare delivery and access in the circumpolar North: important insights for health professionals. Int J Circumpolar Health, 2019;78(1):1571385. doi: 10.1080/22423982.2019.1571385
11. Møller H, Dowsley M, Wakewich P, Bishop L, Burnett K, Churchill M. Qualitative assessment of factors in the uptake of midwifery of diverse populations in Thunder Bay, Ontario. Can J Midwifery Res Pract. 2015;14(3):14–20.
12. Pauktuutit Inuit Women of Canada. Inuit cancer project – year one final report. Ottawa (ON): Pauktuutit Inuit Women of Canada; 2013.
13. Canadian Foundation for Healthcare Improvement. Healthcare priorities in Canada: a backgrounder [Internet]. Ottawa (ON): Canadian Foundation for Healthcare Improvement; 2014 [cited 2020 Jan 10]. Available from: http://www.cfhi-fcass.ca/sf-docs/default-source/documents/harkness-healthcare-priorities-canada-backgrounder-e.pdf
14. Purdon N, Palleja L. Health system neglects northern patients by design: doctor. CBC News [Internet]; 2018 Mar 5 [cited 2020 Jan 10]. Available from: http://www.cbc.ca/news/canada/north/north-health-care-system-problems-1.4523140
15. Office of Audit and Evaluation Health Canada and the Public Health Agency of Canada. Evaluation of Health Canada's First Nations Health Facilities Program 2010–2011 to 2014–2015 [Internet]. Ottawa (ON): Office of Audit and Evaluation Health Canada and the Public Health Agency of Canada; 2017 [cited 2020 Jan 10]. Available from: http://www.canada.ca/en/health-canada/corporate/transparency/corporate-management-reporting/evaluation/first-nations-health-facilities-program-2010-2011-2014-2015.html
16. Exner-Pirot H. Introduction: nursing education in the circumpolar north. North Rev. 2016;43:1–10.
17. Møller H. "You need to be double cultured to function here": toward an anthropology of Inuit nursing in Greenland and Nunavut [dissertation]. Edmonton (AB): University of Alberta; 2011.
18. Møller, H. Culturally safe communication and the power of "language" in Arctic nursing. Etudes Inuit. 2016;40(1):85–104.
19. Statistics Canada. Nunavut [territory] and Canada [country] (table); Census profile, 2016 census [Internet]. Ottawa (ON): Statistics Canada; 2017 Nov 29 [cited 2020 Jan 10]. Catalogue No.: 98-316-X2016001. Available from https://www12.statcan.gc.ca/census-recensement/2016/dp-pd/prof/index.cfm?Lang=E

20. Møller H. "Double culturedness": the "capital" of Inuit nurses. Int J Circumpolar Health. 2013;72:21266. doi: 10.3402/ijch.v72i0.21266
21. Skutnabb-Kangas T, Phillipson R, and Dunbar R. Is Nunavut education criminally inadequate? An analysis of current policies for Inuktut and English in education, international and national law, linguistic and cultural genocide and crimes against humanity [Internet]. Iqaluit (NU): Nunavut Tunngavik Incorporated; 2019 Apr [cited 2020 Jan 10]. Available from: https://www.tunngavik.com/files/2019/04/NuLinguicideReportFINAL.pdf
22. Thompson Rivers University [Internet]. Kamloops (BC): Thompson Rivers University. Aboriginal pathways to health careers; 2020 [cited 2020 Jan 10]. Available from: https://www.tru.ca/nursing/aboriginal-nursing/pathways.html
23. Lakehead University [Internet]. Thunder Bay (ON): Lakehead University. Native nurses entry program; 2020 [cited 2020 Jan 10]. Available from: http://www.lakeheadu.ca/academics/departments/nnep
24. George J. CamBay moms may soon give birth closer to home: Community getting resident midwives. Nunatsiaq Online [Internet]; 2009 Oct 8 [cited 2020 Jan 20]. Available from: https://nunatsiaq.com/stories/article/1009_Cambay_moms_may_soon_give_birth_closer_to_home/
25. Tesson G, Hudson G, Strasser R, Hunt D, editors. The making of the Northern Ontario School of Medicine: a case study in the history of medical education. Montreal (QC): McGill-Queen's University Press; 2009.
26. Ontario Ministry of Health and Long-Term Care [Internet]. Toronto (ON): Government of Ontario. Ontario improving access to Aboriginal midwifery care; 2017 Feb 9 [cited 2020 Jan 10]. Available from: https://news.ontario.ca/mohltc/en/2017/02/ontario-improving-access-to-aboriginal-midwifery-care.html
27. Association of Ontario Midwives. Bring birth home – voices from the Indigenous Midwifery Summit: a reclamation of community birth through a northern Indigenous vision. Summary Report [Internet]. Toronto (ON): Association of Ontario Midwives; 2019 Feb [cited 2020 Jan 10]. Available from: http://www.ontariomidwives.ca/sites/default/files/2019-07/Indigenous%20Midwifery%20Summit%20Report%202019.pdf
28. George, J. Nunavut's health minister vows increased support for midwifery. Nunatsiaq News [Internet]; 2019 Jun 10 [cited 2020 Jan 10]. Available from: https://nunatsiaq.com/stories/article/nunavuts-health-minister-vows-increased-support-for-midwifery/
29. Miller-Mifflin T, McNeil C, Driedger D, Fricke M, Achtemichuk M, Bzdell M, & Robison J. Inuit community therapy assistants: A unique education program and innovative service delivery model for a remote practice context in Nunavut. Physiother Can. 2011 Jul;63(Suppl 1):45.
30. Roots R, Dignum T, Taylor D, French E, Lubino V, Dolgoy L, Leon Torres S. Community-based rehabilitation-workers: Canadian examples of building capacity

in Indigenous communities. Abstract: Canadian Physiotherapy Association Congress, May 28–30 2020.

31. Jong M, Mendez I, Jong, R. Enhancing access to care in northern rural communities via telehealth, Int J Circumpolar Health. 2019;78(2):1554174. doi: 10.1080/22423982.2018.1554174
32. Brown EM. The Ontario telemedicine network: a case report. Telemed J E Health. 2013;19(5):373–6.
33. Johansson AM, Söderberg S, Lindberg I. Views of residents of rural areas on accessibility to specialist care through videoconference. Technol Health Care. 2014;22(1):147–55.
34. Canadian Physiotherapy Association. Access to physiotherapy in rural, remote and northern areas of Canada: an environmental scan [Internet]. Ottawa (ON): Canadian Physiotherapy Association; 2016 [cited 2018 May 1]. Available from: https://physiotherapy.ca/sites/default/files/access_to_physiotherapy_environmental_scan_may2016.pdf
35. Association of Occupational Therapists – British Columbia. Occupational therapists shortage in British Columbia update [Internet]. Vancouver (BC): Canadian Association of Occupational Therapists – British Columbia; 2015 [cited 2018 May 1]. Available from www.caot.ca/document/4602/Jun-2015%20%20Update%20on%20Occupational%20Therapists%20Shortage%20in%20British%20Columbia.pdf
36. Ougler J. Northern Ontario lacks diabetes resources. Sudbury Star [Internet]; 2017 Nov 23 [cited 2018 May 1]. Available from: http://www.thesudburystar.com/2017/11/23/northern-ontario-lacks-diabetes-resources
37. The North needs more doctors. Walrus [Internet]. 2017 Nov 22 [cited 2020 January 20]. Available from: https://thewalrus.ca/the-north-needs-more-doctors/
38. Shah TI, Clark AF, Seabrook JA, Sibbald S, Gilliland JA. Geographic accessibility to primary care providers: comparing rural and urban areas in Southwestern Ontario. Can Geogr. 2019 Aug 8;64(2). doi: 10.1111/cag.12557

7 Recruitment and Retention of Physicians: Physician Supply and Sufficiency

RAYMOND W. PONG

Introduction

In April 2016, the small Indigenous community of Attawapiskat in the far north of Ontario was grappling with a rash of attempted suicides by children and youth. Media reports attributed the crisis to economic deprivation, social desperation, and hopelessness, but it was aggravated by inadequate health care, particularly mental health services. The federal and Ontario governments rushed teams of health workers to Attawapiskat to help the troubled young people. Although other northern communities may not find themselves in such a terrible situation, many experience similar difficulties accessing health services because of a lack of providers.

Shortages of health care providers, particularly physicians, in northern or rural communities have a long history in Canada, though awareness of the problem may have become more acute and complaints more audible after Canada adopted a universal health insurance system, commonly known as medicare, in the 1960s. Medicare was intended to ensure universal access to needed medical and hospital care for all Canadians regardless of ability to pay. But, as it has been noted (1), removal of financial barriers means little if providers are not available and services hard to obtain. Geographic maldistribution of health care providers, particularly physicians, also appears to be an almost universal phenomenon, even in developed nations (2–4). The vast expanse of Canada and the uneven spread of its relatively small population may have accentuated the problem and made it harder to overcome.

This chapter discusses shortages of physicians in many northern and rural communities in Canada and examines some of the strategies used to increase physician availability in those places. The focus on physicians is mostly for practical reasons since it is impossible to cover the entire range of health care providers in a relatively short chapter. But many of the lessons we can learn about physicians in underserved communities are applicable to other practitioners working in similar settings, with appropriate adjustments.

The geographic focus of this discussion is on the North because it is the subject of this book. But because much of the discussion here is based on findings from several studies, the meaning of *the North* varies somewhat depending on how it was understood by the studies cited. The Provincial North is often mentioned, which refers to the northern and sparsely populated parts of a province, though its precise meaning varies from jurisdiction to jurisdiction. It could refer to the three territories or more broadly to rural or remote areas. Although not identical in meaning, the terms *north* (or *northern*), *rural*, and *remote* share some common characteristics such as a small population, geographic isolation, heavy reliance on primary industry, and a lack of infrastructure and services. Also, while rural areas can be found in northern and southern Canada, those in the north (including most of the territories) are likely to be underserved in medical care as northern rural communities tend to be more isolated and farther from major cities.

In this chapter, I knit together a series of studies I and my research collaborators have conducted over a number of years. Although these are independent studies, they share a broad theme, namely, scarcity of physicians in northern or rural communities and ways to attenuate the adverse effects of such shortages. While most of these studies have been published, some findings are presented here for the first time. Some are national in scope, whereas others are about Ontario's Provincial North. For additional information, particularly methodological details, please consult the original publications.

The next section briefly describes the geographic distribution of physicians in Canada based on two sets of analyses. This is followed by an examination of strategies used to deal with physician shortages in northern Ontario over a 35-year period. Although many approaches and programs have been tried, medical education/training specifically designed for rural or northern practice as a health workforce strategy has gained traction in more recent years. Thus, an analysis of where physicians are trained at the postgraduate level is conducted. To determine how effective medical education strategies are, I present some initial findings from a multi-year study of the learners and graduates of the Northern Ontario School of Medicine (NOSM). The last section discusses these studies collectively by asking what we can learn from them and where we go from here.

Where Are Physicians Located in Canada?

Geographic Distribution of Physicians in Canada (5) was published in 1999 – the first national, sub-provincial-level study on where physicians were located. Using data from the Canadian Institute for Health Information

(CIHI), it compared the geographic distribution of the population with that of physicians. The analysis clearly showed that the distribution of physicians did not match that of the population. In 1996, 9.8 per cent of all physicians worked in small towns and rural areas where 22.2 per cent of Canadians resided. The uneven geographic distribution was particularly acute for specialists.

Geographic Distribution of Physicians in Canada: Beyond How Many and Where (6) appeared several years later and represented an update and extension of the earlier study. Using data from CIHI, it found that in 2004, 9.4 per cent of all physicians were located in rural and small-town Canada, compared with 21.1 per cent of Canadians. Just less than 16 per cent of family physicians (including general practitioners) and 2.4 per cent of specialists practised in those areas. Comparing the distribution of all physicians to that of the population across all census divisions resulted in a Gini coefficient – a standard measure of inequality – of 0.25. For family physicians, it was 0.15, but the Gini coefficients for such specialties as psychiatry, orthopedic surgery, and obstetrics and gynecology were much larger, at 0.46, 0.37, and 0.36, respectively. The more recent study also showed that rural family doctors tended to have a wider scope of practice and perform a broader range of clinical procedures than their urban counterparts. The relationships between size and remoteness of a community and family physicians' practice scope were mostly monotonic, indicating that the smaller the community and the farther from a city, the more likely its family physicians had a broader scope of practice. In short, with few or no specialists in small or remote communities, family physicians tend to assume a more comprehensive role in the provision of medical care.

The proportion of rural Canadians has continued to decline and so has the proportion of rural physicians. According to the latest (2016) Canadian census, 18.7 per cent of Canadians resided in a rural area in 2016 (7). But only 8.1 per cent of all physicians worked in rural Canada in that year, representing 13.7 per cent of family physicians and 2.3 per cent of specialists (8). In short, nationally speaking, there was no significant "improvement" in physician distribution relative to population distribution in the 20 years between 1996 and 2016.

What to Do about Physician Shortages?

In response to chronic and often serious shortages of physicians in many northern or rural communities, provinces and territories have taken various measures, with varying degrees of success. With the introduction of the Underserviced Area Program in 1969, Ontario ushered in a complex set of programs in an effort to increase physician supply in northern Ontario – a vast hinterland region with a small and widely dispersed population of about 800,000 people. I examined the policy instruments used over several decades in "Strategies to

Overcome Physician Shortages in Northern Ontario: A Study of Policy Implementation over 35 Years" (1).

The study examined changes in policy instruments used by charting the introduction of new programs between 1969 and 2004, in the belief that a government program is the implementation aspect of a public policy and reflects the policy instrument used. It identified 42 programs introduced over the 35-year period. A detailed analysis of these programs showed that they could be subsumed under nine broad categories of policy instrument (see Table 7.1). A program chronology was then constructed, based on the year in which a program was first put in place.

Several trends can be discerned:

- From the beginning, a variety of strategies were employed. In later years, the range of policy instruments used became even broader. Financial incentives, such as bursaries for medical students and monetary inducements for physicians, were clearly the most popular, followed by programs to bolster rural medical practice, such as locum tenens programs and virtual libraries to support doctors in isolated locations. All this suggests an early awareness that physician-shortage problems were complex and there was no panacea.
- A related development is the emergence of medical education/training as a policy tool in the 1990s and 2000s, culminating in the founding of NOSM.
- Some of the more recent programs were more sophisticated in the sense that they tended to be more complex and have a longer timeframe for yielding results. For instance, earlier programs such as the Medical/Dental Centres Program was intended to quickly attract physicians and dentists by offering a turnkey facility at little cost to any physician or dentist willing to establish practice in the North. Conversely, the medical education/training strategy can be seen as a longer-term investment, since it takes years before a student completes medical training and, even then, there is no guarantee that the new physician will work in northern Ontario.
- Efforts to overcome physician shortages can be broadly divided into recruitment and retention. Recruitment without retention often results in a "revolving door" phenomenon – physicians come and go – which may adversely affect, among other things, patients' continuity of care. Whereas earlier programs focused mostly on recruitment, those in later years, like locum tenens programs, aimed to attract physicians to northern Ontario and keep them there. Many physicians quit isolated communities because of overwork and burnout. Locum tenens programs allow them to take time off for vacations or continuing education.
- In more recent years, attempts were made to address more fundamental issues and not just to provide symptomatic relief. Decisions such as the

Table 7.1 Programs to deal with physician shortages in northern Ontario introduced by the Ontario government by policy instrument type and year, 1969–2004

	Financial incentive	Physician recruitment	Use of alternative providers	Rural medical education	Medical practice support	Medical service outreach	Patient travel assistance	Telehealth	Rural health workforce research
1969	xx		x			x			
1970		x							
1972				x					
1977					x				
1978		x							
1979	x				x				
1982					xx	x			
1985							x		
1991				x					
1992	x								x
1994					xx				
1995	x	x							
1996	xx			x					
1997	x				x				
1998		x			x			x	
1999	x			x		x			
2000	x		x	x					
2001	x								
2002		x		xxx	x				
2004		x							

Note: Each x represents an Ontario government-funded program. Multiple crosses in a cell indicate several programs belonging to the same policy instrument type were introduced in that year.

establishment of NOSM were likely made with the realization that in the long run, northern Ontario needed to "grow" some of its own doctors, instead of relying solely on imports.
- But conspicuous by their absence were directive measures that would require new physicians to work in underserved areas for a period of time as a condition for medical school admission or getting a physician billing number.

This study has shown that while the policy objective of enhancing access to medical services in northern Ontario remained unchanged throughout the study period, the programs and policy tools used evolved over time. It has revealed trial-and-error experimentation and an accumulation of past experiences by the government in dealing with an enduring and vexing problem.

Where to Train Physicians for Rural Practice?

Governments are not the only players in the game. As noted above, medical education has gradually come to be seen as providing a more lasting solution to the problem that plagues many northern or rural regions. More and more studies from different parts of the world have confirmed the roles medical schools could play in increasing the number of physicians willing and able to work in medically underserved areas (9–12). As Curran and Rourke (13) have pointed out, medical schools have control over, among other things, student recruitment, admissions policy, medical curriculum, and the location of learning experience. By emphasizing a rural perspective, medical schools could influence the likelihood of their graduates entering rural practice.

The emphasis here is on locations of learning experience. In the not too distant past, medical learners had little exposure to health care settings outside major urban centres. This is not unexpected since most medical schools in Canada were – and still are – located in big cities, and much of clinical learning took place in large, urban-based teaching hospitals. But the situation started to change in the 1980s, particularly in family medicine, as distributed medical education – delivery of clinical training outside traditional academic health centres – gathered steam, though boosting rural physician supply was just one of its many rationales. According to Krupa and Chan (14), the number of rural family medicine residency programs in Canada rose from 1 in 1973 to 12 in 2002, and the number of rural residency positions quadrupled from 36 to 144 between 1989 and 2002. Other more recent developments include the adoption of a distributed campus model by the University of British Columbia with the creation of three additional medical campuses on Vancouver Island, in northern British Columbia, and in the Okanagan region, and the opening of a new medical school in northern Ontario.

To examine the current state of distributed medical education at the postgraduate level, I conducted a geographic analysis of all residency programs in all 17 Canadian medical schools using 2013 information from the Canadian Resident Matching Service (CaRMS),[1] which is an independent agency that matches medical school graduates with residency programs throughout the country. The CaRMS website provides information on every residency program, including training locations. I perused and analysed program descriptions. If the website information was deemed insufficient or unclear, I and research staff attempted to contact the program directors for clarification.

Specialties were grouped into three broad categories: family medicine, generalist specialties (i.e., general surgery, internal medicine, obstetrics and gynecology, pediatrics, and psychiatry), and all other specialties and sub-specialties (e.g., dermatology, ophthalmology, public health, and cardiac surgery). Many programs had multiple streams. For instance, some streams were for Canadian graduates while others were for international graduates. Some programs had multiple streams in different locations. A classification of geographic types was developed based on the location of a residency program/stream and the nature and extent of its rural exposure:

- Exclusively in large cities (A)
- Mostly in large cities but with some mandatory or optional exposure in rural communities or small cities (B)
- Exclusively or mostly in small cities with some exposure in other geographic types (C)
- Exclusively or mostly rural with some urban exposure (D)
- More or less equal exposure in two or more geographic types (E)

The findings are presented in Table 7.2.

While slightly over 50 per cent of all residency programs (including streams) were located exclusively in large urban centres, close to half provided some exposure in smaller or more remote communities, including some placements in the territories. Family medicine was the most varied in terms of training locations. About 17 per cent took place exclusively in large urban centres. Although only nine family medicine programs took place exclusively in rural areas, most of the others had varying degrees of rural exposure. Almost 70 per cent of generalist specialty training took place mostly in large cities, but with some mandatory or optional exposure in smaller cities or rural communities. Not surprisingly, clinical learning in the other specialties and sub-specialties took place almost exclusively in big cities. Only about 20 per cent provided some learning experience in other geographic types, but most of this was optional and short. It is possible that locations other than large cities have neither the population base nor the necessary facilities or equipment to support highly specialized training.

Table 7.2 Residency programs (including streams) in Canada by broad specialty category and geographic type, 2013

	A	B	C	D	E	Total
Family medicine	27 17.2%	51 32.5%	42 26.8%	9 5.7%	28 17.8%	157 100.0%
Generalist specialties	44 31.2%	96 68.1%	1 0.7%	–	–	141 100%
Other specialties/ sub-specialties	255 78.5%	70 21.5%	–	–	–	325 100%
Total	326 52.3%	217 34.8%	43 6.9%	9 1.4%	28 4.5%	623 99.9%

Source: CaRMS website

In 2002, Hutton-Czapski and Thurber (15) asked, "Who makes Canada's rural doctors?" Their research showed that the proportion of rural practice locations of graduates two years after completing residency varied tenfold between medical schools and residency programs. For instance, whereas Memorial University and Université Laval produced a disproportionate number of rural family physicians, only a handful of rural family doctors were from the University of Toronto. What about the situation in 2013? Because the data I used were about residency programs, not graduates, it is impossible to tell which rural doctor was from which medical school. But an examination of family medicine programs shows that the great majority of medical schools did not train their family doctors exclusively or mostly in big cities. Instead, they typically offered options in the form of multiple programs or streams in locations belonging to different geographic types. For example, the Dalhousie University family medicine program offered residency positions in geographic types B, C, and D, and those at the University of Manitoba were in geographic types B, C, and E. Thus, at least in family medicine, an effort has been made by many medical schools to make genuine rural-based training available.

Does Rural Training Lead to Rural Practice?

It has often been said that physicians tend to practise where they train. Most Canadian studies supporting this claim are informed opinions or are research based on small samples or practice location intentions rather than actual behaviours. The opening of NOSM in 2005 afforded researchers a rare opportunity to test the hypothesis that rural medical training leads to rural practice, albeit at just one medical school.

NOSM is one medical school at two universities – Laurentian University in Sudbury and Lakehead University in Thunder Bay (16). To fulfil its mandate to prepare physicians for northern or rural practice, this relatively small medical school – with a current enrolment of 64 first-year students – has adopted various strategies, including an emphasis on family medicine and generalist specialties; a curriculum that incorporates topics like northern and rural health, social and population health, and Indigenous health; an admissions policy that actively encourages those with a northern, rural, or Indigenous background to apply; and, above all, a community-based, distributed medical education approach, including a requirement that all undergraduates spend their third year living and learning in one of about a dozen smaller northern Ontario communities.

Sensing a unique opportunity to conduct a natural experiment on the impact of rural-friendly medical education on physicians' practice locations, I and my colleagues at the Centre for Rural and Northern Health Research (CRaNHR) at Laurentian University, in cooperation with NOSM, launched a program of research with a view to understanding how NOSM's medical education programs and approaches shaped its graduates' specialty choice, practice location, and practice profile. The research was multi-year, multi-cohort, multi-method, and multi-data sourced. It started in 2005 and is still ongoing. Each cohort of students was surveyed multiple times from the time they entered NOSM, through their four-year undergraduate medical education and two- to five-year postgraduate residency training, to the early phase of their medical career. The research involved quantitative analysis of the survey data and administrative data from other sources and qualitative analysis of in-depth interviews of some learners. A detailed description of the methodology and sequencing of the tracking surveys is available (17).

The first publication based on an analysis of the survey data appeared in 2016 (18). This study was based on 131 graduates who had completed family medicine training between 2011 and 2013. They included 49 family physicians (37.4 per cent) who had completed their MD degree at NOSM but did residency elsewhere; 31 (23.7 per cent) who had obtained their MD degree elsewhere but did residency at NOSM; and 51 (38.9 per cent) who did both their undergraduate and postgraduate training at NOSM. International medical graduates and graduates of specialist residency programs were not included in the analysis.

The outcomes that are of interest here are the graduates' primary practice locations: rural northern Ontario, northern Ontario, and rural Ontario. Practice location information as of September 2014 was obtained from provincial/territorial medical licensing bodies, such as the College of Physicians and Surgeons of Ontario.

Slightly over 16 per cent of the NOSM graduates located their primary practice in rural northern Ontario, 45 per cent practised in urban northern Ontario, and 5 per cent worked in rural southern Ontario. The number of rural-background years was a statistically significant predictor of practice locations in rural northern Ontario and rural Ontario. Those with rural background were 1.16 times and 1.12 times more likely to practice in rural northern Ontario and rural Ontario, respectively. But locations of medical education/training were the most powerful predictors. For instance, those who completed both NOSM undergraduate and NOSM postgraduate residency training were 8.62 times more likely to practise in rural northern Ontario. A significantly higher proportion of family physicians who did both their undergraduate and postgraduate training at NOSM worked in rural northern Ontario (26 per cent) or northern Ontario (94 per cent), compared with those with only NOSM undergraduate education (6 per cent and 20 per cent, respectively). Those with only NOSM residency were somewhere in between. Sex, French-language ability, northern background, marital status, and other factors were not found to be related to practice location. In sum, approximately 61 per cent of the family physicians who had completed at least some of their training at NOSM practised in northern Ontario. Slightly more than a quarter of them located their medical practice in rural northern Ontario.

Looking Back, Looking Ahead

The Canada Health Act assures all Canadians access to needed medical and hospital care regardless of their financial wherewithal. But ready access is often contingent on where one resides because health care practitioners, especially physicians, and their services are not equitably distributed. Northern and rural residents often find it difficult to obtain the care they need. Several studies conducted by me and my research colleagues have been presented above. Together, they tell a story about the extent of physician maldistribution in Canada and the efforts and changing approaches taken to redress the balance. They offer some insights.

First, physician shortages in rural or northern areas are a persistent and pervasive phenomenon. Generally speaking, physician availability is inversely proportional to geographic remoteness or isolation. Although physician maldistribution is a fact of life in many countries, Canada, possibly because of its universal health care system and professed adherence to the principle of health equity, has the impetus to do something about it and, in fact, has strived hard to confront the problem, as the case study on dealing with doctor shortages in northern Ontario has attested.

Second, physician maldistribution in Canada stayed mostly unchanged at the national level between the 1990s and the 2010s (and possibly longer), but views regarding what to do about it have evolved over time. While financial incentives are still widely used to entice physicians to underserved areas, they are now generally seen as stopgap measures with no lasting retention effects. Increasingly, policymakers have turned to strategies that do not necessarily bring immediate relief but may address more fundamental issues and have a more enduring impact. A case in point is the decentralized, community-based approach to preparing family doctors and, to a much lesser extent, other types of physicians.

Third, the analysis of NOSM graduates' practice locations lends impressive, though tentative, support to the physicians-practice-where-they-train hypothesis. The support is tentative because only the first few cohorts of NOSM graduates and only those in family medicine were examined, and those graduates had been in practice for just a short time, mostly because NOSM is a young school and medical education is a lengthy process. Hopefully, as the CRaNHR surveys track more learners and for more years, the accumulated evidence will become more convincing. The growing trend of residency training taking place outside metropolitan areas offers another opportunity to test the hypothesis nationwide. In the future, a "big data" analysis could be done, correlating training locations with physicians' practice locations.

What needs to be done? There are no silver bullets that could solve the physician maldistribution problem, but there are many potential strategies, each of which may be more or less suitable for a particular situation. Each region or community needs to find the solutions that are most workable, given its unique circumstances, and it can learn from the experiences of others about what works, what doesn't, and why. While government policies and programs are crucial, other institutions and organizations, such as medical schools and non-governmental organizations, also have useful roles to play. Instead of concentrating all their efforts in one area, concerned individuals or communities should work with as many stakeholders as possible. Similarly, a multi-pronged strategy is likely to be more effective than a single-barrel approach as physician maldistribution is a multifaceted problem.

There is a growing body of research evidence on the effectiveness of physician-shortage-related interventions, but the strength of the evidence is not uniform. Before recommending how to increase health workforce supply in remote and rural areas, the World Health Organization (2) conducted a systematic review of such interventions worldwide and found wide variations in the quality of the evidence. To ensure that their decisions are evidence-based, policymakers should work with researchers to sort through the evidence to determine what interventions to adopt when, where, and how.

Medical educators should apply the distributed medical education model to specialist training, at least to such generalist specialties as internal medicine and psychiatry.[2] Some baby steps have been taken by some medical schools, but they are not enough. Northern and rural communities should also consider playing a more active role in rural medical education efforts by, for instance, becoming clinical teaching and learning sites.

Last, rural and northern regions are not the only medically underserved areas. Some poor inner-city neighbourhoods and ethnic minority enclaves face similar predicaments, perhaps for very different reasons. Rural and northern residents would be wise to join forces with their urban counterparts to fight for their rights. Together and united, their voices would be that much louder when demanding a fair share of health resources and services. As Martin Luther King, Jr. reportedly said, "Of all the forms of inequality, injustice in health is the most shocking and inhumane" (20). Lack of ready access to needed medical care due to physician unavailability, regardless of location and cause, should be treated as a health equity issue. Individuals and communities experiencing similar plights could be brought together under the banner of equity in health for all.

Is there anything to look forward to? Given the nature of our health care system, the general reluctance of governments to stand up to organized medicine on behalf of citizens, and the eroding political power base of rural Canada because of depopulation, a major transformation of our health workforce that would bring long-term relief to rural and northern communities does not appear to be in the cards. However, small remedial measures and incremental improvements are always possible. As I have previously observed (1 p7), "Apparently, physician maldistribution is not like a disease that can be cured, but is more akin to a chronic condition that needs to be managed."

ACKNOWLEDGMENTS

The author wishes to acknowledge the helpful comments on earlier drafts provided by Drs. Roger Pitblado and Geoffrey Tesson.

NOTES

1 This analysis was conducted for the Canadian Post-MD Education Registry (CAPER). CAPER has kindly given the author permission to present the findings in this chapter. The 2013 data for the analysis was obtained from the CaRMS website (https://phx.e-carms.ca), For a brief description of CaRMS, see https://medapplications.com/canadian-resident-matching-service/.

2 A study I and my colleagues conducted (19) has provided some initial evidence of a positive association between postgraduate specialty training in northern Ontario and specialists' eventual practice in northern and smaller communities.

REFERENCES

1. Pong RW. Strategies to overcome physician shortages in northern Ontario: a study of policy implementation over 35 years. Hum Resour Health [Internet]. 2008 Nov 11;6:24. Available from: https://human-resources-health.biomedcentral.com/articles/10.1186/1478-4491-6-24

2. World Health Organization. Increasing access to health workers in remote and rural areas through improved retention: global policy recommendations. Geneva (CH): World Health Organization; 2010.
3. European Commission. Recruitment and retention of the health workforce in Europe. Brussels (BE): European Commission; 2015.
4. Ono T, Schoenstein M, Buchan J. Geographic imbalances in the distribution of doctors and health care services in OECD countries. In: Health workforce policies in OECD countries: right jobs, right skills, right places [Internet]. Paris (FR): OECD Publishing; 2016 [cited 2018 Jun 28]. p. 129–61. Available from: http://www.oecd-ilibrary.org/social-issues-migration-health/health-workforce-policies-in-oecd-countries_9789264239517-en
5. Pitblado JR, Pong RW. Geographic distribution of physicians in Canada. Ottawa (ON): Health Canada; 1999.
6. Pong RW, Pitblado JR. Geographic distribution of physicians in Canada: beyond how many and where. Ottawa (ON): Canadian Institute for Health Information; 2005.
7. Bollman, RD. Rural demographic update: 2016 [Internet]. Guelph (ON): Rural Ontario Institute; 2017 [cited 2018 Jun 28]. p. 152. Available from: http://www.ruralontarioinstitute.ca/file.aspx?id=26acac18-6d6e-4fc5-8be6-c16d326305fe
8. Canadian Institute for Health Information [Internet]. Ottawa (ON): Canadian Institute for Health Information; 2017 Sep 28. Data table: Supply, distribution and migration of physicians in Canada, 2016; 2017 Sep 28 [cited 2018 Jun 28]. Available from: http://www.cihi.ca/en/access-data-reports/results?query=Data+table per cent3A+Supply per cent2C+distribution+and+migration+of+physicians+in+Canada per cent2C+2016&Search+Submit=
9. Rabinowitz HK. Evaluation of a selective medical school admissions policy to increase the number of family physicians in rural and underserved areas. New Engl J Med. 1988;319:480–6.
10. Rolfe IE, Pearson SA, O'Connell DL, Dickinson JS. Finding solutions to the rural doctor shortage: the roles of selection versus undergraduate medical education at Newcastle. Aust N Z J Med. 1995;25(5):512–17.
11. Rosenblatt RA, Whitcomb ME, Cullen TJ, Lishner DM, Hart LG. Which medical schools produce rural physicians? J Am Med Assoc 1992;268(12):1559–65.
12. Wang L. A comparison of metropolitan and rural medical schools in China: which schools provide rural physicians? Aust J Rural Health. 2002;10:94–8.
13. Curran V, Rourke J. The role of medical education in the recruitment and retention of rural physicians. Med Teach. 2004;26(3):265–72.
14. Krupa LK, Chan BTB. Canadian rural family medicine training programs: growth and variation in recruitment. Can Fam Physician. 2005;51(6):852–3.
15. Hutten-Czapski P, Thurber AD. Who makes Canada's rural doctors? Can J Rural Med. 2002;7(2):95–100.

16. Tesson, G, Hudson G, Strasser R, Hunt D, editors. The making of the Northern Ontario School of Medicine: a case study in the history of medical education. Montreal (QC): McGill-Queen's University Press; 2009.
17. Hogenbirk JC, French MG, Timony PE, Strasser RP, Hunt D, Pong RW. Outcomes of the Northern Ontario School of Medicine's distributed medical education programmes: protocol for a longitudinal comparative multicohort study. BMJ Open [Internet]. 2015 [cited 2018 Jun 28];5:e0008246. Available from: http://bmjopen.bmj.com/content/5/7/e008246.full
18. Hogenbirk JC, Timony TE, French MG, Strasser R, Pong RW, Cervin C, Graves L. Milestones on the social accountability journey: family medicine practice locations of Northern Ontario School of Medicine graduates. Can Fam Physician [Internet] 2016 [cited 2018 Jul 6];62(3):e138–45. Available from: http://www.cfp.ca/content/62/3/e138.full
19. Hogenbirk JC, Mian O, Pong RW. Postgraduate specialty training in northeastern Ontario and subsequent practice location. Rural Remote Health [Internet]. 2011 Mar 2 [cited July 6, 2018];11(1):1603. Available from: http://www.rrh.org.au/journal/article/1603
20. Moore A. Tracking down Martin Luther King, Jr.'s words on health care. Huffington Post [Internet]. 2013 Jan 18 [updated 2013 Mar 20; cited 2019 Dec 2019]. Available from: http://www.huffpost.com/entry/martin-luther-king-health-care_b_2506393

8 Nursing in the North: Recruitment and Retention of Nurses

HELLE MØLLER

Introduction

Working as a health professional in one of the many small communities in northern Canada has been described as tremendously rewarding and satisfying professionally, personally and financially. It has also been described as challenging, demanding, very independent, and at times professionally isolated work. It requires the ability to be flexible, patient, and tolerant, and to perform to the limits of the nursing or nurse practitioner scope of practice (1). All this can make recruiting and retaining health professionals, whether nurses, physicians (see Pong, chapter 7, this volume), dentists, physiotherapists, occupational therapists (2), nutritionists and dietitians (3), or mental health professionals (Kassam, chapter 11, this volume), very challenging for northern communities. In addition, very few institutions of higher education are located in northern Canadian communities, which makes it difficult for northerners to train in these professions. For northerners to access the training available, extensive water, air, or road travel is often necessary. These barriers make it harder to create "home-grown" health professionals.

The professionals of focus in this chapter, nurses, are often the health professionals that are most present if not continuous in northern communities. The chapter starts with a historical review of nurses' presence, their roles, working conditions, and issues regarding recruitment and retention in the Canadian North. It continues with an appraisal of the current situation of recruitment and retention of nurses in the North using Nunavut as a case study. The chapter concludes with a discussion of what has been and should be done to ensure that communities in northern Canada are able to attract, recruit, and retain nurses and provide an appropriate level of health care.

A Brief History of Early Health Care in Northern Canada

The northernmost regions of Canada (currently Yukon, Northwest Territories, and Nunavut) have unique formal health and nursing care histories. One of the earliest health care facilities on record in Yukon is St. Mary's Hospital, erected at the beginning of the gold rush by Father (Fr.) William Judge. Fr. Judge was a Jesuit priest from Forty Mile, Yukon. He died in 1899, a year after St. Mary's was established. The Sisters of St. Anne then took over running the hospital. None of them were formally trained as nurses, but they soon had the practical training through experience – if not the adequate tools – to perform in the role. Four trained nurses, likely the first in the territory – Georgia Powell, Rachel Hanna, Margaret Payson, and Amy Scott – were recruited to join the surgeon at the police barracks hospital in Dawson and serve at the first two hospitals in Yukon: St. Mary's and the other in Bonanza Creek just south of Dawson. Lady Ishbel Aberdeen, the wife of the then governor-general of Canada, recruited the four nurses. Lady Aberdeen had founded the Victorian Order of Nurses (VON) in 1897 (4). Apart from the individual nurses employed at Whitehorse General Hospital, built in 1901, no major influx of nurses occurred in Yukon until World War II, during the building of the Alaska Highway. These nurses were hired by the US army, which built its own hospital (5). With the advent of VON, the early outpost nursing programs in Canada started. It would, however, be the mid-1900s before the populations in Yukon or the Northwest Territories saw any nursing stations.

The Northwest Territories, as opposed to Yukon, did not have any residing Western medical doctors until well into the 1900s, and nurses were absent. The Church, industry, and police largely provided the medical care and support (6,7), and the hospitals that did exist were mission hospitals. These included one built close to Pangnirtung on Blacklead Island in 1902 (8), one in Aklavik built in 1920 (9), one built in Chesterfield Inlet in 1929, and one built in collaboration with the federal government in Coppermine in 1929 (10). St. Luke's Hospital in Pangnirtung was built and received its first patients in 1931 (9). As of 1830, there were six medical officers in the Northwest Territories (9). Where there were hospitals and doctors, there inevitably were women performing in nursing-like roles and eventually trained nurses. Unfortunately, these female care providers are not often mentioned in the literature.

Apart from St Luke's, most other mission hospitals that opened subsequently closed a few years after. This included the ones in Aklavik, Chesterfield, and Coppermine (11). The medical officers of these hospitals were often federally employed (7), and the federal government supported the hospitals financially to some degree (8). However, "medical care and culture change were often viewed by the Euro-Canadian caregivers to be interrelated" (7 p199) and medical aid was used as an attempt to Christianize the Inuit. In 1943 in the Northwest

Territories, there were 11 hospitals, nine owned by missions and two by mining companies, and in 1946 there were nine physicians employed (12). The number of nurses appears to not have been recorded.

Despite appalling accounts from doctors, traders, and explorers into the early 1940s, nothing much was done by the Canadian government to help Inuit improve living conditions and overcome severe health issues (11,13,14). VON and other organizations described below had, however, called for and started implementing outpost nursing stations in other areas of northern Canada. Still, in Canada's most northern areas, money and effort spent by the government and others in the North was aimed mainly at assuring sovereignty (13,15); documenting for posterity these "strange, happy and naive people" (14 p77) and their cultural curiosities before they became extinct; pursuing commercial endeavours that would enrich people from elsewhere (13); and ideologically transforming the Inuit to conform to the dominant religion, beliefs, and values of Euro-Canadian society (11,13,15,16).

Sovereignty concerns accelerated government control of health care in the Arctic after World War II. The eastern Arctic patrol boat *Nascopie*, and then the *CD Howe*, were commissioned to fight the tuberculosis (TB) epidemic from the mid-1940s. The ships visited all Arctic settlements and camps, and medical professionals examined and X-rayed most inhabitants during the ice-free months of the year, shipping those with disease to southern hospitals (11,13,17). Not only did the *CD Howe* serve as a sailing TB clinic, but it also delivered a number of other health care services. The medical staff on *CD Howe*'s inaugural journey included a medical doctor, a medical attendant, a dentist, and an X-ray technician, and the group was enlarged with a nurse and another medical doctor midway in the journey. The number and variety of medical staff, including the number of nurses, steadily increased during the operation of the vessel; social workers and translators were also added. These additions enabled staff to report back to community members about their families in the south and to address concerns about the welfare of both patients and their family members who were left in the community, easing the journey for the patients and the pain of separation for both (11). Although conditions improved greatly over time, and the campaigns were seen as a success from an administrative perspective, they were a cultural and social disaster for many Inuit (11,13,17).

Government Involvement and the Introduction of British Nurse Midwives and Nursing Stations

With the increase in government control of Canadian Arctic health care, the remaining missionary hospitals were eventually taken over or shut down by the federal government and replaced with nursing stations. The first opened in 1947 in Inukjuak, then called Port Harrison, situated in Nunavik, and the second in Kugluktuk, then called Coppermine, situated in the Kitikmeot region of Nunavut (12). Because of the work started by VON and carried on by the Canadian Red Cross and other organizations in Alberta, Quebec, and Newfoundland and Labrador, British nurse-midwives were hired by the federal government to serve in the North specifically for their dual training. However, while the British nurse-midwives provided much needed assistance to pregnant and birthing mothers, their mandate was to care for the whole person and for the whole community (18). They were not recognized in authority or in pay for their midwifery qualifications. Midwifery was not legal in Canada until 1993. The Canadian Medical Association was unwilling to relinquish responsibility for childbirth, and physicians saw labour and births as belonging under the auspices of medical doctors (19,20).

In the early 1960s, nursing stations were operating in 12 major Inuit settlements and servicing another 14 smaller outposts (18). Although these nurses provided excellent health care, many often simultaneously fostered "a situation where the Inuit were dependent on their services for all aspects of their well-being" (21 p286), resulting in a medicalization of community life with a nurse who monitored community members as if they were "patients on a hospital ward" (21 p286). This fact at times created challenging relationships between nurses and community members (9).

Some Inuit worked in the nursing stations as caretakers and in other support positions. Some who worked for many years in a nursing station received onsite training to enable them to serve a triage function to determine whether a client had to see a nurse. Some Inuit in the small settlements, where there was no nursing station, would receive six weeks of intensive instruction in basic medicine and then serve as the settlement's lay dispenser of medicine (21). While little or no encouragement in general was given to Inuit to become trained medical professionals (22), for one Inuk who worked at St. Luke's Hospital in Pangnirtung, this was different. She reminisced to Cowall and Aklivaktuk (23) when they interviewed her that she and another Inuk hospital worker were asked to go to Aklavik to be trained as nurses by the missionaries. They did not end up going, however, as they were not able to get their parents' consent. Another former hospital staff member recounted to Cowall and Aklavik how she would relieve the nurses for them to "visit," "go for a walk," or otherwise just "do their things." This would give her a chance to be the one "to look after everything" (23).

The little evidence of Inuit having been encouraged to train to become nurses, nurse's aides, or medically trained midwives can be seen in the context of other Canadian realities. Indigenous people, people of colour, and Asian immigrants had been barred from nursing education until World War II. Even well into the 1960s, it was difficult for anyone who was not of European descent to receive nursing training in many Canadian provinces (24). After World War II, some Indigenous people were educated in southern Canada as nurses, although the records provided no differentiation between Inuit, First Nations, and Métis people (24). In 1951, 15 Inuit and Indian students were enrolled in nursing programs in Canada; by 1961, the number had increased to 38 (24).

By 1970, a majority of communities with more than a hundred inhabitants had fully equipped nursing stations (21). The nurses in Arctic Canada were expected to take the role of sole health care provider. They had contact, although unreliable, with physicians who visited very sporadically. Medical evacuations and transportation to southern hospitals for more extensive treatment became more common (10), and evacuation for birthing became the norm (25). Currently, the 24 communities in Nunavut that are without a hospital all have nursing stations that employ varying numbers of nurses (called community health nurses) depending on the size and needs of the community. Nursing stations or community health centres similar to those in Nunavut are also found in the remote, generally Indigenous communities in the Northwest Territories (26 communities) (26) and in Yukon (14 communities) (27). What follows provides a more in-depth examination of contemporary nursing, using Nunavut as a case study, including an exploration of current issues in the recruitment and retention of nurses in the North.

Contemporary Nursing in Nunavut

With its inauguration in 1999, the new Government of Nunavut assumed immediate responsibility for health care and education. It took over an already established health care system that was developed and governed by Euro-Canadians or southerners and predominantly staffed by southern health care professionals who most often did not (and most often still do not) speak the local language. About 85 per cent of residents in Nunavut are Inuit, and about 85 per cent of them speak Inuktitut as their mother tongue. Therefore, it is often necessary to have interpreter support during clinical encounters between community members and health professionals. Even with an interpreter present, the margin for misunderstanding is large, both linguistically and culturally (28–31). Many medical terms and concepts do not exist in Inuktitut, and not only what is said but also body language and what is not said can be highly relevant (27,28). As Stephen Lewis stated after a TB fact-finding visit to Nunavut in the fall of 2017, "How do you keep track of the subtleties and complications of a disease like Tuberculosis if you can't speak the language of the people?" (32 para11). This problem affects quality of care. As noted by Prime Minister Trudeau (33 soundclip 5, line 8) in his apology for Canada's mistreatment of Inuit during the TB epidemics of the 1940s, 1950s, and 1960s, "the colonial mindset that drove the government's actions" has led to some Inuit not trusting the health care system and has affected Inuit perceptions of the quality and accessibility of the health care available. It can result in care not being sought until an illness has taken a big toll on an individual. If the illness is TB, the delay in seeking care may impact a whole community, regardless of how well-intentioned, dedicated, and well-educated current health care providers, including community health nurses, are (34,35).

The community health nurses working in Nunavut have an expanded scope of practice that "requires specialized skills, knowledge, and competencies that are beyond traditional nursing education programs. With proper in-service training and education, community health nurses can also perform certain medical functions delegated to them by a physician" (36 para13). They examine patients, diagnose illnesses, and prescribe, conduct, and evaluate some tests. They initiate some treatment on their own or in consultation with a doctor over the phone. They also offer general public health programs and provide emergency care. With the support of telehealth, the nurses in the remote communities in Nunavut (as well as the Northwest Territories and Yukon) are able to provide communities with a wide range of health care, social programs, and services through teleconferencing both within and outside the territory that would not otherwise be available (37,25,26,).

In theory, one full-time community health nurse is hired for approximately every 200 people in the community. In addition, some communities have one or more mental health nurses, TB nurses, and homecare nurses. When community health nurses encounter patients whose conditions they are not able to deal with in the nursing centres, even with physician support over telephone or telehealth, patients will be medevacked (flown) to the nearest hospital where a physician can deal with the condition. At times, however, critical decisions need to be made "with limited support from other health-care professionals, which may pressure nurses to act beyond their licensed scope" (38 p21).

As part of the Nursing Practice in Rural and Remote Canada II study, MacLeod and colleagues (38) analysed rural and remote nurses' perceptions of their scope of practice and found that almost 10 per cent felt they were working beyond it. The authors noted that nurses working in fly-in communities, particularly those working more than 1000 kilometres from an advanced referral centre; those who worked in centres where staffing was an issue; younger nurses; and male nurses more often than other nurses felt they worked beyond their scope of practice (38). The researchers added that the perception of working past scope of practice could have many causes, including not having been introduced to the scope practised in remote areas and instead relying on the scope of practice governing nursing in other jurisdictions. The relevance of this in Nunavut is discussed in more detail below as a case study of contemporary recruitment and retention issues in northern nursing (38).

Recruitment and Retention of Nurses in Nunavut

Nunavut, similar to other northern regions nationally and internationally, has historically had difficulty recruiting and retaining health care professionals, including nurses, despite higher salaries, bonuses, and allowances than it would be possible to earn in most other places in Canada. Over the last couple of decades, however, many of these benefits and bonuses have dwindled, affecting recruitment and retention further and contributing to the fact that in March 2016, 62 per cent of Nunavut's community health nurse positions were vacant (36). The auditor general of Canada (36) wrote in his report about Nunavut's health care system that retention rather than recruitment was the primary issue in Nunavut and that the factors impeding retention include housing shortages, the climate, the high food costs, the remoteness from family and home community coupled with the expense of travel, a lack of infrastructure, and for some the difficulty for a spouse or partner to secure employment (36). In addition, Inuit nurses who practise in their home communities and even nurses who come from southern communities and take employment in remote or northern regions may find it challenging to separate personal and professional roles as they are caring for friends, families, neighbours, and colleagues (29). This intertwinement can result in nurses not participating in the social aspects of the community to maintain professionalism, or it can impact community members' belief about whether confidentiality is being maintained (39,40). Either scenario may compromise the nurse's well-being and may prevent them from remaining employed in a northern community or even from applying for a position there (39,40).

Some nurses specifically seek employment in the North because of nurses' expanded roles and responsibilities and the independent nature of the work, as discussed above (1). Unfortunately, the latter may also affect retention. Bauman and colleagues (40) note that after nurses are employed in remote and northern communities, they are frequently "required to apply their knowledge and skill without the resources often found in urban settings" (40 p16). They often practise entirely autonomously, to the limits of their scope of practice (41). This autonomy may be of particular concern for younger nurses beginning their careers and looking for mentorship or clinical supervision in demanding and difficult emergency situations, contributing to younger nurses choosing not to practise in the territory or not staying. In addition, many recent graduates stay only until they have children or until their children reach school age. Often the nurses who do take employment in the territory are at the older end of the age continuum (42). Their children have left home, and the higher salaries allow them to top up their retirement payment over a limited number of years. MacLeod and colleagues (42) reported that income was the primary reason for seeking employment in the territories for almost 62 per cent of nurses, and that of the nurses who stay for longer periods, 70 per cent do so because of the income. Unfortunately, this means that while some nurses hired from the south are very invested in the communities where they work and consider Nunavut their primary home, a majority may not (42).

Of those who do not consider Nunavut home, some take a permanent position and stay for one to five years or more, and others take positions that, although permanent, allow them to work a certain number of months on and off in the same community. These nurses are flown between Nunavut and their southern home three or four times a year. Still others are hired as casual nurses and take shorter periods of employment in different communities, either as Government of Nunavut hires or as agency nurses. The latter are much more expensive and add to the high turnover rates, which can lead to decreased work satisfaction and burnout among the nurses who are employed in permanent positions (36).

In addition to high turnover rates, nurses' work satisfaction and ability to provide optimal health care are affected by the high number of vacant positions (36,41). When a community health centre has only two or three nurses (when it should have five), they are forced to prioritize emergency care. Capacity and time to provide health promotion and illness prevention can then be limited, and screening programs may suffer. For example, the continuity of care that expectant mothers (43) and individuals living with chronic diseases (44) often desire and get the most benefit and best outcome from may not be possible. At times it may even be necessary to close the health centres for anything but emergencies, because there simply are not enough nurses to operate fully. Still, many nurses who choose to work in the territories thrive and report positively about many aspects of this work. Aspects highlighted include the "opportunity to make a difference in communities where nurses may be the only health care provider," the intersection of the practice and community experience and "the opportunity to enact a broad scope of practice … and practice with considerable autonomy and responsibility" (1 Findings para 2).

Recent Approaches to Improve Recruitment and Retention of Nurses in Northern Canada

"Home-Grown" Nurses

To improve quality of care and Inuit health and well-being, and mitigate the historical recruitment and retention issues in the Northwest Territories, a nursing school was created in Aurora College in Yellowknife in 1994. With the advent of Nunavut, the college split into two territorial colleges: Aurora College and Nunavut Arctic College in Iqaluit, Nunavut. With the split into two territorial colleges, the nursing program also split, with the program at Nunavut Arctic

College under the auspices of Dalhousie University (45) and the nursing program at Aurora College under the auspices of the University of Victoria (46). Thus, although the program is offered in the Inuit territory of Nunavut, it is, as is the health care system, largely based on a Euro-Canadian model and language.

While some teaching allegedly takes place in Inuktitut in Nunavut (45), the vast majority takes place in English, teaching materials are in English, and no teachers are Inuit. Almost all Inuit students' mother tongue, on the other hand, is Inuktitut, and the vast majority of the people they will care for are Inuit whose mother tongue is Inuktitut. Some Inuit nurses and students find this challenging when they care for Inuit patients because they do not master a medical vocabulary in Inuktitut. Some resort to interpreter support, which they state adds a layer of distance and possibility of misunderstanding, as discussed above (28–32,34,35). In addition, working with non-Inuit nurses may add to Inuit nurses' workload: many Inuit clients prefer a care provider who can speak their language, and non-Inuit nurses at times need help to interpret subtle linguistic or behavioural signals they are unfamiliar with. As observed by one Inuk nurse:

> The patients do not understand the Southern nurses, which means that misunderstandings often occur. It also means that we as Inuit have to explain to the patients afterwards and that creates double work for us. (29 p148)

The nursing program in Iqaluit has a capacity of 14 students annually, and while a majority are northern residents, far from all are Inuit. Between 2004 and 2016, 51 nurses graduated, 20 of whom were Inuit (47). At Aurora College, there is a discrepancy between the number of Indigenous and non-Indigenous students and the number of each who graduate, with more non-Indigenous persons graduating (48). Some Inuit students believe the reasons for this difference include that the language of instruction is English rather than Inuktitut and that the program caters to southern ways of learning rather than Inuit ways, both of which add to an already challenging program (29,30). Historically, students in Nunavut, particularly high school students, have been taught curricula that were developed in the south for southern students and taught by southern teachers who may come from backgrounds that are both linguistically and culturally dissimilar to those of the northern students (29,30, also see Walton, chapter 1, this volume) – facts that, combined with other determinants, contribute to fewer Inuit graduating high school than other Canadian students. Other determinants that have historically impacted educational attainment in Nunavut include colonization, continued colonialism, racism, and discrimination (29,46,49), and some argue that this is still the case (49).

Being aware of the colonial history of health care and education, Aurora College has partnered with the University of Victoria, Camosun College, Selkirk

College, and the College of the Rockies and is striving to decolonize its nursing program. Some of the methods include emphasizing cultural safety, attempting to transform the curriculum and pedagogy to better reflect Indigenous ontology, inviting Indigenous Elders to teach in the program, focusing on attracting Indigenous faculty, and advocating for childcare to be available and children to be allowed into the classroom. The faculty have encountered barriers to some of these efforts, which they interpret as a perpetuation of Eurocentric nursing discourses and premises and thus colonial processes (46).

In addition to the program in Iqaluit, a nursing access program focused on educating Inuit specifically ran in Nunatsiavut in the 2000s. In 2005, 19 students started; six graduated in 2010 and one in 2011 (50). However, even the students who did not graduate as nurses are still success stories. Attending the access program prepared them for further education in other fields, such as practical nursing or early childhood education, or for a degree in education. In other words, both students and communities benefit (50).

Most Inuit and non-Inuit students who have graduated as nurses stay in the North, although not all, particularly Inuit, will be employed in nursing positions. In Nunavut, where there are few university-prepared professionals, graduates may be sought for these qualifications and be pulled into other government or Indigenous organizations. Inuit who have graduated and are employed as nurses add tremendous value to the nursing force in the territories because they are both bilingual and double cultured in addition to being university-prepared nurses. Those who choose to work in their own or another Inuit community are also invaluable to their fellow community members. Still, there are not yet enough of them to have a significant impact on the issue of recruitment and retention (29). In the 2000s, the Nunavut government tried to remedy the nursing need by recruiting international nurses as discussed next.

International Nurses

In 2004, Nunavut's Department of Health signed a contract with Trillium Talent Resource Group, a Toronto-based consulting and recruitment firm, in its effort to address the nursing shortage. The essence of the contract was that Trillium should recruit 100 international nurses on behalf of Nunavut (51). During 2005, 17 nurses from India and 21 from the Philippines arrived in the territory. The nurses were allegedly experienced nurses who left jobs and families at home with the idea of bringing their families to Canada once they had settled (52). Unfortunately, the majority of the nurses failed their exams several times. Finally, 23 of 34 passed their qualifying exams in the fall of 2006 (there is no mention of the other four). It was not part of Nunavut's contract that Trillium should pay the salaries of nurses who initially failed their exams while they continued to receive training and study to retake it. Therefore, the undertaking ended up being more costly to the Nunavut government than initially projected. In 2007, the government abandoned the plan to hire international nurses and the contract with Trillium was changed to focus their recruitment efforts on Canadian nurses instead. News articles and Hansards between 2007 and 2017 attested to the continued challenges with recruitment and retention and the shortage of nurses in Nunavut (51–54), Yukon (55,56), and the North West Territories (57,58).

Recent Recommendations

With a national shortage of nurses that the Canadian Nurses Association has estimated will grow over the next several years (59,60), it is likely that the territories will continue to struggle with recruitment and retention issues, and the ensuing issues of continuity and quality of care (61), and that this struggle will impact the northern areas of the Canada's provinces as well (62).

Although commendable attempts have been made to address the challenges that exist, including government interventions to entice nurses to consider rural practice, "efforts have largely been a patchwork approach that has been ineffective towards a broader goal of enabling a sustainable workforce" (40 p9).

This statement was included in the report by the Registered Nurses' Association of Ontario (RNAO), "Coming Together, Moving Forward: Building the Next Chapter of Ontario's Rural, Remote and Northern Nursing Workforce" (40). The organization subsequently made numerous recommendations, most of which apply to recruiting and retaining nurses in remote and northern areas of Canada overall. The Canadian Nurses Association (59) reiterated many of the recommendations to the Canadian government through the 2016 pre-budget consultations. They were also highlighted by the auditor general in his 2017 review of Nunavut's Department of Health (36) and by Steven Lewis after his TB fact-finding visit to Nunavut (32). The recommendations included the following very relevant one: "Invest in early, secondary and post-secondary education for Indigenous students and in continuing professional development for healthcare providers who serve Canada's Northern rural and remote communities" (59 p5).

Elaborating on this recommendation, the Canadian Nurses Association (59 p6) wrote that the following steps are needed:

- Enrolling students with a rural background and/or Indigenous descent in health professional education programs (e.g., nursing) and offering rurally based clinical rotations to enhance the competencies
- Creating postsecondary schools and introducing satellite programs in rural locations
- Providing high-quality, safe, supportive working environments to make northern nursing careers and postings professionally attractive

- Implementing outreach activities, including widespread telehealth and high-fidelity simulation capabilities, to facilitate cooperation between health care professionals across settings and distances
- Designing continuing education and professional development programs that meet the unique population health and practice needs of rural health care providers
- Offering a combination of fiscally sustainable financial incentives that outweigh the opportunity costs associated with working in rural areas
- Increasing career development programs and providing senior posts in rural areas to create enduring, meaningful career paths

Conclusion

While these recommendations are only part of those made by the Canadian Nurses Association, the RNAO, Steven Lewis, and the auditor general, they may be among the most important. They remind us again about the influence of the social determinants of health on equity in access to basic quality health care and the determinants that need to be considered to get us there. The changes that are needed are substantial and will be both costly and challenging. They are also tasks that, ideally, Canada's northern territories and communities should not have to address alone (31,32). As Stephen Lewis noted after his visit to Nunavut, "My issue is with the federal government. I didn't know that would be the case when I came to Nunavut, I certainly know that now" (32 para20). Among other things, he called on the government to deal with the underlying social issues that hinder Inuit students from entering and graduating the local nursing program in order to train Inuktitut-speaking nurses and increase the education, recruitment, and retention of Indigenous and non-Indigenous nurses in Canada's North. It will take time and requires a change in thinking about what the individual responsibilities of provinces, territories, and regions should be. It is encouraging, then, that the Canadian government has pledged to implement the recommendations from the Truth and Reconciliation Commission, in this connection particularly the seven calls to action focusing on health generally and on call 23 specifically. This call to action

> call[s] upon all levels of government to:
>
> i. Increase the number of Aboriginal professionals working in the health-care field.
> ii. Ensure the retention of Aboriginal health-care providers in Aboriginal communities. (63, para6)

Time will tell whether the funding allocated will be enough to make a significant difference.

REFERENCES

1. MacLeod M, Garraway L, Jonatansdottir S, Moffit P. What does it mean to be a nurse in Canada's northern territories? In: Exner-Pirot H, Norbye B, Butler L, editors. Northern and Indigenous health and health care [Internet]. Saskatoon (SK): University of Saskatchewan; 2018 [cited 2019 Aug 7]. Chapter 35. Available from: https://openpress.usask.ca/northernhealthcare/chapter/chapter-31-what-does-it-mean-to-be-a-nurse-in-canadas-northern-territories/
2. Roots RK, Li LC. Recruitment and retention of occupational therapists and physiotherapists in rural regions: a meta-synthesis. BMC Health Serv Res. 2013;13(59):59. doi: 10.1186/1472-6963-13-59
3. Dietitians of Canada. Dietitians of Canada submission to the House of Commons Standing Committee on Finance 2017 pre-budget recommendations [Internet]. Toronto (ON): Dietitians of Canada; 2016 [cited 2018 May 1]. Available from: http://www.ourcommons.ca/Content/Committee/421/FINA/Brief/BR8398234/br-external/DietitiansOfCanada-e.pdf
4. Gates M. Early days in Yukon no picnic. Yukon News [Internet]. 2013 May 10 [cited 2017 June 20]. Available from: http://yukon-news.com/letters-opinions/early-days-of-nursing-in-the-yukon-were-no-picnic/
5. Women's Directorate, Government of Yukon. October is women's history month … Yukon nurses: a history of compassion and caring. Whitehorse (YK): Women's Directorate, Government of Yukon; 2002.
6. Wenzel GW. Inuit health and the health care system: change and status quo. Etudes Inuit. 1981;5(1):7–15.
7. Waldram JB, Herring DA, Young TK. Aboriginal health in Canada: historical, cultural, and epidemiological perspectives. 2nd ed. Toronto (ON): University of Toronto Press; 2007.
8. Farrell EC. Longings of the heart: the women of St. Luke's Mission Hospital, Pangnirtung, 1930–1972. J Can Church Hist Soc. 2004;46(2):129–50.
9. Copeland DM, Myles EL. Remember nurse. Toronto (ON): Ryerson Press; 1960.
10. Jenness D. Eskimo administration: II Canada. Arctic Institute of North America Technical paper No. 14. (Original publication 1964). Ottawa (ON): Arctic Institute of North America; 1972.
11. Grygier PS. A long way from home: the tuberculosis epidemic among the Inuit. Montreal (QC): McGill-Queen's University Press; 1984.
12. Duffy RQ. The road to Nunavut: the progress of the Eastern Arctic Inuit since the Second World War. Montreal (QC): McGill-Queen's University Press; 1988.
13. Tester FJ, Kulchyski P. Tammarniit (mistakes): Inuit relocations in the Eastern Arctic 1939–63. Vancouver (BC): UBC Press; 1994.
14. Vanast WJ. The death of Jennie Kanajuq: tuberculosis, religious competition, and cultural conflict in Coppermine. Etudes Inuit. 1991;15(1):75–104.
15. Brody H. The people's land: Inuit, whites and the eastern Arctic. Toronto (ON): Douglas & McIntyre; 1991.

16. McNicoll P, Tester F, Kulchyski P. Arctic abstersion: the Book of Wisdom for Eskimo, modernism and Inuit assimilation. Etudes Inuit. 1999;23(1–2):199–220.
17. Tester FJ, McNicoll P, Irniq P. Writing for our lives: The language of homesickness, self-esteem and the Inuit TB epidemic. Etudes Inuit. 2001;26(1–2):121–40.
18. Dodd D, Elliot J, Rousseau N. Outpost nursing in Canada. In: Bates C, Dodd D, Rousseau N, editors. On all frontiers: four centuries of Canadian nursing. Ottawa (ON): University of Ottawa Press; 2005. p. 135–52.
19. Dodd DE, Gorham D, editors. Caring and curing: historical perspectives on women and healing in Canada. Ottawa (ON): University of Ottawa Press; 1994.
20. Mitchinson W. Giving birth in Canada, 1900–1950. Toronto (ON): University of Toronto Press; 2002.
21. O'Neil JD. The politics of health in the fourth world: A northern Canadian example. In: Coates KS, Morrison WR, editors. Interpreting Canada's north: selected readings. Toronto (ON): Copp Clark Pitman Ltd; 1989. p. 279–98.
22. Jenness D. Eskimo administration IV. Greenland. Arctic Institute of North America Technical Paper No. 19. Ottawa (ON): Arctic Institute of North America; 1967.
23. Cowall EES, Alivaktuk M. The work we have done: relationships, investment and contribution – the Inuit workers of St. Luke's Hospital, Panniqtuuq, 1930–1972. 2015. doi: 10.13140/RG.2.1.1291.5685
24. McPherson KM. Bedside matters: the transformation of Canadian nursing, 1900–1990. Toronto (ON): University of Toronto Press; 2003.
25. Kaufert P, O'Neil J. Cooptation and control: the reconstruction of Inuit birth. Med Anthropol Q [Internet]. 1990 [cited 2019 Aug 7];4(4):427–42. Available from: http://www.jstor.org/stable/649225
26. Government of the Northwest Territories Health and Social Services [Internet]. Yellowknife (NT): Government of the Northwest Territories Health and Social Services; 2021. Health and Social Services Authority – regional portals; [cited 2021 Feb 15]. Availablable from: https://www.nthssa.ca/en/regional-portals
27. Government of Yukon Health and Social Services [Internet]. Whitehorse (YT): Government of Yukon Health and Social Services; 2017 Mar 30. Health centres – communities; 2017 Mar 30 [cited 2017 Jun 29]. Available from: http://www.hss.gov.yk.ca/healthcentres.php
28. O'Neil JD, Kaufert P. Irniktakpunga!: Sex determination and the Inuit struggle for birthing rights in northern Canada. In Ginsburg F, Rapp R, editors. Conceiving the new world order: the global politics of reproduction. Berkeley (CA): University of California Press; 1995. p. 59–74.
29. Møller H. "You need to be double cultured to function here": toward an anthropology of Inuit nursing in Greenland and Nunavut [dissertation]. Edmonton (AB): University of Alberta; 2011.
30. Møller, H. Culturally safe communication and the power of "language" in Arctic nursing. Etudes Inuit. 2016;40(1):85–104.

31. Inutiq S. Final report of the Office of the Languages Commissioner – Qikiqtani General Hospital, 2015. Iqaluit (NU): Office of the Languages Commissioner of Nunavut; 2015.
32. Lewis S. Press statement by Stephen Lewis on TB in Nunavut [Internet]. Iqaluit (NU): AIDS-Free World; 2017 Sept 9 [cited 2018 Feb 18]. Available from: https://aidsfreeworld.org/commentary/2017/9/9/statement
33. Lynch L [host]. The Current transcript for March 8, 2019 [Internet]. [Prime Minister Trudeau's speech included in soundclips]. Toronto (ON): CBC Radio, The Current; 2019 Mar 8 [cited 2021 Feb15]. Available from: https://www.cbc.ca/radio/thecurrent/the-current-for-march-8-2019-1.5048220/friday-march-8-2019-full-transcript-1.5049439#segment1
34. Møller H. "A problem of the government?" Colonization and the socio-cultural experience of tuberculosis in Nunavut [master's thesis]. Copenhagen (DK): University of Copenhagen, Institute of Anthropology; 2006.
35. Møller H. "Double culturedness": the "capital" of Inuit nurses. Int J Circumpolar Health. 2013;72. doi: 10.3402/ijch.v72i0.21266
36. Ferguson M. Report of the Auditor General of Canada to the Legislative Assembly of Nunavut – 2017: Health care services – Nunavut [Internet]. Ottawa (ON): Her Majesty the Queen in Right of Canada, as represented by the Auditor General of Canada; 2017 Mar 7 [cited 2018 Jan 12]. Available from: https://www.oag-bvg.gc.ca/internet/English/nun_201703_e_41998.html
37. Registered Nurses Association of the Northwest Territories and Nunavut. Scope of practice for registered nurses and nurse practitioners, 2019. Yellowknife (NT): Registered Nurses Association of the Northwest Territories and Nunavut; 2019.
38. MacLeod MLP, Stewart NJ, Kosteniuk JG, Penz KL, Olynick J, Karunanayake CP, Kilpatrick K, Kulig JC, Martin-Misener R, Koren I, Zimmer LV, Van Pelt L, Garraway L. Rural and remote registered nurses' perceptions of working beyond their legislated scope of practice. Nursing Leadersh. 2019;32(1):20–9. doi: 10.12927/cjnl.2019.25851
39. Møller H, editor. Grønlandske sygeplejersker fortæller: om sygepleje og sygeplejersker i Grønland [Greenlandic nurses' voices: about nursing and nurses in Greenland]. Copenhagen (DK): Gramma Publishing; 2014.
40. Registered Nurses' Association of Ontario. Coming together, moving forward: building the next chapter of Ontario's rural, remote and northern nursing workforce report. Toronto (ON): Registered Nurses' Association of Ontario; 2015.
41. MacLeod MLP, Kulig JC, Stewart NJ, Pitblado JR. The nature of nursing practice in rural and remote Canada. Ottawa (ON): Canadian Health Services Research Foundation; 2004.
42. MacLeod MLP, Stewart NJ, Kulig JC, Anguish P, Andrews ME, Banner D, Garraway L, Hanlon N, Karunanayake C, Kilpatrick K, Koren I, Kosteniuk J, Martin-Misener R, Mix N, Moffitt P, Olynick J, Penz K, Sluggett L, Van Pelt L, Wilson E, Zimmer L. Nurses who work in rural and remote communities in

Canada: a national survey. Hum Resour Health. 2017;15:34. doi: 10.1186/s12960-017-0209-0

43. Møller H, Dowsley M, Wakewich P, Bishop L, Burnett K, Churchill M. Qualitative assessment of factors in the uptake of midwifery of diverse populations in Thunder Bay, Ontario. Can J Midwifery Res Pract. 2015;14(3):14–20.
44. Health Quality Ontario. Continuity of care to optimize chronic disease management in the community setting an evidence-based analysis. Ont Health Technol Assess Ser. 2013;13(6):1–41.
45. Murray-Arnold T. SON, Nunavut Arctic College celebrate their 20-year successful, collaborative partnership [Internet]. Halifax (NS): School of Nursing, Dalhousie University; 2019 Jun 28 [cited 2019 Jul 8]. Available from: http://www.dal.ca/faculty/health/nursing/news-events/news/2019/06/28/son__nunavut_arctic_college_celebrate_their_20_year_successful__collaborative_partnership.html
46. Moffit P. Mobilizing decolonized nursing education at Aurora College: historical and current considerations. North Rev. 2016;43:67–81.
47. Wang P. "Believe yourself": Inuk nursing student to graduate Nunavut Arctic College after a decade of dedication. CBC North Online [Internet]. 2017 Apr 30 [cited 2019 July 6]. Available from: http://www.cbc.ca/news/canada/north/inuk-nursing-student-graduates-nubiya-enuaraq-1.4090380
48. Burke E. Being a nurse in the North is challenging, but there are salary perks – big ones. Maclean's [Internet]. 2015 Nov 30 [cited 2018 Mar 1]. Available from: http://www.macleans.ca/education/college/being-a-nurse-in-the-north-is-challenging-but-there-are-salary-perks-big-ones/
49. Skutnabb-Kangas T, Phillipson R, Dunbar R. Is Nunavut education criminally inadequate? An analysis of current policies for Inuktut and English in education, international and national law, linguistic and cultural genocide and crimes against humanity. Iqaluit (NU): Nunavut Tunngavik Incorporated; 2019.
50. Turner G. Nurses for Nunatsiavut. Presentation at: Cultural competency and cultural safety: A knowledge translation symposium [Internet]. Canadian Association of Schools of Nursing; 2012 Mar 12–13 [cited 2018 May 16]; Toronto (ON). Available from: http://www.casn.ca/2014/10/cultural-competence-cultural-safety-knowledge-translation-symposium/
51. Government of Nunavut. Legislative Assembly of Nunavut, 3rd session, 2nd assembly, Hansard, official report, day 32 [Internet]. Iqaluit (NU): Government of Nunavut; 2006 Jun 12 [cited 2018 Feb 28]. Available from: http://www.assembly.nu.ca/sites/default/files/Hansard_20060612.pdf
52. Government of Nunavut. Legislative Assembly of Nunavut, 4th session, 2nd assembly, Hansard, official report, day 10 [Internet]. Iqaluit (NU): Government of Nunavut; 2007 Mar 7 [cited 2019 Jul 10]. Available from: http://www.assembly.nu.ca/sites/default/files/Hansard_20070320.pdf
53. George J. GN abandons recruiting of international nurses. Nunatsiaq News Online [Internet]. 2007 Mar 30 [cited 2018 Feb 28]. Available from: http://www.nunatsiaq.com/stories/article/gn_abandons_recruiting_of_international_nurses/

54. Scura E. Nunavut aims to save money with new nursing agency contracts. CBC News [Internet]. 2016 Mar 22 [cited 2017 Jun 26]. Available from: http://www.cbc.ca/news/canada/north/nunavut-agency-nurse-contracts-1.3501317
55. Yukon nurse shortage compromises safe competent and ethical care, says nursing association. CBC News [Internet]. 2017 Oct 16 [cited 2018 Feb 28]. Available from: http://www.cbc.ca/news/canada/north/yukon-nurses-shortage-yrna-yeu-1.4357108
56. O'Connor A. Rural nurses are working 15–20 days alone. Whitehorse Daily Star [Internet]. 2015 Oct 27 [cited 2017 Jun 26]. Available from: http://whitehorsestar.com/news/rural-nurses-are-working-15-20-days-alone
57. Study explores reason behind N.W.T's low cancer screening rates. CBC News [Internet]. 2015 Nov 3 [updated 2015 Nov 3; cited 2018 Mar 1]. Available from: https://www.cbc.ca/news/canada/north/nwt-low-cancer-screening-rates-1.3300827
58. Cohen S. "It's very stressful": Yellowknife nurse says short staffing is impacting patient safety: N.W.T.'s largest hospital had 37 vacant full-time-equivalent nursing positions on June 5. CBC News [Internet]. 2019 Jul 5 [updated 2019 Jul 5; cited 2019 Jul 10] Available from: https://www.cbc.ca/news/canada/north/stanton-nurse-shortage-yellowknife-1.5200589
59. Canadian Nurses Association. 2016 pre-budget consultations: submission to the Standing Committee on Finance [Internet]. Ottawa (ON): Canadian Nurses Association; 2016 [cited 2018 Feb 18]. Available from: http://www.cna-aiic.ca/~/media/cna/page-content/pdf-en/cna-2016-pre-budget-submission-to-standing-committee-on-finance_feb2016.pdf?la=en
60. Canadian Federation of Nurses Union. Canada's nurses commission study of nurse staffing in face of growing crisis [Internet]. Ottawa (ON): Canadian Federation of Nurses Union; 2019 Jul 5 [cited 2019 Jul 10] Available from: https://nursesunions.ca/nurses-commission-staffing-study/
61. Playford D, Wheatland B, Larson A. Does teaching an entire nursing degree rurally have more workforce impact than rural placements? Contemp Nurse. 2010;35(1):68–76. doi: 10.5172/conu.2010.35.1.068.
62. Trépanier A, Gagnon MP, Mbemba GI, Côté J, Paré G, Fortin JP, Duplàa E, Courcy F. Factors associated with intended and effective settlement of nursing students and newly graduated nurses in a rural setting after graduation: A mixed-methods review. Int J Nur Stud. 2013;50(3):314–25.
63. Crown-Indigenous Relations and Northern Affairs Canada. Delivering on Truth and Reconciliation Commission calls to action: health [Internet]. Ottawa (ON): Government of Canada; 2019 Sep 5 [cited 2020 Jan 10]. Available from: http://www.rcaanc-cirnac.gc.ca/eng/1524499024614/1557512659251

9 Maternal Health Care: Maternal Health in Manitoba Northern First Nations Communities – Challenges, Barriers, and Solutions

JAIME CIDRO AND STEPHANIE SINCLAIR

Introduction

Maternal and child health care in Canada has dramatically changed over the last century. Pregnancy and birth for Indigenous communities is considered to be a special ceremonial time, where the person is supported by loved ones. Birth is the first rite of passage, marking the transition from the spiritual world to the physical world (1). Traditionally, Canadian women, particularly First Nations women, gave birth in their home communities, among friends and extended family (2). Cultural practices established strong community roots for the mother, the infant, and the family. The children born in the community developed a clear sense of identity that helped them become resilient and responsible members of that community. This way of welcoming a new life into the community resulted in the child having a strong identity with connections to family, friends, culture, and language from birth (3).

Currently, travelling for birth from northern remote and rural communities is a typical experience for many women in Canada and in particular for Indigenous women. After a history of outpost nurses providing maternal and obstetric care in Indigenous communities throughout the first half of the twentieth century (4), in the 1970s, the efforts to decrease maternal mortality and morbidity in the general population led to a move towards hospital deliveries for all women. Criteria were established for evacuating mothers with high-risk pregnancies from northern and remote communities to tertiary centres. By the 1980s, not just high-risk but essentially all deliveries occurred outside northern and remote communities (5). For northern Indigenous women, this led to being transferred out of their home community weeks before their due date, an event that often resulted in a cascade of negative social consequences (6,7). In this chapter, we explore the role of Indigenous doulas in supporting northern First Nations women and families who must temporarily relocate to deliver their babies away from their community.

This chapter starts with a review of the challenges maternal health care faces in the Canadian north. The chapter continues with a discussion of the medicalization of birth, which demonstrates the gaps that continue to place expectant women and their families in precarious circumstances. Then the impacts experienced by northern First Nations women who travel for birth to tertiary care centres are described. This is followed by a discussion of the specific role of doulas as one way to better support women and families with the long-term goal of returning birthing back to communities. This chapter focuses specifically on work being done in northern Manitoba, Canada, with First Nations.

Challenges in Northern Maternal Health Care

While access to adequate health care generally is a challenge in the North, access to maternal care is particularly difficult. Specifically, it is a challenge to train and retain qualified, culturally competent staff (see Pong, chapter 7, and also Møller, chapter 8, this volume) and to provide access to other specialized maternal care providers, such as midwives, anaesthesiologists, lactation consultants, and mental health care providers. Although maternal health care services are available in the province, 11.5 per cent of Manitoba women receive inadequate prenatal care, and "the northern regions of the province and inner-city areas in Winnipeg … have the highest rates of inadequate prenatal care, and are known to be more socioeconomically deprived" (8 p10). In addition to living on low income, receiving income assistance, and living in a low-income neighbourhood, several other social determinants of health have been associated with inadequate prenatal care, including northern or rural residence, a young maternal age, being a lone parent, parity at four or more, a short inter-pregnancy interval, and the highest attained education being high school or lower (8). Maternal medical conditions, such as hypertensive disorders, antepartum hemorrhage, diabetes, and prenatal psychological distress, have also been associated with lower odds of receiving adequate prenatal care (9). Low prenatal care access and use can have significant detrimental impacts. In Manitoba, Heaman et al. (10) associated low prenatal care access and use with increased odds of stillbirth, preterm births, and low birth weight and size for gestational age, after adjusting for maternal age group, region of residence, income quintile, parity, maternal diabetes, hypertension, prenatal depressive/anxiety disorder, and antepartum hemorrhage. The health of the mother does have a direct impact on health outcomes for the child.

One of the ways to ascertain maternal and child health status is infant mortality. Elias et al. (9) note that in Manitoba, the First Nations crude annual infant mortality rate was 10.7/1000, which is almost double that of all other Manitobans (5.73/1000) (9). For First Nations populations in northern rural Manitoba, the rate was 10.5/1000, compared to a rate of 6.36/1000 for rural northern

Manitoba as a whole (9 p290). Elias et al. found that there were further distinctions in the rural north. For example, the rate of infant mortality on reserve was 11.6/1000, compared to a rate of 6.8/1000 off reserve (9). In other words, the rate of infant mortality in the rural north is much higher than it is in the rest of Manitoba, and on rural northern reserves, the rate of infant mortality is almost twice that of the rural north off reserve (9 p290).

Health care for First Nations people in Canada is influenced by the jurisdictional issues between federal and provincial or territorial governments. The main issue is defining who is responsible for funding care services for First Nations people living on reserve. The Canadian Constitution outlines the responsibilities of the federal and provincial or territorial governments. The health of Canadians generally is a provincial or territorial responsibility as outlined in the Canada Health Act. The health supports for First Nations are seen to be the responsibility of the federal government as designated in the Indian Act. A lack of clarity about providing health services to First Nations in existing policies has been used by both levels of governments to justify not providing coordinated health care services to First Nations, including maternal health care (11). Jurisdictional health issues for First Nations people have been highlighted through Jordan's Principle, a child-first principle that is intended to "address … the needs of First Nations children by ensuring there are no gaps in government services to them" (12). A private Member's motion in support of Jordan's Principle was passed unanimously in the House of Commons of Canada on 12 December 2007. The implementation of Jordan's Principle by the Canadian government has, however, been very limited, leading to the Canadian Human Rights Tribunal issuing a third set of non-compliance orders in 2017.

Furthermore, the provision of on-reserve health care in northern First Nations is largely provided by federally funded nursing stations, whereas in southern communities, health care is provided through health centres. The nursing station model, which exists in 21 remote and isolated communities in Manitoba, delivers a limited scope of primary health care services that are provided by nurses with an expanded scope of practice, supplemented by visiting physicians. First Nations communities that are not isolated, who theoretically should be able to access provincially delivered health services off reserve, are served by health clinics staffed with part-time employees, including nurses, health care aides, and community wellness workers providing preventive care only. Many of the specialized services required for maternal care, such as midwives, obstetricians, and mental health care providers, are located outside the community. There is an additional burden of coordination of care and transportation for families located in the North.

Experience of racism is an additional and very significant determinant related to why northern rural and remote First Nations women are not accessing maternal health care. Research suggests that racism impacts health even when other confounding factors, such as socio-economic status, employment, marital status, and education, are controlled for (13). Unfortunately, many examples of racism as a determinant of health and its detrimental impact on health care delivery have been reported in Manitoba (14,15). Culturally appropriate health care that addresses the holistic health of the mother, including mental, emotional, physical, and spiritual needs while pregnant, is necessary (16).

Medicalization of Birth

Many life and biological events have been medicalized; Zadoroznyj (17) argues, however, that women's experiences with pregnancy epitomize the process of medicalization. Where historically pregnancy was a natural, normal event with women at the centre, today pregnancy "is conceptualized as a dangerous time wherein a woman and her fetus are at risk and in need of constant medical monitoring and intervention" (18 p785). The Canadian Institute for Health Information reported that in 2016–17, 28 per cent of deliveries were by caesarean section (19). Ironically, the medicalization of birth is particularly prominent in the communities that have least access to medical care and services. In Canada, these communities are often located in northern, rural, and remote areas, and many are Indigenous. Leanne Simpson, a renowned Indigenous anti-colonial scholar and activist, underscores that for First Nations, "the Western medicalization of birth replaced our ceremony ... By undermining our most sacred and powerful ceremony and or most sacred responsibilities of mothers, our colonizers thought they could achieve the destruction of our nations" (20 p28).

The role of midwives and number of home births decreased for all Canadian women concurrently, and Western medicine has been the predominant approach used across Canadian mainstream and Indigenous communities for decades. The key message that was, and is often still, given to women, whether Indigenous or non-Indigenous, is that it is safer for both mother and baby to deliver using modern technology and conveniences (21). Historically, Western medical providers purported that First Nations midwives, their medicines, and their ceremonies were superstition and senseless, and furthermore, promoted that Western medicine was the only safe way for expectant mothers. The result for Indigenous peoples in Canada was an imposition of colonial policies and practices that transferred births and maternal care from the home to nursing stations and, subsequently, to hospitals located outside the community. The transfer of responsibility for maternal care and birthing from traditional midwives located within the community to external service providers located outside the community diminished and eventually led to the discontinuation of traditional midwifery and traditional doula care in First Nations communities (3). With this, the process of practising and passing important Indigenous

Knowledge about pregnancy and birthing from one generation to the next was seriously damaged.

In addition to, and in some ways supported by, the evacuation policy, the imposition of the Western health care system served as an attack on Indigenous women's ability to bear children and create new life through forced sterilization. Pegoraro (22) estimates that the sterilization of tens of thousands of Indigenous women in the United States and Canada was funded and mandated by the two nations' respective governments. Indigenous women were sterilized well into the 1970s in Canada, with Alberta and British Columbia establishing Sterilization Acts (23). A recent news article (24) stated that 60 Indigenous women in Saskatchewan are filing a class action lawsuit alleging forced sterilization. There are other instances of unnecessary medical procedures being performed on Indigenous women during birth, which has resulted in fear being the dominant emotion during childbirth (11). Still, travelling for birth remains a factor that impacts almost all Indigenous women living in northern and remote communities.

Health Impacts of Travel for Birth

The rationale for continuing the evacuation process, discussed above, has largely focused on the risks of birthing outside the medical setting. To date, discussions of risk have focused exclusively on the physical aspects of pregnancy, ignoring risks associated with dislocating the birthing event from its sociocultural context. Women are faced with choosing culture or risk, resulting in "diminishing birthing choices, with loss of connection to family, clan and culture when they [leave] their communities to give birth" (25 p7). Often unaccompanied, women must leave their communities to experience labour and delivery in a distant referral centre, where they reside in short-term boarding houses for weeks.

First Nations women who travel for birth experience a range of stressors, such as insecurity, loneliness, disconnection from community and culture, isolation from and missing family and children, and discrimination, in addition to the stress and anxiety of managing family life while away. Many women live with financial hardships before being relocated for birth. This is exacerbated by the added costs of relocating. Maintaining connections to their families through phone calls, buying extra food, supporting family members to stay for the delivery, and paying for childcare for the children left at home all place a great deal of financial stress on expectant families (7,25,26). These stressors may exacerbate existing pregnancy issues and subsequent infant health conditions (27; see also 21,25). Women with limited resources associate their postpartum depression with economic stress and a lack of family support (25), such as that experienced when being evacuated for birth. This can affect the mother's capacity to bond with and nurture the baby and subsequently impact the health and well-being of both (25). Compounding this is the poorer nutrition many mothers experience when away from home in the last weeks before delivery (21,27). Further, children of First Nations mothers who were evacuated for birth felt distress and sadness when their mothers left them to give birth outside the community. Teenage girls may be particularly vulnerable when left without their mothers/caregivers for weeks at a critical time in their development (7). It increases the potential for experiences of racism and for creating susceptibility to trafficking (28). In addition to cultural, socio-economic, emotional, and mental health detriments before birth, relocation for birth has also been shown to be detrimental for birth and postpartum outcomes for both mother and child. Medical relocation for birth increases maternal and newborn complications, increases postpartum depression, and decreases breastfeeding rates (29–33)

Forcing women to leave their communities for birth is a costly practice that adversely affects families, deprives the community of a reason for celebration, and ignores – and thereby hastens the loss of – traditional birthing knowledge. This evacuation policy has been opposed by academics, policymakers, and communities since its implementation in the 1980s (5, 34–36). Despite the negative impacts and opposition, maternal evacuation remains a current practice and a common experience for First Nations women. In Manitoba, an estimated 1100 prenatal women relocate temporarily from rural and remote northern First Nations communities to Winnipeg or other urban tertiary centres to give birth each year (37). In a response to the impacts of maternal evacuation, the development of a doula program was initiated along with a research project. Doula, or birth support worker, is not a new caregiving role. This supportive role was often provided by family members or a local woman who was experienced in pregnancy and birth (38). Because pregnant women are often living away from their families, they need further support. The contemporary doula care provider, discussed below, emerged as a formal birth companion role. While not providing medical, midwifery, or nursing care, a doula provides continual physical, emotional, and advocacy support during labour and birth (38).

Maternal and Birth Support

Support is an important factor for a positive birth experience for women and is associated with shorter labour; a decreased need for the use of analgesics, oxytocin, forceps, and caesarean sections; and an overall higher level of satisfaction with the birth experience. Continual support has the greatest benefits when the support begins early in labour and when the person providing support is a peer rather than health care staff (39). Avoiding psychosocial stressors and poor health outcomes associated with negative birthing experiences for patients is an important challenge facing primary care providers. To work successfully in First Nations communities, health care providers must be culturally competent, be able to apply their knowledge, have self-awareness, and have personal attributes and attitudes that facilitate respectful partnerships with communities (40). Continual emotional and social support to women during childbirth, as often provided by midwifes whether traditional or contemporary, has positive impacts, not only for labour and delivery but also for breastfeeding rates and attachment (40). Midwifery is not available in most northern Canadian contexts, and this is particularly true in Manitoba.

Culturally Based Support through Doulas

The caregiving and supportive role that doulas have in relation to birthing is not new; however, traditionally the responsibility to provide this care and support rested with family members or an experienced local woman (41). Because women often need to live away from their families, the role of the contemporary doula includes being a maternal care provider and formal birth companion. A doula provides continual physical, emotional, and advocacy support during labour and birth but does not provide medical, midwifery, or nursing care (41). For First Nations women, the move away from births in communities has meant a loss of traditional birthing knowledge and mentors. The role of an older female relative (i.e., a traditional Aunty) is documented as an important component of pregnancy and childbirth because it ensures the transfer of critical cultural practices that are essential to establishing and revitalizing the strong cultural connection and spiritual path for First Nations children (40). In an Alberta First Nation, it was recommended that the role of doulas be recognized as key to addressing childbirth and infant health and that women should be trained to accompany the pregnant women through the entire process, providing prenatal teaching, connections, and support and liaising with health care professionals as needed (40).

Many northern First Nations communities have programs and services for prenatal and postnatal women, such as the Maternal Child Health Strengthening Families program, and, in exceptional cases, midwives; however, it is increasingly recognized that a trained birth companion, such as a doula, can have significant positive impacts on some of the psychological and social stressors experienced by women, as well as on birth and health outcomes, especially for women who travel for birth (6).

In 2017, the University of Winnipeg, the First Nations Health and Social Secretariat of Manitoba, and the Manitoba Indigenous Doula Initiative (MIDI) created a joint project to begin to identify ways to address these stressors experienced by First Nations women who travel for birth. Three northern Cree communities are currently involved in the project, including Pimicikamak Cree Nation (Cross Lake) (latitude: 54.622° N), Nisichawayasihk Cree Nation (Nelson House) (latitude: 55.789° N), and Misipawistik Cree Nation (Grand Rapids) (latitude: 53.1846° N). This project is implementing a culturally and community-driven Indigenous doula program designed for women who are required to travel for birth. Expectant mothers in these communities are paired with a local Indigenous doula who has undergone culturally specific doula training from MIDI, along with mentorship from an Indigenous doula/midwife team in Winnipeg, Thompson, or The Pas. The expectant mothers receive doula care from pregnancy to postpartum from their doula team, which consists of two doulas.

The research team is measuring a variety of outcomes related to psychological and social stressors and health outcomes using a variety of qualitative, quantitative, and clinical evaluation. These prenatal measurements include quality of prenatal care (42), interpersonal processes of care (43), stress (6,25) and postpartum depression (44). This project is assessing whether health, social, and cultural outcomes for mothers and newborns improve with the use of First Nations culturally based doulas for women from northern First Nations who travel for birth. Underpinning this project is the concept of resilience. Despite years of having traditions of birthing and midwifery replaced by biomedical notions of risk and safety, communities have developed pathways of resiliency. This project supports resiliency and is "reflective of the larger response to domination faced by evacuated First Nations communities" (45 p62).

MIDI developed the curriculum for Indigenous doula training with Knowledge Keepers, families, and service providers. The five-day training provides both Western and Indigenous knowledge about pregnancy, birth, and healing. In 2016–17, MIDI, in partnership with the Winnipeg Boldness Project, the First Nations Health and Social Secretariat of Manitoba, and Mount Carmel Clinic, trained a group of Indigenous women as part of an initial pilot project focusing on providing care and support to expectant mothers in Winnipeg's north-end community. Twelve women were trained and provided doula care for Indigenous women in Winnipeg and northern Manitoba. Interviews conducted with the doulas about their experiences identified several key themes, including prior negative birthing experiences, clashes with mainstream health and social services, the understanding of doulas as advocates, and empowerment and disempowerment. One interview participant identified that "the doulas are able to serve as teachers and facilitators, helping women and their families to discover or restore these teachings" (3 p5).

Some of the key aspects of MIDI's work is its culturally based curriculum and the ongoing support they provide to the trained doulas. The curriculum is customized for every community through local Knowledge Keepers, delivering components of the training with local birth knowledge and traditions. The key components of the training include the following:

1. Scope of Indigenous birth helpers (practice and ethics)
2. Impacts of colonization on birthing
3. Rites of passage and teachings of the life stages
4. How to integrate traditional knowledge into practice
5. Building of positive relationships with others (clients, staff, families)
6. Facilitation of prenatal and postpartum visits
7. Labour support techniques
8. Support for initial chest/breastfeeding
9. Resource access
10. Postpartum care
11. Building of trust and client confidentiality (1)

The training provides an overview, but doulas are also encouraged to add to their birthing knowledge by seeking out Knowledge Keepers and attending further specialized training. They are also mentored by MIDI while they support families. Training Indigenous doulas is one step towards revitalizing Indigenous birthing knowledge and returning birth to northern communities.

Reducing Social and Health Issues with Indigenous Doulas

One motivation for this research was to address some of the direct causes of the many social and health issues facing northern Indigenous populations. Knowledge Keepers and Western academics have stated that the first five years of life are key to development and health. Supporting mothers and families to get the best start for new life is expected to result in children having better health and social outcomes. One of the most urgent issues among First Nations people is the continued apprehension and separation of children from their families by child and family services (CFS). This is a country-wide issue, and Manitoba specifically has an overwhelming overrepresentation of Indigenous children in the child welfare system. Indigenous children make up almost 90 per cent of children in CFS care (46). The role of doulas in supporting pregnant Indigenous women who themselves may have been in CFS custody or may have had other children in care has been taken up by the Government of Manitoba through a social impact bond program (47). This two-year pilot project called Restoring the Sacred Bond matches doulas with expectant Indigenous women who are considered at risk of having their infants apprehended through CFS.

With the first Winnipeg cohort of doulas, the doulas themselves indicated that the birth work they engage in represents a more profound role than simply facilitating a healthy physical pregnancy, birth, and postpartum; it encourages the establishment and maintenance of relationships with the expectant mothers that "sustain and support the mothers no matter what they go through" (3 p4). The creation of safe spaces for Indigenous women to give birth was considered an integral part of the doula's role in "defending these mothers and babies from CFS workers" (3 p4). In northern Manitoba, the threats of CFS still loom large for Indigenous women, as does the experience of racism in the health care system, which may play a role in the low number of women accessing prenatal care.

This research and research generally around mothers, babies, and families is intensely personal to us. Both of us are Indigenous mothers (Anishinawbe), and this work is about improving our own children's pregnancies and births and developing strong families where culture is not an afterthought but instead is a central component of who they are. For me (Cidro), being a pregnant woman, a mother, and a parent has provided me with the opportunity to understand some of the essence of growing up in spirit. Working in an academic field that has long been grounded in uncovering the stories of the "other," this work has provided me with an opportunity to understand the optimal way to do research with community, starting with spirit and binding people together with friendship. For me (Sinclair), as an Indigenous student in Native studies and a policy analyst for an Indigenous organization, I wanted to conduct research to provide the community with the evidence they need to implement the solutions they know will work. As an Indigenous researcher, it is important that the research projects focus on community priorities, that we take direction from spirit, and that the relationships are the focus. When working with Indigenous communities, it is important to be flexible and regularly communicate to address issues as they arise. My research world view is that the research has to be useful to the community; they must be able to use it and want the knowledge created in the research project. Indigenous knowledge is the basis for a research project as it contains the current community realities and context within the teachings.

Conclusion

Pregnancy and birthing are important times in a woman's life and in the life of her family and community. In Indigenous communities across Canada and across the world, the interruption of traditional women's knowledge through medical intervention has not improved health and social outcomes for either mothers or babies. Western medical knowledge has overtaken traditional birth knowledge and, in many cases, has replaced important intergenerational wisdom. In recent years, communities have called for a return to birthing and traditional birth practices from Indigenous communities across Canada. They have recognized that many of the challenges facing Indigenous people are not being overcome because of the need to "go back to the beginning." The beginning is birth.

Birthing in the community creates lifelong connections. When the community is involved in welcoming a new life, it affirms relationships and renews the responsibility of each person to teach, guide, and support the child and their family. It is vital that communities reclaim Indigenous women's rights to have a safe, culturally appropriate space in which to give birth, where the involvement of their loved ones and community is welcomed and recognized as necessary to restore wellness among families. Training Indigenous doulas in First Nations is a first step in revitalizing Indigenous birth knowledge and creating a path to returning birth to communities. Returning birthing also means returning to pregnancy and birthing knowledge and ceremony. This chapter discussed this return within a larger discussion of the impact of colonial structures on birth. The focus of the authors' research is northern Manitoba First Nations communities, and the chapter discussed the specific challenges, barriers, and solutions to improving maternal care in this region; however, the content and the research have application to northern Canada generally.

REFERENCES

1. Manitoba Doula Initiative. Sacred circle of life: Indigenous doula training curriculum manual. Winnipeg (MB): Manitoba Doula Initiative; 2018.
2. Anderson K. Life stages and Native women: memory, teachings, and story medicine. Winnipeg (MB): University of Manitoba Press; 2011.
3. Cidro J, Doenmez C, Phanlouvong A, Fontaine A. Being a good relative: Indigenous doulas reclaiming cultural knowledge to improve health and birth outcomes in Manitoba. Front Women's Health [Internet]. 2018 [cited 2019 Aug 7];3(4):2–8. Available from: http://www.oatext.com/being-a-good-relative-indigenous-doulas-reclaiming-cultural-knowledge-to-improve-health-and-birth-outcomes-in-manitoba.php doi: 10.15761/FWH.1000157
4. Dodd D, Elliot J, Rousseau N. Outpost nursing in Canada. In: Bates C, Dodd D, Rousseau N, editors. On all frontiers: four centuries of Canadian nursing. Ottawa (ON): University of Ottawa Press; 2005. p. 135–52.
5. Kaufert P, O'Neil J. Cooptation and control: the reconstruction of Inuit birth. Med Anthropol Q [Internet]. 1990 [cited 2019 Aug 7];4(4):427–42. Available from: http://www.jstor.org/stable/649225
6. Society of Obstetricians and Gynaecologists of Canada. Returning birth to Aboriginal, rural, and remote communities. J Obstet Gynaecol Can [Internet]. 2010 [cited 2019 Aug 7];32(12):1186–8. Available from: http://www.jogc.com/article/S1701-2163(16)34744-2/pdf doi: 10.1016/S1701-2163(16)34744-2

7. Chamberlain M, Barclay K. Psychosocial costs of transferring indigenous women from their community for birth. Midwifery [Internet]. 2000 [cited 2019 Aug 7];16(2):116–22. Available from: http://www.midwiferyjournal.com/article/S0266-6138(99)90202-4/pdf doi: 10.1054/midw.1999.0202
8. Heaman M, Martens P, Brownell M, Chartier M, Thiessen K, Derksen S, Helewa M. Inequities in utilization of prenatal care: a population-based study in the Canadian province of Manitoba. BMC Pregnancy Childbirth [Internet]. 2018 [cited 2019 Aug 7];18. Available from: https://bmcpregnancychildbirth.biomedcentral.com/track/pdf/10.1186/s12884-018-2061-1 doi: 10.1186/s12884-018-2061-1
9. Elias B, Hart L, Martens P. "Just get on with it": linking data systems to report on infant mortality and the First Nations population in Manitoba (Canada). Statistical J IAOS [Internet]. 2014 [cited 2019 Aug 7];30(3):285–95. Available from: https://content.iospress.com/download/statistical-journal-of-the-iaos/sji00827?id=statistical-journal-of-the-iaos%2Fsji00827 doi: 10.3233/SJI-140827
10. Heaman M, Martens P, Brownell M, Chartier M, Derksen S, Helewa M. The association of inadequate and intensive prenatal care with maternal, fetal, and infant outcomes: a population-based study in Manitoba, Canada. J Obstet Gynaecol Can [Internet]. 2019 [cited 2019 Aug 7];41(7): 947–59. Available from: http://www.jogc.com/article/S1701-2163(18)30702-3/fulltext doi: 10.1016/j.jogc.2018.09.006
11. National Collaborating Centre for Aboriginal Health. An overview of Aboriginal health in Canada [Internet]. Ottawa (ON): National Collaborating Centre for Aboriginal Health; 2013 [cited 2019 Sep 10]. Available from: https://www.ccnsa-nccah.ca/docs/context/FS-OverviewAbororiginalHealth-EN.pdf
12. Government of Canada [Internet]. Ottawa (ON): Government of Canada; 2018. Definition of Jordan's Principle from the Canadian Human Rights Tribunal; 2018 Jun 11 [cited 2019 Jul 28]. Available from: https://www.sac-isc.gc.ca/eng/1583700168284/1583700212289
13. Allan B, Smylie J. First peoples, second class treatment: the role of racism in the health and well-being of Indigenous peoples in Canada [Internet]. Toronto (ON): Wellesley Institute; 2015 [cited 2019 Sep 10]. Available from: http://www.wellesleyinstitute.com/wp-content/uploads/2015/02/Summary-First-Peoples-Second-Class-Treatment-Final.pdf
14. McCallum MJ, Perry A. Structures of indifference: an Indigenous life and death in a Canadian city. Winnipeg (MB): University of Manitoba Press; 2018.
15. Sinclair Working Group. Ignored to death – out of sight: interim report of the Sinclair Working Group [Internet]. Winnipeg (MB): Sinclair Working Group; 2017 [cited 2019 Sep 10]. Available from: http://ignoredtodeathmanitoba.ca/index.php/2017/09/15/out-of-sight-interim-report-of-the-sinclair-working-group/
16. Abma S. Racism a barrier to prenatal health care, midwives say. CBC News [Internet]. 2018 Oct 18 [cited 2019 Sep 10]. Available from: http://www.cbc.ca/news/canada/ottawa/midwife-racism-prenatal-health-care-conference-1.4867236

17. Zadoroznyj M. Social class, social selves and social control in childbirth. Sociol Health Illn [Internet]. 1999 [cited 2019 Aug 7];21(3):267–89. Available from: https://onlinelibrary.wiley.com/doi/abs/10.1111/1467-9566.00156 doi: 10.1111/1467-9566.00156
18. Parry DC. "We wanted a birth experience, not a medical experience": exploring Canadian women's use of midwifery. Health Care Women Int [Internet]. 2008 [cited 2019 Aug 7];29(8–9):784–806. Available from: http://www.tandfonline.com/doi/full/10.1080/07399330802269451 doi: 10.1080/07399330802269451
19. Canadian Institute for Health Information [Internet]. Ottawa (ON): Canadian Institute for Health Information; 2018. Press release, C-section rates continue to increase while birth rates decline; 2018 Apr 19 [cited 2019 Sep 10]. Available from: https://web.archive.org/web/20180711212414/http://www.cihi.ca/en/c-section-rates-continue-to-increase-while-birth-rates-decline?utm_source=crm&utm_medium=emailmedemb&utm_campaign=hospch&utm_content=mediareleaseEN
20. Simpson L. Birthing an Indigenous resurgence: decolonizing our pregnancy and birthing ceremonies. In: Memee Lavell-Harvard D, Corbiere Lavell J, editors. Until our hearts are on the ground: Aboriginal mothering, oppression, resistance and rebirth. Bradford (ON): Demeter Press; 2006. p. 25–33.
21. Olson R, Couchie C. Returning birth: The politics of midwifery implementation on First Nations reserves in Canada. Midwifery [Internet]. 2013 [cited 2019 Aug 7];29(8):981–7. Available from: http://www.midwiferyjournal.com/article/S0266-6138(12)00246-X/fulltext doi: 10.1016/j.midw.2012.12.005
22. Pegoraro L. Second-rate victims: the forced sterilization of Indigenous peoples in the USA and Canada. Settl Colon Stud [Internet]. 2015 [cited 2019 Aug 7];5(2):161–73. Available from: http://www.tandfonline.com/doi/abs/10.1080/2201473X.2014.955947 doi: 10.1080/2201473X.2014.955947
23. Stote K. An act of genocide: colonialism and the sterilization of Aboriginal women. Winnipeg (MB): Fernwood; 2015.
24. Soloducha A. Sask. Indigenous women file lawsuit claiming coerced sterilization. CBC News [Internet]. 2017 Oct 10 [cited 2019 Aug 3]. Available from: http://www.cbc.ca/news/canada/saskatchewan/sask-indigenous-women-file-lawsuit-claiming-coerced-sterilization-1.4348848
25. Cidro J, Neufeld HT, editors. Indigenous experiences of pregnancy and birth. Bradford (ON): Demeter Press; 2017.
26. Varcoe C, Brown H, Calam B, Harvey T, Tallio M. Help bring back the celebration of life: a community based participatory study of rural Aboriginal women's maternity experiences and outcomes. BMC Pregnancy Childbirth [Internet]. 2013 [cited 2019 Aug 7];13(26):1–10. Available from: https://bmcpregnancychildbirth.biomedcentral.com/articles/10.1186/1471-2393-13-26 doi: 10.1186/1471-2393-13-26
27. National Aboriginal Health Organization. Exploring models for quality maternity care in First Nations and Inuit communities: a preliminary needs assessment: final report on findings [Internet]. Ottawa (ON): National Aboriginal Health

Organization; 2006 [cited 2019 Aug 7]. Available from: https://ruor.uottawa.ca/bitstream/10393/30538/1/Models_Maternity_Care_Needs_Assessment_2006.pdf

28. Sethi A. Domestic sex trafficking of Aboriginal girls in Canada: issues and implications. First Peoples Child Fam Rev [Internet]. 2007 [cited 2019 Aug 7];3(3):57–71. Available from: http://journals.sfu.ca/fpcfr/index.php/FPCFR/article/view/50
29. O'Neil J, Kaufert P, Postl B. Study of the impact of obstetric policy on Inuit women and their families in the Keewatin region, NWT. Winnipeg (MB): University of Manitoba; 1990.
30. Smith D. Maternal-Child Health Care in Aboriginal communities. Can J Nurs Res [Internet]. 2003 [cited 2019 Aug 7];35(2):143–52. Available from: http://cjnr.archive.mcgill.ca/article/viewFile/1838/1832
31. Klein MC, Christilaw J, Johnston SMB. Loss of maternity care: the cascade of unforeseen dangers. Can J Rural Med. 2002 [cited 2019 Aug 7];7(2):120–1.
32. Lawford K, Giles A, Bourgeault I. Canada's evacuation policy for pregnant First Nations women: resignation, resilience, and resistance. Women Birth [Internet]. 2018 [cited 2019 Aug 7];31(6):479–88. Available from: http://www.womenandbirth.org/article/S1871-5192(17)30201-9/pdf doi: 10.1016/j.wombi.2018.01.009
33. Kornelsen J, Kotaska A, Waterfall P, Willie L, Wilson D. The geography of belonging: the experience of birthing at home for First Nations women. Health Place [Internet]. 2010 [cited 2019 Aug 7];16(4):638–45. Available from: http://www.sciencedirect.com/science/article/abs/pii/S1353829210000109?via%3Dihub doi: 10.1016/j.healthplace.2010.02.001
34. Guse L. Maternal evacuation: a study of the experiences of northern Manitoba Native women. Winnipeg (MB): University of Manitoba; 1982.
35. Hiebert S. The utilization of antenatal services in remote Manitoba First Nations communities. Int J Circumpolar Health [Internet]. 2001 Jan [cited 2019 Aug 7];60(1):64–71.
36. Eni R. An articulation of the standpoint of peer support workers to inform childbearing program supports in Manitoba First Nation communities: institutional ethnography as de-colonizing methodology [dissertation on the Internet]. Winnipeg (MB): University of Manitoba; 2005 [cited 2019 Aug 7]. Available from: http://hdl.handle.net/1993/29670
37. Phillips-Beck W. Development of a framework of improved childbirth care for First Nation women in Manitoba: a First Nation family centred approach [master's thesis on the Internet]. Winnipeg (MB): University of Manitoba; 2010 [cited 2019 Aug 7]. Available from: http://hdl.handle.net/1993/3985
38. Schmonsky, JR. Holding the space: the reemerging role of the doula [dissertation on the Internet]. San Francisco (CA): San Francisco State University; 2016 [cited 2019 Sep 10]. Available from: http://sfsu-dspace.calstate.edu/handle/10211.3/173408

39. Hodnett ED, Gates S, Hofmeyr GJ, Sakala C. Continuous support for women during childbirth. 2013 July 15 [cited 2019 Aug 7]. In: Cochrane Database of Systematic Reviews [Internet]. Hoboken (NJ): John Wiley & Sons, Ltd. c1999 - . Available from: https://www.cochranelibrary.com/cdsr/doi/10.1002/14651858.CD003766.pub5/epdf/full/en doi: 10.1002/14651858.CD003766.pub5
40. Wiebe AD, Barton S, Auger L, Pijl-Zieber E, Foster-Boucher C. Restoring the blessings of the morning star: childbirth and maternal-infant health for First Nations near Edmonton, Alberta. Aborig Policy Stud [Internet]. 2015 [cited 2019 Aug 7];5(1):47–68. Available from: https://journals.library.ualberta.ca/aps/index.php/aps/article/view/23823 doi: 10.5663/aps.v5i1.23823
41. Campbell-Voytal K, McCornish JR, Rowland CA, Kelleher J. Postpartum doulas: motivations and perceptions of practice. Midwifery [Internet]. 2011 [cited 2019 Aug 7];27(6):214–21. Available from: http://www.midwiferyjournal.com/article/S0266-6138(10)00149-X/fulltext doi: 10.1016/j.midw.2010.09.006
42. First Nations and Inuit Health Branch (FNIHB) adult care: clinical practice guidelines for nurses in primary care [Internet]. Ottawa (ON): Health Canada; 2012 Nov 22. Chapter 12, Obstetrics; [modified 2013 May 8; cited 2016 Sept 28]. Available from: http://www.canada.ca/en/indigenous-services-canada/services/first-nations-inuit-health/health-care-services/nursing/clinical-practice-guidelines-nurses-primary-care/adult-care/chapter-12-obstetrics.html
43. McShane K, Smylie J, Adomako P. Health of First Nations, Inuit, and Métis children in Canada. In: Smylie J, Adomako P, editors. Indigenous children's health report: Health assessment in action. Toronto (ON): University of Toronto; 2009. p. 11–65.
44. Lalonde AB, Butt C, Bucio A. Maternal health in Canadian Aboriginal communities: challenges and opportunities. J Obstet Gynaecol Can [Internet]. 2009 [cited 2019 Aug 7];31(10):956–62. Available from: http://www.jogc.com/article/S1701-2163(16)34325-0/fulltext doi: 10.1016/S1701-2163(16)34325-0
45. Kornelson J, Kotaska A, Waterfall P, Willie L, Wilson D. Alienation and resilience: the anxiety of birth outside of the their community for rural First Nations Women. J Aborig Health [Internet]. 2011 Mar [cited 2019 Aug 7];7(1):55–64. Available from: https://journals.uvic.ca/index.php/ijih/article/view/12353 doi: 10.18357/ijih71201112353
46. Government of Manitoba. Review of child welfare legislation in Manitoba [Internet]. Winnipeg (MB): Government of Manitoba; 2017 [cited 2019 Sep 10]. Available from: http://www.gov.mb.ca/fs/child_welfare_reform/pubs/discussion_guide.pdf
47. Government of Manitoba. Manitoba announces first social impact bond [Internet]. Winnipeg (MB): Government of Manitoba; 2019 Jan 7 [cited 2019 Sep 10]. Available from: https://news.gov.mb.ca/news/index.html?item=44895

10 Elder Health and Long-Term Care: Northern Indigenous Elders and Long-Term-Care Services

BONITA BEATTY AND JOSEPHINE MCKAY

Introduction

This chapter explores continuing care services (distribution, access, delivery) in the North, specifically for Indigenous Elders seniors). The introduction provides a short overview of the issue and its importance. We then situate who we are as authors, followed by a brief description of terms used. This chapter also provides a general description of the organization and delivery of continuing care services in the North, including formal and informal (family) care. It then discusses the challenges in long-term care and illustrates some of these through a case study. The chapter concludes with a discussion of the strengths and gaps of Elders/senior care services in the North and makes some recommendations.

Before Euro-Canadian colonization, northern Indigenous people occupied diverse northern subarctic and Arctic homelands that shaped distinct kinship cultures, beliefs, and land-based ways of life. Early accounts describe northern Indigenous people as being generally healthy (1,2). Their traditional health systems were embedded in holistic world views and resourced by kinship networks, land-based knowledge, nature medicines, and traditional medicine experts (3,4). This changed for the worse with the onset of Western diseases (tuberculosis, small pox, measles, influenza) and the suppression of traditional health systems under the larger Western political and economic systems (1).

Today, like other Indigenous Elders in Canada, northern Indigenous seniors face higher poverty levels and more health problems than the general population of seniors in Canada (5,6), and the challenge of living well is especially difficult because of issues of remoteness and high costs (7). While this is a growing concern for governments and health providers (5,6), it is especially so for Elders and their families. Many fear that they will eventually lose the ability to look after themselves and become dependent on others or even become homeless (2,8,9).

In my own (Bonita) personal and work experience with frail Elders, I found that abandonment, isolation, and being unable to afford necessities are very real fears. As a First Nation Cree from northern Saskatchewan, I remember visiting my widowed aunt in a hospital; she spoke only Cree, and she worried about what would happen to her after she left the hospital, who would take care of her, and where she would live. Further, having helped take care of my own parents before they died and having worked in a health manager position in the North for many years, I know that my late aunt's concerns are a common anxiety among Indigenous Elders. They often live without stable health care supports or are placed in long-term-care facilities away from their home communities and without the appropriate cultural supports (3,7,10). My co-author, Josephine, also a Cree from northern Saskatchewan, shares similar issues in her family. We are not unique. In one of our northern research projects working with Indigenous Elders and caregivers, a participant caregiver also described the same concerns, saying, "modern society assumes that you have everything, like a roof over your head and stuff like that and a caring, giving family. When that's not true. There are some of those homes on reserve ... that are not built for mobility for someone in a wheelchair" (11).

The importance of addressing gaps in stable support services, including long-term care, in the North is crucial and growing. While the issue is gaining greater political profile (6) and positive efforts are being made in some northern regions (12), there remains a need for stable, appropriate funding to build and maintain long-term-care facilities in northern Indigenous communities and in areas closer to home that take in northern factors like population growth, inflation, and remoteness. Furthermore, there is a need for a northern Indigenous Elder/senior care strategy that covers the Far North as well as Provincial Norths.

Briefly Situating Ourselves

We situate ourselves as First Nation authors with a northern Indigenous focus, and while we cannot possibly cover the distinct richness of cultures in the northern Indigenous communities and their health services, we hope to highlight the urgency to improve continuing care services (home care, long-term-care services, palliative and respite care) in northern communities and regions. Situating oneself or *positionality* is a relatively new term that appears to be an emerging requirement in scholarly writing relating to Indigenous peoples, but I (Bonita) use it here as a conversation piece to tell you who we are. My PhD was on First Nations health governance, with much of it based on my own work experiences in the community and in broader levels of government, both provincial and First Nations. Thanks to my now-late parents, I am fluent in the woodland Cree language and also have a Cree linguistics degree from the First Nations University of Canada. My current focus at the university and in my research still relates to northern government policies and service delivery, training, and Indigenous health governance and administration, especially focusing on services that relate to vulnerable populations. First Nations seniors/Elders in care are an example. I helped both my parents at their end-of-life season with things they could no longer do themselves, a role commonly referred to as *care-giving*. My mother who only spoke Cree called it partnership, *wechewitowin*, or walking together – a term denoting equality. I still prefer that term. It took many hands to help both parents, including family members and health professionals, both northern local and urban. Much of the care was about helping to navigate the health care system with all of the seemingly uncoordinated jurisdictional quandaries and rules between programs and services in different locations. Nonetheless, the partnerships forged with health care professionals at various levels were invaluable as far as establishing innovative mechanisms of solving problems together.

My co-writer, Josephine McKay, a former research assistant, is also a Cree First Nation northerner. In her words, she is both a northern Indigenous educator and a researcher, with experience in health care service administration and delivery. She worked with several provincial health regions and a First Nation health authority. She was also a caregiver for several elderly loved ones, who have and continue to receive continuing care services. She has a bachelor of commerce in human resources management, followed by six years of health care human resources experience. She also has a master of business administration (MBA) specializing in Indigenous leadership and health care administration, followed by several years of service in postsecondary education supporting students pursuing health care professions. Furthermore, she also has a master's in northern governance and development, followed by several years as a research associate in health care administration. She is currently with the University College of the North (UCN), which services northern Manitoba, where she started as a college instructor and is now an Indigenous education specialist, supporting all of UCN's program areas, including health.

Terms Used

Northern Indigenous Elders or seniors – These terms are used interchangeably and broadly here to refer to those northerners over 65 years of age (in line with the general reference in the Canada Pension Plan). Notably, some may consider ages 55+ to be a better reflection of the term *senior* in Indigenous communities because of the generally poor health status of Indigenous populations (3,8).

Long-term care – Again as defined by Indigenous Services Canada, "long-term care" is part of "continuing care" but refers solely to "facility-based care" (6 p13) for those needing 24/7 supervised health care and can no longer take care of themselves. This includes medical care, personal care, and other services like meals, laundry, and housekeeping. This term includes nursing homes (13,14).

Continuing care services – As defined by Indigenous Services Canada, this term refers to a spectrum of services, including "home care, community support services, supportive and assisted living and long-term facility-based care, as well as respite services and palliative and end-of-life care" (6 p13; see also 15,16).

Issues of a Growing Elder Population

The Indigenous population in Canada as a whole is growing fast and is young, but it is also aging. This is likely reflective of the Indigenous North as well. According to the 2011 National Household Survey, the Indigenous Elder population (ages 65 and older) made up about 6 per cent of the estimated 1.4 million Indigenous people in Canada (17). By 2016, the Statistics Canada population census reported a growth in the Elder population to 7.3 per cent of the estimated 1.7 million Indigenous people in Canada (18). It also projected the Indigenous Elder population will more than double by 2036 (18). The broad growth trends suggest more pressure on an already pressured health care system in Canada, and this will likely be higher in the North. In most cases, Indigenous families care for their Elders as best they can, but they need support (3,19).

Continuing care services for Indigenous Elders are fragmented in Canada, but are especially so in the North (3,7,20,21). The lack of appropriate and accessible health care services and long-term-care facilities for Elders is a critical issue for the northern regions (3,9,10). For example, current homecare programs have capped hours (weekdays only) thus leaving Elders with limited or no services after hours and on weekends (2), and increasingly Elders are having to leave home to access care (3,6,10). Northern residents, especially Indigenous people, face distinct regional challenges, including poverty, substandard housing, under-resourced health care, lack of long-term-care facilities in communities, limited Elder health services, and lack of needed caregiving supports for families (3,9,10). Shortages of housing, limited homecare, lack of long-term care, jurisdictional barriers, and problems accessing medical technology, equipment, needed supplies, and medications were similarly identified in a 2013 Health Council of Canada Report as the most pressing health needs of First

Nations, Inuit, and Métis seniors (9). Similar issues emerged as key concerns in a 2018 House of Commons report by the Standing Committee on Indigenous and Northern Affairs. It identified challenges of delivering continuing care in First Nation communities (6), and while it addressed First Nations broadly, it included First Nations living in northern remote and isolated regions.

Organization and Delivery of Long-Term-Care Services in Canada: Formal and Informal

Formal Care – An Introduction to the Continuing Care System

The continuing care system is Canada's formal system of care for Elders. It includes home and community care services (homecare), long-term care, respite, and palliative care. It is delivered by a blend of jurisdictions including federal, provincial and territorial, and some municipal governments (15,20,22,23). The federal government also funds the on-reserve First Nations and Inuit health care systems through various health transfer arrangements. For example, in Saskatchewan, since the health services transfers in 1988, the majority of First Nations Bands have designed and delivered their own health services in their communities (24). Health Canada plays a national role in funding, research, and policy analysis through the Canada Health Transfer (13,15,22,23,25). Continuing care is not publicly insured like hospital-based care (26,27). Home care services, for example, are mostly delivered through provincial and territorial government health systems through federal transfer arrangements for health and social services.

Continuing care involves a spectrum of services, which in general include professional health supports that can be delivered at home (homecare), in retirement homes, in long-term-care homes (private and public), and in other assisted living residences. There are three main types of service: home living care (homecare), assisted living, and long-term care. Homecare includes formal support services that enable seniors to stay at home for as long as they are able (26). It includes nursing services, personal care, cleaning, meal preparation, access to adult day programs (meals on wheels, friendly visitor programs), and other supports (28). Assisted living is similar but is provided to those in assisted living residences and retirement homes. Long-term-care homes (or nursing homes) are those facilities that provide 24-hour medical care year-round for those who require high-level care, respite, palliative, and end-of-life care. Access to the publicly funded (subsidized) services occurs through client assessment processes. These processes and the subsequently subsidized services can vary depending on jurisdiction of the health authority. Long-term care is not universally covered, falling outside the Canada Health Act, and is buried in the mix of federal health funding transfers to the provinces (13,14). Like the provinces, each of the three northern territories (Nunavut, Yukon, Northwest Territories) provides its own continuing care services, which are described in more detail below.

COMMUNITY CARE PROGRAMS IN THE TERRITORIES

In Nunavut, the Territorial Home and Continuing Care Program is available to Nunavummiut with a valid Nunavut health care card who have been formally assessed as needing level 2–3 care. For those with higher-level care needs (level 4–5 care), the Department of Health has three continuing care facilities for a total of 28 long-term-care beds in Cambridge Bay, Igloolik, and Gjoa Haven (19,29). There are also assisted living facilities (for those with lower care needs) in Iqaluit, Baker Lake, and Arviat (10,29). Those with significant and complex needs like dementia are referred out of Nunavut to a specialized facility: the Embassy West Senior Living Centre in Ottawa (29). In 2017, Nunavut political leaders from Rankin Inlet pressed the premier and government to find solutions to take better care of Elders at home rather than sending them to residential care facilities located thousands of kilometres from Nunavut (10). The lack of federal resources to build the more specialized long-term-care facilities in Nunavut was reported as the key issue. Recently, the Government of Nunavut proposed the addition of 156 beds spread over all three Nunavut regions, with new long-term-care facilities in Kivalliq, Kitikmeot, and Iqaluit (serving the Qikiqtani region), to address its waiting list and to address higher levels of care, such as for those living with dementia (12).

The *Nunavut Seniors' Information Handbook* produced by the premier of Nunavut, who at the time was also Nunavut's seniors' advocate, provides overviews of the support services available for seniors in the region, ranging from information about pensions, the seniors' fuel subsidy, and housing options to home and continuing care and property tax relief (29). Nunavut, with its large service area and the lower health status of its members, will continue to be challenged in delivering its health services (30). Nunavut has the geographically largest area of all territories and provinces, with its 25 isolated and geographically diverse communities (30). The size of the area, the dispersion of its small communities, the weather, and the reliance on air transportation were some of the key challenges noted in a March 2017 report of the auditor general of Canada on health services in Nunavut (30). Key recommendations in the report included improvements in staffing and staff training, and the need to consult Nunavummiut in the design and delivery of health services and programs (30).

In the Northwest Territories, continuing care services fall under the Department of Health and Social Services, and they include "but are not limited to, nursing care, personal care, supervised or supported living, respite care, palliative care, and care in a facility. Continuing care also includes acute care services related to early discharge from the hospital" (16 para4). The Government of the

Northwest Territories 2017 *Seniors' Information Handbook* provides an overview of seniors' services, including continuing care services: home and community care, long-term care, and supported living (31). The Northwest Territories has nine long-term-care facilities, with one each at Behchokǫ, Fort Simpson, Fort Smith, and Inuvik; two in Hay River; and three in Yellowknife, including the Territorial Dementia Facility and the Stanton Territorial Hospital Extended Care Unit (16). The occupancy rate of the long-term-care facilities in 2013 was estimated at over 95 per cent, with most residents being Elders over 70 years old (19). The challenges in delivering continuing care in the Northwest Territories are also geographically unique to the North, and there is strong reliance on community agencies, such as the NWT Seniors' Society, to provide important social and health advocacy work for Elders (31).

In Yukon, the Department of Health and Social Services provides continuing care services, including long-term care, homecare, and regional therapy services (32). It has five continuing care facilities – four in Whitehorse (Birch Lodge, Copper Ridge Place, Thomson Centre, Macaulay Lodge) and one (McDonald Lodge) in Dawson City (32). The homecare program includes essential homecare services, palliative care, and regional therapy programs. Respite care services are included. A brochure for the *Yukon Home Care Program* has contact information for the various services it offers (32). Elder/senior health care delivery in Yukon faces its own challenges as a northern region. A November 2017 news article reflects some of the concerns raised by a seniors' advocacy group, Seniors Action Yukon, about issues relating to health care, housing, and social services (33). Some key concerns included the relocation of Elders away from their homes and communities without their informed consent and inadequate homecare in the communities by caregivers. Some solutions offered included increasing homecare supports to families in the communities to help people stay home longer, training staff in rural areas, and engaging seniors in the long-term plans to look at the future needs of older adults (33).

Informal Care (Unpaid Family Care)

There is also a lesser known, but increasingly vital, informal family-care health system in the North, which involves families, friends, and other caregivers (3). Homecare was designed to assist Elders and their families with support services that are determined through assessments so that Elders can remain independent and at home for as long as possible (26,27). Indigenous people value and still use the kinship systems in their communities, but all caregivers, regardless of who they are, can become overtaxed and need help at times, especially those caring for loved ones with high-level care needs (11,34,35). Family caregivers provide significant *informal* (meaning unpaid) health care supports to their chronically ill Elders, with often limited support from federal or provincial or territorial governments and health care agencies. This is also increasingly evident for the general population (27). A 2012 Statistics Canada report estimated that over eight million Canadians (about 48 per cent of family members) provided various types of care (transportation, household work, meal preparation, appointment escorts) to their parents and other chronically ill loved ones (36). Another 2012 report by the Health Council of Canada on homecare and the needs of seniors and caregivers used a study sample of five regions (including northern areas like Yukon and the northern health authority in BC) and estimated that family caregivers provided more than three-quarters of required care to seniors and that homecare (professional services) provided the remaining one-quarter (37). If caregiver burnout is a real risk for those caring for high-needs Elders in the general population, with more support resources and more homecare hours to enable appropriate care being recommended (37), then it is even more so for northern caregivers, as evidenced by the few available care facilities discussed above.

In our own case study in 2017 (11) on the caregiving experiences of a sample of First Nation family caregivers (those who managed the care of a parent or grandparent) from northeast Saskatchewan, participants expressed issues and ideas consistent with emerging literature on Elder care. The growing literature on caregiving issues in general suggests patterns that emphasize the significant role that families play in the health care of Elders, and this is no different for Indigenous family caregivers. The help of their families, especially the 24/7 caregivers living with them, is critical for Indigenous seniors in northern regions. It continues to be important to tell their story from their perspective. Fortunately, Indigenous health professionals and researchers working in their communities are starting to fill that gap.

Beatty and McKay – 2017 Case Study of Caregiver Perspectives in Northeastern Saskatchewan

Our caregiver study findings in northeastern Saskatchewan (11) illustrated several common concerns among the interviewed caregivers. Supported by the Canadian Institutes of Health Research Strategy for Patient-Oriented Research, preliminary findings from this small study, as noted above, explored the caregiving experiences of a sample of First Nation family caregivers (those who managed the care of a parent or grandparent) from three reserve communities in northeast Saskatchewan. The communities are part of the northern administrative district in Saskatchewan. While the sample reserves have road access, many of them are several hundred kilometres from the nearest hospital. Caregiver participants were asked to identify what they felt were leading priorities and gaps in the health care services provided to the Elders in the area. The research highlighted an urgency for governments and health agencies to better address Elder care services in the area.

The available health care services identified in the reserves included the primary care nursing services and the First Nation homecare and continuing care programs offered by the First Nations' health centres. Other more specialized health care services were provided in the cities (Flin Flon, Manitoba, 160 kilometres away; and Prince Albert, Saskatchewan, 400 kilometres away) by provincial/regional authorities and included hospital services, homecare services, and, for those eligible, residential 24/7 long-term-care facilities. There are several on-reserve First Nation personal care homes in northern Saskatchewan (not to be confused with the nursing homes that offer subsidized, specialized care) that offer residential care for those generally needing light to medium care (levels 1, 2, and low 3). There are no similar community and reserve-based care facilities in the northeast area, which is of great concern because it means that seniors requiring high-level (3–4) medical care usually have to leave home and family to access that care. Most eligible frail Elders from the northeast area who need higher levels (3–4) of medical care are placed hundreds of kilometres away from their communities in available nursing home facilities or, in some cases, hospitals.

Our overall survey findings suggested that family caregivers wanted to honour the wishes of their loved ones to stay at home, close to family, and be provided with the needed supports from health care professionals and other community services. They also wanted improved and culturally respectful services in hospitals and long-term-care facilities for Indigenous elderly, such as translators to help them communicate with health care providers. Other key recommendations included the need to build long-term-care facilities in or near their communities to better support northern Indigenous seniors, and to develop sustainable and targeted support programs for Indigenous seniors and caregivers, including advocacy services, language supports, culturally responsive care, consistent medical care among rotating physicians who treat the Elder, monitored health care, communication, and health education. All levels of government were advised to enhance existing homecare resources and services in the communities so that they could provide the needed specialized health care services for Elders. Study participants also expressed a need to better link health services across jurisdictions, especially between community health care providers and those working in urban-based hospitals and long-term-care facilities. Overall, the key theme was the desire to ensure that Indigenous Elders are better treated and supported and not made to feel unwelcome as Indigenous people and as Elders.

Summary of the Challenges in Eldercare/Senior Care in the North

As suggested above, health care systems for northern Indigenous peoples are challenged on many fronts (20). According to a 2013 Health Council of Canada report on improving health care for Indigenous seniors, Elders have significant health and social challenges (9). Most are low income and in poor health with multiple chronic health conditions, which can often make it more difficult to access the health services they need. The administration requirements of the federal programs are onerous and can often create problems for Indigenous seniors in northern communities who have to negotiate their care needs in and out of regional, provincial, territorial, and federal health care systems for services that are not available in their home communities (9,11,20). Various barriers such as language and other communication issues such as the *medicalese* used in prescribing medications, can often leave seniors vulnerable to fear and shame for not understanding health professionals, especially when they do not have family members or compassionate health professionals helping them navigate the process (11). This can be a very isolating experience for an Elder. Initial findings from our 2017 study of Indigenous caregivers in northern Saskatchewan suggested similar barriers in health care delivery, including limited health services in the community, language barriers, lack of communication, and lack of proper care (11). One participant noted the constant rotation of doctors who would often prescribe different levels of medication, but they had to deal with "whoever was on call." Much appreciation, however, was indicated for health professionals and staff who addressed the needs of their loved ones respectfully and kindly (11). A health system navigator is one idea that is becoming more common. In the Northwest Territories, for example, a health and social systems navigator helps people navigate the health care and social services system by connecting them to appropriate resources and helping with forms (31).

Strengths, Gaps, and Recommendations

Trends in northern Indigenous health determinants, such as lower incomes, education, housing, jurisdictional issues, and unemployment pressures, will undoubtedly continue to increase the burden on Elders to properly care for themselves (3,6,10,12,34,35,37). Indigenous caregivers are also directly affected, especially those living in remote and isolated northern regions where costs of living are higher. Our caregiver study (11) also highlighted similar concerns about the need to support families caring for parents or grandparents and to invest in building First Nation long-term-care facilities on reserve and in nearby towns and cities to keep Elders at home or close to home. Family visits and support care were considered critical but were often unaffordable for many, with the high transportation costs, accommodation costs, and time off work (especially if travel is more than three hours one way). Other things could be done to help support Elders and families. One is to invest in enhancing home care programs on reserve to cover evenings and weekends and to add palliative and respite care (3,7,9,26,37). Another is to develop transition support programs that link resources and services between the community and the health care facilities so that the Elder does not fall through gaps in care caused by fragmented communication between service providers, including family. Essentially, the continuum of holistic health care should follow the Elders, ensuring dignity of care instead of stopping at the northern community and reserve door. The provision of respectful, sustainable health care should be a common standard and a human right for northern Indigenous Elders wherever they go to access needed health care services (3,6,7,9,21).

It is evident that "northern factor" adjustments should be a part of the funding equations and program designs for northern First Nation and Inuit continuing care services. The lack of long-term-care facilities in First Nation reserves and in northern areas is reflected in most of the northern research relating to continuing care. It is not being appropriately addressed in Canada, and not doing so is increasingly placing northern Indigenous Elders at risk at home without adequate supports for them, as well as for their families (3,10,33,38). It will also increase the costs of health care overall, which will spill over to the broader Canadian community. There is a need for a northern strategy on continuing care for Elders and others in need of such services.

The strengths of continuing care, especially homecare, include its philosophy and practical support services to keep Elders as independent as possible in their homes for as long as they can. It also coincides with Indigenous values of kinship and working together to support the Elders and the vulnerable in society. The weaknesses of continuing care are capped and under-resourced budgets and capped services to the Elders. Enhancing supports at the community level – on the frontlines – is the answer, but it also comes with a need for an appropriate investment of fiscal and human resource supports. While funding is not always considered the answer, when it comes to under-resourced health providers (both formal and informal), it is the needed solution for many of the concerns relating to continuing care. The lack of long-term-care facilities for high-level specialized care, such as for dementia, is a case in point. We are not suggesting unnecessary institutionalization of Indigenous Elders living in northern Canadian communities; rather, a complement of services is needed to allow those who are able to age in place with the continuing care and support they need. However, the messaging across the North is the same: Elders and their family caregivers do not want to forcibly relocate vulnerable Elders to access appropriate care, especially since many experienced similar forced relocations as children to residential schools and other government institutions (39,6,9,12,19). For this to stop, the federal government needs to expand and fund long-term-care services for higher levels of care on reserve and in northern regions (3,14).

REFERENCES

1. Obomsawin R. Traditional medicine for Canada's First Peoples [Internet]. Vancouver (BC): University of British Columbia; 2007 [cited 2019 Aug 7]. Available from: http://lfs-indigenous.sites.olt.ubc.ca/files/2014/07/RayObomsawin.traditional.medicine-1.pdf
2. Young TK. Health care and cultural change: the Indian experience in the central subarctic. Toronto (ON): University of Toronto Press; 1988.
3. Beatty B, Weber-Beeds A. Mitho-pimatisiwin for the elderly: the strength of a shared caregiving approach in Aboriginal health. In: Newhouse D, FitzMaurice, K, McGuire-Adams, T, Jetté, D, editors. Well-being in the urban Aboriginal community. Toronto (ON): Thompson Educational Publishing; 2013. p. 113–30.
4. Inuit Tapiriit Kanatami. Social determinants of Inuit health in Canada [Internet]. Ottawa (ON): Inuit Tapiriit Kanatami; 2014 Sep [cited 2019 Aug 7]. Available from: https://itk.ca/wp-content/uploads/2016/07/ITK_Social_Determinants_Report.pdf
5. Dyck D. Aging Aboriginals pose new fiscal, social challenge for government. CTV News [Internet]. 2017 Oct 25 [cited 2019 Mar 3]. Available from: https://www.ctvnews.ca/canada/aging-aboriginals-pose-new-fiscal-social-challenge-for-government-census-1.3647899
6. Mihychuk MA. The challenges of delivering continuing care in First Nation communities: report of the Standing Committee on Indigenous and Northern Affairs [Internet]; 42nd Parliament, 1st Session; Ottawa (ON): Speaker of the House of Commons (CA); 2018 Dec [cited 2019 Sep 7]. Available from: https://www.ourcommons.ca/Content/Committee/421/INAN/Reports/RP10260656/inanrp17/inanrp17-e.pdf
7. Moffitt P, Timpson B. Influences on quality of life of the older adult in the Northwest Territories [Internet]. Inuvik (NT): Aurora Research Institute and NWT Seniors' Society; 2015 Jan 7 [cited 2019 Aug 4]. Available from: https://nwtresearch.com/sites/default/files/influences_on_qol_of_older_adults_in_the_nwt_report.pdf
8. Assembly of First Nations, Environmental Stewardship Unit. Environmental health older adults and seniors (elders) [Internet]. Ottawa (ON): Assembly of First Nations; 2009 Mar [cited 2017 Oct 10]. Available from: https://www.afn.ca/uploads/files/rp-enviro_health_and_older_adults_and_seniors.pdf
9. Health Council of Canada. Canada's most vulnerable: improving health care for First Nations, Inuit, and Métis seniors [Internet]. Toronto (ON): Health Council of Canada; 2013 [cited 2017 Oct 14]. Available from: https://healthcouncilcanada.ca/files/Senior_AB_Report_2013_EN_final.pdf
10. Sponagel J. Nunavut struggles to care for elders closer to home. CBC News [Internet]. 2017 Jun 5 [cited 2018 Feb 17]. Available from: https://www.cbc.ca/news/canada/north/nunavut-seniors-plan-1.4145757

11. Beatty B; McKay J. Northern Aboriginal caregivers project. 2017. Unpublished manuscript. Available through the first author.
12. Rogers S. Nunavut government moves on plans for long-term care in all three regions. Nunatsiaq News [Internet]. 2019 May 9 [cited 2019 Aug 20]. Available from: https://nunatsiaq.com/stories/article/gn-moves-on-plans-for-long-term-care-in-all-three-regions/
13. Health Canada [Internet]. Ottawa (ON): Health Canada; [modified 2004 Oct 1]. Long-term facilities-based care; [cited 2017 Oct 14]. Available from: https://www.canada.ca/en/health-canada/services/home-continuing-care/long-term-facilities-based-care.html
14. Banerjee A. An overview of long-term care in Canada and selected provinces and territories [Internet]. Toronto (ON): Women and Health Care Reform; 2007 [cited 2017 Oct 17]. Available from: http://www.womenandhealthcarereform.ca/publications/banerjee_overviewLTC.pdf
15. Health Canada [Internet]. Ottawa (ON): Health Canada; [modified 2016 Apr 13]. Home and community health care; [cited 2018 Mar 3]. Available from: https://www.canada.ca/en/health-canada/services/home-continuing-care/home-community-care.html
16. Government of Northwest Territories, Health and Social Services. Continuing care services [Internet]. Yellowknife (NT): Health and Social Services; [cited 2018 Feb 20]. Available from: https://www.hss.gov.nt.ca/en/services/continuing-care-services
17. Statistics Canada [Internet]. Ottawa (ON): Statistics Canada; 2013. Aboriginal peoples in Canada: First Nations people, Métis and Inuit; [modified 2018 Jul 25; cited 2017 Jan 17]. Available from: http://www12.statcan.gc.ca/nhs-enm/2011/as-sa/99-011-x/99-011-x2011001-eng.cfm
18. Statistics Canada [Internet]. Ottawa (ON): Statistics Canada; 2017 Oct 25. Aboriginal Peoples in Canada: Key results from the 2016 census; 2017 Oct 25 [cited 2018 May 17]. Available from: https://www.statcan.gc.ca/daily-quotidien/171025/dq171025a-eng.htm
19. Legislative Assembly of Nunavut (CA). Continuing care in Nunavut, 2015 to 2035 [Internet]. Iqaluit (NU): Legislative Assembly of Nunavut; 2015 Apr [cited 2019 Aug 29]. Available from: https://assembly.nu.ca/sites/default/files/TD%2078-4(3)%20EN%20Continuing%20Care%20in%20Nunavvut,%202015%20to%202035_0.pdf
20. Kelly, MD Toward a new era of policy: health care service delivery to First Nations. Int Indig Policy J [Internet]. 2011 [cited 2018 Feb 1];2(1). Available from: http://ir.lib.uwo.ca/cgi/viewcontent.cgi?article=1017&context=iipj
21. Canadian Health Coalition. Ensuring quality care for all seniors [Internet]. Ottawa (ON): Canadian Health Coalition; 2018 Nov [cited 2019 Aug 4]. Available from: https://www.healthcoalition.ca/wp-content/uploads/2018/11/Seniors-care-policy-paper-.pdf

22. Madore O. The Canada Health Act: overview and options [Internet]. Ottawa (ON): Parliament of Canada, Economics Division; 1995 Jan [revised 2003 Jun 16; cited 2017 Oct 18]. Available from: http://www.publications.gc.ca/Collection-R/LoPBdP/CIR/944-e.htm
23. Allin S, Rudoler D. The Canadian health care system: international health care system profiles [Internet]. New York (NY): The Commonwealth Fund; 2016 Jan. [cited 2018 Feb 17]. Available from: https://www.commonwealthfund.org/sites/default/files/documents/___media_files_publications_fund_report_2016_jan_1857_mossialos_intl_profiles_2015_v7.pdf
24. First Nations and Inuit Health Branch, Saskatchewan Region (CA). Strategic plan, 2014–2019 [Internet]. Ottawa (ON): Health Canada. 2014 [cited 2019 Sep 19]. Available from: http://publications.gc.ca/collections/collection_2014/sc-hc/H34-275-2014-eng.pdf
25. Government of Canada [Internet]. Ottawa (ON): Health Canada; [modified 2016 Aug 22]. Canada's health care system; [cited 2017 Oct 17]. Available from: https://www.canada.ca/en/health-canada/services/canada-health-care-system.html
26. Government of Canada. First Nations and Inuit home and community care (FNIHCC) 10-year plan (2013–2023) [Internet]. Ottawa (ON): Health Canada; 2015 Apr [cited 2017 Oct 17]. Available from: http://publications.gc.ca/collections/collection_2016/sc-hc/H34-282-2015-eng.pdf
27. Canadian Healthcare Association. Home care in Canada: from the margins to the mainstream [Internet]. Ottawa (ON): Canadian Healthcare Association; 2009 [cited 2018 Feb 18]. Available from: https://www.healthcarecan.ca/wp-content/themes/camyno/assets/document/PolicyDocs/2009/External/EN/HomeCareCanada_MarginsMainstream_EN.pdf
28. Stonebridge C, Hermus G, Edenhoffer K. Future care for Canadians seniors: a status quo forecast [Internet]. Ottawa (ON): Conference Board of Canada; 2015 Nov 3 [cited 2018 Feb 17]. Available from: https://www.conferenceboard.ca/e-library/abstract.aspx?did=7374
29. Government of Nunavut [Internet]. Iqaluit (NU): Department of Health; 2018. Home and continuing care; 2018 [cited 2018 Feb 17]. Available from: https://www.gov.nu.ca/health/information/home-and-continuing-care
30. Office of the Auditor General of Canada [Internet]. Ottawa (ON): Office of the Auditor General of Canada; 2017. 2017 March report of the auditor general of Canada: health care services – Nunavut; 2017 Jan 10 [cited 2018 Feb 17]. Available from: https://www.oag-bvg.gc.ca/internet/English/nun_201703_e_41998.html
31. Government of Northwest Territories, NWT Seniors' Society. Seniors' information handbook [Internet]. Yellowkinfe (NT): Department of Health and Social Services; 2017 Sept [cited 2018 Feb 20]. Available from: http://www.hss.gov.nt.ca/sites/hss/files/seniors_information_handbook.pdf

32. Yukon Health and Social Services [Internet]. Whitehorse (YK): Department of Health and Social Services; 2017. Continuing care; 2017 [cited 2018 Feb 17]. Available from: https://www.hss.gov.yk.ca/continuing.php
33. Maguire LN. The Yukon's health care crisis cannot continue. Yukon News [Internet]. 2017 Nov 23 [cited 2018 Apr 20]. Available from: https://www.yukon-news.com/opinion/the-yukons-health-care-crisis-cannot-continue/
34. Parrack S, Gillian MJ. The informal caregivers of Aboriginal seniors: perspectives and issues. First Peoples Child Fam Rev. 2007;3(4):106–11.
35. Health Canada. Continuing care in First Nations and Inuit communities: evidence from research [Internet]. Ottawa (ON): Health Canada; 2007 [cited 2017 Oct 4]. Available from: http://publications.gc.ca/collections/collection_2012/sc-hc/H34-182-2007-eng.pdf
36. Sinha M. Portrait of caregivers, 2012 [Internet]. Ottawa (ON): Statistics Canada; 2013 [modified 2015 Nov 30; cited 2018 Feb 19]. Available from: https://www.statcan.gc.ca/pub/89-652-x/89-652-x2013001-eng.htm
37. Health Council of Canada. Seniors in need, caregivers in distress: what are the home care priorities for seniors in Canada? [Internet]. Toronto (ON): Health Council of Canada; 2012 Apr [cited 2018 Apr 10]. Available from: https://healthcouncilcanada.ca/files/HCC_HomeCare_FA.pdf
38. Cram S. First Nation Family forced off reserve for health care. CBC News [Internet]. 2016 Nov 29 [cited 2018 Apr 10]. Available from: https://www.cbc.ca/news/indigenous/first-nation-family-uprooted-from-reserve-for-health-1.3819879

11 Mental Health and Addictions Care: A Path towards Mental Health Care with Northern Indigenous Peoples

AZAAD KASSAM

Akilak fears that she will never be able to complete her journey. But her grandmother's spirit accompanies her and replaces that fear – with hope. "Caribou looked at Akilak and said with a smile, 'Your destination did not run away, you will reach it soon.'" (1 p6)

This chapter hopes to illuminate challenges in mental health services in Canada's North and offer potential directions for culturally relevant mental health care. I approach this subject as a non-Indigenous, non-white scholar and cultural psychiatrist who has worked clinically with Indigenous and non-Indigenous peoples in the North for two decades. The communities from which I derive these insights are located in northeastern Ontario, including the Cree Nations of the James Bay Coast and Inuit communities of Nunavik (northern Quebec). I highlight some vignettes from my own clinical encounters, as well as innovative projects pertinent to mental health with northern Indigenous communities. The chapter begins with a brief review of essential background history and determinants of mental health, which have been expounded in more detail elsewhere in this book, followed by a discussion of inequities in mental health care in the North. I then explore directions toward better mental health care in the North, including professional development and northern innovation. Last, I offer clinical approaches based on principles of cultural mental health, which are imperative to providing culturally safe and effective mental health care to northern peoples. The "Clinical Encounters" in the boxes in this chapter highlight different stories, each with a unique contribution to describing the importance of cultural safety in northern Indigenous mental health and addictions care.

Historical Context and Contemporary Landscape of Mental Health Care in the North

Northern Indigenous communities in Canada have been deeply affected by colonization (2), a history that has been referred to as "the social murder of the Indigenous body" (3). Beliefs and value systems were stripped away rapidly and violently, disrupting the very foundations of cultural existence. Former Supreme Court of Canada chief justice Beverley McLachlin acknowledged this history as an attempt at "cultural genocide" (4 p7). It is well established that historical trauma is largely responsible for the mental health issues in northern Indigenous communities (5,6). Many communities are suffering with significant psychosocial issues, including suicide, substance use, depression, abuse, violence, intergenerational trauma, and neglect (7,8–13). Youth suicide rates in some northern communities are among the highest in the world (7,14,15). These afflictions represent not only individual pathologies but also interrelational forms of social suffering affecting entire communities (7,13,16).

The North can be defined beyond geography alone by a diversity of northern Indigenous and local cultures, particular local economies, and variability in the way northern communities live, work, and play. Both the commonalities and the variations of northern life influence mental health and well-being, as well as the way services are developed and experienced. Many factors affecting mental health extend beyond the scope of health services and require integration and collaboration among a number of sectors, including health, education, law, social services, and others (17). However, development of mental health care systems remains critically important to addressing the needs of northern Indigenous peoples.

Clinical Encounter 1

A psychiatric consultation was requested for a young Inuk man who had been transported to a southern hospital from his community without family or community members. He was suffering from a terminal illness, and the medical team was concerned that he might require antidepressant medication. The consulting psychiatry resident assessed that he was struggling with the reality of his health situation but that he was not clinically depressed and would not likely benefit from psychotropic medication. The patient felt that he would be best served by consuming traditional Inuit country food, such as caribou and fresh raw fish, but this was viewed with skepticism by the medical team. The psychiatry resident advocated with the medical unit to facilitate access to these foods and to arrange for his family to join him. As a result, therapeutic alliance with the team improved and mutual understanding and respect developed. Consumption of country food helped him to gain strength and healing. Supportive psychotherapy helped both the young man and his parents to grieve the illness and ultimate loss (14). In this example, it was important to recognize the connection with the land and its healing power, based on the Inuit concept of ecocentrism – an intimate connection to the land as a living and sustaining being (5,18).

Determinants of Mental Health in the North

Many social factors are powerful determinants of mental health and span the levels of individual, family, community, and society. Determinants of mental health align with many of the social determinants of health for Indigenous peoples, such as those described by Reading and Wien (17), and include the following (5,3,12–14,18–39):

- Public health infrastructure
- Stable, secure, and safe housing
- Employment and economic stability
- Food security and nutrition
- Personal or family history of residential school attendance
- Personal or family history of mental illness and addiction
- Effective parenting and intergenerational communication
- Access to education and early childhood development opportunities
- A safe school environment and freedom from bullying and abuse
- Social inclusion and positive personal relationships
- Freedom from discrimination and racism
- Health equity and access to culturally safe health services
- Cultural continuity, local control of services, and self-determination
- Access to land and land-based traditional activities
- Climate change

These determinants intermingle in complex ways and should be conceptualized as fluid, rather than discrete. Among these determinants, the influence of historical factors and cultural change is striking, many representing the negative impacts of colonialism. The variety of factors that determine mental health in northern and Indigenous communities is, thus, extensive in breadth and depth.

Clinical Encounter 2

A man was transferred to a hospital acute psychiatry unit after presenting himself to local police in his remote northern community. He had been feeling that he had committed a grave sin and that certain people in the community were sending him telepathic signals. He was convinced that the devil would come to get him and that he would soon go to hell, which made him contemplate suicide and try to obtain a firearm. He had been clear of any substance use over the past year and had been working in a skilled trade. On the mental health unit, he was quite afraid of punishment, which he felt he deserved. He was withdrawn and felt very confined. As per legal requirements for safety, he had to remain in hospital. The psychiatrist explored with him what might help him with his distress, and the man asked for a priest. In the past, he had also benefited from Indigenous spiritual traditions. The hospital Native Services Department was consulted. Antipsychotic medication had been started at the referring hospital. Usual protocol would not allow for a new patient to leave the mental health unit until there was some certainty that he could manage and remain safe. Recognizing the patient's intolerable feelings of confinement and his culture's value of open space as potentially healing, the psychiatrist facilitated time off the unit. The man benefited from time with his family members away from the hospital ward, and trust with the mental health team improved.

Mental Health Care Inequity

Access to mental health care in northern Indigenous communities compared to southern settler communities is not equitable (40,41). Access to mental health professionals and healers is limited, and facilities are often inadequate (12,42). Clients with mental health issues are supported by community members, nurses, social workers, and community mental health workers often working in isolation (14). Northern communities have suffered from a lack of investment in mental health and addiction services (43,44). Funding is often transient and inadequate, making sustainable programming precarious (20).

Fluctuations in government and health system leadership have led to the building of mental health care infrastructure that are then decimated some time later. As a result, northern mental health professionals provide care in a system that is often unstable, overwhelmed, and poorly designed to meet the needs of those suffering from mental illness. Support is limited for interdisciplinary services, including Indigenous-led, culture-based intervention.

Clinical Encounter 3

An Indigenous man in a northern community sought medical attention for mental distress associated with finances and marital issues. He had developed symptoms of clinical depression and had recently been turning to cannabis to cope with worry and insomnia. He presented as intelligent and thoughtful but quite dysthymic. He had a past history of depression, his father had died from suicide many years earlier, and his mother had longstanding depression and had benefited from antidepressant medication. During difficult and depressed times in the past, he had engaged with Indigenous healing methods, including sweat lodge, sage, sweet grass, tobacco, and cedar. However, he had become so low, withdrawn, and preoccupied with his worldly problems that he had lost his connection to his cultural practices and spiritual existence. The consulting psychiatrist suggested re-engaging in traditional healing, the possibility of marital counselling, and referral to social work to explore financial issues. Motivational interviewing explored culturally safe programs for substance use. Given the longstanding, persistent depression with a significant family history, the psychiatrist offered an explanation of how brain chemistry might be relevant and described the potential benefits and risks of antidepressant medication. In this way, the patient was able to pursue both psychiatric and traditional remedies for his condition.

Many hospitals in the North and elsewhere house Indigenous service programs that are supposed to meet the needs of Indigenous clients. However, these often operate with minimal human and other resources, which can lead to disappointing results. For the client, this system can then become another source of trauma, rather than a source of healing and recovery.

When northern communities don't have the financial, architectural, and professional resources to provide care for a person experiencing mental illness, the alternative is to transfer the individual to a larger hospital centre located far from home (45). Likewise, addiction centres are often located far from clients' home communities, and the client returns from treatment to the same situations and stressors with little or no aftercare (46). Although there is a role for centralized, specialized service, institutions often fail to appreciate the local circumstances of the client and do not facilitate the supports necessary for culturally safe care (14). Even in large centres, the mainstream mental health system is often disjointed and unable to meet the needs of its proximal population. Having areas in the North feed into these inadequate systems (or try to mimic them) can result in poor outcomes.

A Journey towards Better Mental Health Care in the North

Based on in-depth and collaborative research discussion, the Mental Health Commission of Canada offers strategic direction to improve mental health and well-being in northern Indigenous populations (47,48). The commission emphasizes the need to heal the intergenerational impacts of colonization and to respond to the intergenerational trauma associated with residential schools, in particular. It recommends addressing poor living conditions, increasing funding, closing gaps in services, providing incentives to attract mental health service providers to the North, enhancing local job opportunities, supporting contextually appropriate mental health programs, ensuring cultural safety, strengthening coordination and communication with communities and health system structures, and increasing access to tele-mental health and e-mental health.

The following describes some of these issues in more detail, with a focus on the importance of recruiting and retaining northern mental health professionals, valuing local knowledges and northern innovation for the improvement of mental health services, and providing culturally safe care.

Northern Mental Health Professionals

Clinical Encounter 4

A young man from a remote northern Indigenous community sought help for suicidal thoughts after his wife left him. He had been struggling with use of multiple substances over a number of years. Further exploration revealed that many of his family members had died in a tragic accident when he was a teenager. In his grief, he had turned to drugs and alcohol to cope and often fantasized about ending his life so that he might join his family. The marital breakup had triggered feelings of loss, abandonment, fear, and anger. The psychiatrist acknowledged the trauma and the resilience the man had shown in surviving a horrific event, provided a physically and emotionally safe space, offered a small amount of medication for acute relief of anxiety and withdrawal, and explored with him the notion of spiritual reconnection. It was suggested that he might want to consider culturally based addiction programs and a consultation with an Indigenous traditional healer.

Educational institutions play a critical role in the development of culturally sensitive professionals who will work with communities to ultimately transform mental health care in the North. Culture-based mental health training, including in Indigenous history, health, and healing, remains inadequate across most medical schools, psychiatry residencies, and other mental health training programs (49). Training students from northern communities in health and healing professions can have a significant impact on access to mental health care (50). Indigenous mental health professionals in Canada are few, and the need is great for such individuals to be developed and supported in leading change in northern communities (51). The training of Indigenous health professionals in Canada has been limited, primarily because of racism and historical lack of opportunity (52). The medical community has recently made efforts to address this disparity. The University of British Columbia trains medical students in its Northern Medical Program each year, including a cohort of Indigenous students, many of whom go on to serve northern Indigenous communities (53). The Northern Ontario School of Medicine focuses on locally relevant innovation and training. Many of its graduating doctors stay in northern Ontario and provide primary and specialized mental health care to rural, remote, and urban northern communities (54).

Recruitment and retention of mental health professionals is an important source of service provision. Incentives such as student loan repayments, benefits, and academic opportunities can attract well-trained professionals to northern communities. Such recruits need to be provided with opportunities to develop local knowledge and cultural competence in the areas in which they work. Retention of such professionals depends on how well they integrate into the community, the opportunities for career growth and contribution, how their personal circumstances develop, and the opportunities available for their families (54). As discussed by Møller in this volume (chapter 8), professionals who add the greatest value to the North and can work effectively are those who are able to develop longer relationships with communities and understand local customs and cultural nuances.

Northern Innovation

Clinical Encounter 5

A northern Indigenous woman is admitted to intensive care after accidental overdose with opiates and alcohol. She had been in foster care as a child and has a history of childhood sexual abuse. Her parents were both survivors of residential school and had subsequently struggled with their own mental health and addiction issues. She has longstanding issues with self-esteem, identity, and relationships, as well as unstable moods and impulsivity. The doctor asks her about her cultural background and practices, but she has been disconnected from Indigenous traditions and faith. The question triggers her recollection of her mother engaging in the practice of smudging and the patient has a positive association with this memory. The patient suggests that she could visit a healing centre close to her community. She had tried to see a mental health professional for depression and attend an addiction program specialized in opiate dependence but was still on the very long waitlist for services.

Northern innovation is essential to the development of effective mental health care in northern Canada. Mental health services tend to be more successful when initiated and based in the community (14). Yet many decisions about northern health care services and their funding occur at a great distance from the regions for which they are intended. Decisions are often made by administrators who have never lived or worked in the North; few are made by Indigenous leaders (19). Frequently, northern institutions hire "expert" consultants from the south whose primary frame of reference is large, urban, and southern.

Their recommendations often fail because they have not been able to fully appreciate the local challenges that can only be understood by living in the North. Good decisions require an understanding of the history, cultures, values, strengths, and challenges of a community (21). A salient example of northern leadership is the National Inuit Suicide Prevention Strategy, an Inuit-led mental health initiative grounded in appreciating Inuit culture, history, health, and context. It highlights six priority areas of focus: creating social equity, creating cultural continuity, nurturing healthy Inuit children from birth, ensuring access to a continuum of mental wellness services for Inuit, healing unresolved trauma and grief, and mobilizing Inuit knowledge for resilience and suicide prevention (26). Partnerships between northern institutions, local communities, Indigenous organizations, civil society, and government are critical if efforts to improve mental health services are to succeed (34).

Technology, the internet, and social media play an evolving and somewhat unpredictable role in reaching, connecting, and influencing northern populations. Greater connectivity does not necessarily lead to greater interpersonal connection. Indeed, technology can be isolating, reducing real social contact with community and land (32). However, when engaged on a foundation of cultural values and ethical, thoughtful implementation, technologies can be an innovative way to offer services to remote and underserviced communities. Videoconferencing is now a well-established method of providing mental health consultation. Telehealth research suggests that many clients and providers find it to be a useful modality to receive service that would otherwise require travel (55–57). Whether via technology or in person, the standard medical-psychiatric model of consultation has significant limitations, including assumptions about its validity, usefulness, and cultural relevance (14). Effective mental health consultation requires a humble approach to listening, an appreciation of local culture, and thoughtfulness about what recommendations will be helpful and achievable in the patient's northern context (14).

Culture and Spirituality: The Foundation for Healing

Cultural safety is a necessary foundation for working with northern Indigenous clients (13,47–48). Yet many Indigenous people continue to feel unsafe in mainstream health services (58). Culture forms the backdrop for the expression of distress. It offers explanations of why someone is suffering, as well as direction on how to alleviate it. Mental health professions based in Western biopsychosocial theories ascribe to a particular world view, with its own values and ways of communicating. We tend to implicitly consider our own professional knowledge to be superior to other ways of understanding (epistemological hegemony). We tend to talk about what we "know" about something, but what others "believe" (59). Might there be other ways of understanding an experience? Is it possible to view an issue through both a psychiatric and a spiritual lens? We must give our professional narcissism a dose of cultural humility. Listening respectfully to understand clients' narratives, the meaning of their experiences, and their social context can help to create a safe clinical environment. Self-examining biases, including unconscious racism, is an important part of working with culture. Useful clinical tools, such as the Cultural Formulation, can assist clinicians to better comprehend their client's predicament and approach intervention from a more culturally informed perspective (59).

Mental health practitioners and decision makers working with northern Indigenous peoples must be guided by the voices of the communities they are serving. Culture refers not only to "otherness" in ethnicity, race, and religion but to local norms, values, histories, and ways of living (59, 60). In a notable study, a broad group of Indigenous Elders highlighted the importance of community involvement and cultural identity: "The beginning of any journey in Indigenous communities is to situate oneself – who are you and where do you come from?" (16 p21). Culturally safe programs are grounded in Indigenous knowledge and recognize cultural diversity and the influence that social inequalities and imbalances in power have on relationships between service provider and service user (47,48). All mental health practice is cultural. All healing is spiritual (16 p20).

Cultural Safety and Pluralism in Mental Health Care: Integration of Indigenous and Western Knowledge

Intergenerational and personal trauma is all too common among northern Indigenous peoples. When working with individuals and families, clinicians must be sensitive to the likelihood that clients have experienced trauma, and they must apply the core principles of trauma-informed care, including trauma awareness, safety and trust, empowerment, choice and collaboration, and cultural awareness (61). Culturally consonant psychotherapy can be useful but must understand local and historical context, as well as challenges of the modern world, such as social media and technologies. The First Nations Mental

Health Continuum Framework provides a useful model of empathic mental health care and recovery. It brings together knowledge of multiple Indigenous traditions and emphasizes four important outcomes for mental well-being: hope, meaning, purpose, and belonging (34). These critical elements have proven invaluable in therapies with both northern Indigenous and non-Indigenous patients.

A variety of culture-based therapies have been successful in improving mental wellness in northern communities, including sweat lodge, smudging, cedar baths, soul retrieval, powwow, hunting camps, fishing camps, equine therapy, culture-based counselling, creative arts therapies, and traditional plant-based medicines (19). Land-based healing can be particularly effective in youth (7,14). As well, creative arts therapies, such as theatre, dance, visual arts, and music, may have particular resonance with the youth population (14,62) and have been shown to have positive impacts in promoting health, positive relationships, mental wellness, community building, and resilience with northern youth (62).

Indigenous peoples, however, including those in various regions of northern Canada, have a diversity of cultures. Individuals and families may diverge in how they conceptualize issues and how best to approach healing journeys. Models of mental health assumed to be universal may not resonate with some families or individuals, and Western-based therapies have limits in what they can achieve (13,14). Engaging with Indigenous knowledge requires going beyond narrowly defined evidence-based practice to appreciating a more holistic understanding of evidence: "Indigenous epistemologies and other forms of evidence offer additional and equally important ways of understanding interventions" (63 p2). It can be helpful to view mental health struggles through multiple lenses – diagnostic, psychodynamic, existential, and spiritual – drawing on Western and Indigenous knowledge. Some Indigenous Knowledge Keepers refer to this as two-eyed seeing. Help may come from Western disciplines; from traditional Indigenous knowledge, faith, and ceremony; and from the development of novel and creative forms of healing. Pluralism values diversity, respect, fairness, and exchange and enhances cultural safety.

True integration of Indigenous and Western healing traditions is more effective than adding an Indigenous component to an institution that otherwise operates entirely on Western methods. In Yukon, Whitehorse General Hospital houses a robust First Nations health program where a team of over a dozen individuals with various Indigenous-based skills provide services to all patients who want to use them. Traditional foods, such as bannock and meats such as caribou and moose obtained by local hunters, are served. Physicians work with Native medicine practitioners in an integrative model in which both Western and traditional Native medicines are provided (64).

Towards a Path of Healing

Mental wellness in northern Indigenous communities will require broad, community-driven efforts that include, but extend well beyond, the provision of adequate mental health care. Clinicians, administrators, politicians, and the public must understand the traumatic history of colonization, disempowerment, and the challenges of northern mental health and addiction services. Truth and reconciliation are foundational to healing for mental health and wellness in the North. Leaders from the south and the North must care for the spirit of the people and invest time, energy, and resources into mental health and addiction care. Failing to properly fund mental health initiatives from the community level through to tertiary care will only worsen an epidemic crisis and increase financial and human cost. Northern and Indigenous communities need the opportunity to take charge of their own recovery and lead change in developing local approaches towards research, prevention, and healing. Invariably, this involves reappropriation and renewal of traditional cultural values. Northern institutions play a pivotal role in empowering and facilitating long-term change that is equitable, responsive, and innovative. Genuine collaboration between government, community, and civil society is necessary to shift historically oppressive structures and empower northern Indigenous communities (3,18,19–21). Northern Indigenous world views envision a holistic shift: "We have to do something assertive with our societal foundations" (18).

Mental health practices must be rethought and adapted to the local social and cultural realities of the North. Cultural safety, idioms of distress, and social conditions must be considered. Pluralism in mental health care offers greater choice and opportunity to draw upon different traditions for health and healing. Viewing mental health and addiction through multiple lenses facilitates an integrated, culturally informed approach to care. Engaging with Indigenous knowledge with genuine curiosity and openness will facilitate progression from mere tolerance of other forms of knowing to the integration of health systems.

Northern Indigenous peoples deserve the opportunity to develop positive assets, such that resilience prevails in the face of adversity. With an increasing juxtaposition of traditional culture with modern global citizenry, it will be crucial for northerners to discover a sense of belonging, a purpose with which to move forward, a spiritual meaning for existence, and the inspiration of hope. Mental health clinicians can draw upon their own culture and spirit to serve their clients' healing journey. Recognize that no one is alone in dealing with the hardships of people; like the title character in Deborah Kigjugalik Webster's *Akilak's Adventure* (1), we are guided by the ancestors of our patients and of ourselves (21). All mental health practice is cultural. All healing is spiritual. It may be in the Creator's gift where we ultimately find mental health: "Go to the bush, listen to the trees" (21).

REFERENCES

1. Kigjugalik Webster D. Akilak's adventure. Iqaluit (NU): Inhabit Media Inc; 2016.
2. United Nations declaration on the rights of Indigenous peoples. Geneva (CH): United Nations; March 2008.
3. Lavallee B. Removing culture from cultural safety: structural challenges to addressing Indigenous health in Canada. Keynote speech at: Towards health and reconciliation. Annual University of Toronto Faculty of Medicine Indigenous Health Conference; 2016 May 26–27; Toronto, ON.
4. McLachlin B. Reconciling unity and diversity in the modern era: Tolerance and intolerance. Lecture presented at: Annual Pluralism Lecture of the Global Centre for Pluralism; 2015 May 28; Toronto, ON.
5. Boksa P, Joober R, Kirmayer L. Mental wellness in Canada's Aboriginal communities: striving toward reconciliation. J Psychiatry Neurosci. 2015;40(6):363–5.
6. Culhane D. Narratives of hope and despair in downtown eastside Vancouver. In: Kirmayer L, Valaskakis G, editors. Healing traditions: the mental health of Aboriginal peoples in Canada. Vancouver (BC): UBC Press; 2009. p. 221–48.
7. Kirmayer J, Fletcher C, Watt R. Locating the ecocentric self: Inuit concepts of mental health and illness. In: Kirmayer L, Valaskakis G, editors. Healing traditions: the mental health of Aboriginal peoples in Canada. Vancouver (BC): UBC Press; 2009. p. 289–314.
8. Young TK, Rawat R, Dallmann W, Chatwood S, Bjerregaard P, editors. Circumpolar health atlas. Toronto (ON): University of Toronto Press; 2012.
9. Chachamovich E, Kirmayer L, Haggarty J, Cargo M, McCormick R, Turecki G. Suicide among Inuit: results from a large, epidemiologically representative follow-back study in Nunavut. Can J of Psychiatry. 2015;60(6):268–75.
10. Public Health Agency of Canada. The human face of mental health and mental illness in Canada 2006 [Internet]. Ottawa (ON): Public Health Agency of Canada. 2016 [cited 2017 Nov 27]. Available from: https://www.phac-aspc.gc.ca/publicat/human-humain06/pdf/human_face_e.pdf
11. Kielland N, Simeone T. Current issues in mental health care in Canada: the mental health of first nations and Inuit communities (in brief) [Internet]. Ottawa (ON): Library of Parliament; 2014 Jan 6 [cited 2017 Nov 27]. Publication No.: 2014-02-E. Available from: https://lop.parl.ca/staticfiles/PublicWebsite/Home/ResearchPublications/InBriefs/PDF/2014-02-e.pdf
12. Kirmayer L, Brass G. Addressing global health disparities among Indigenous peoples. Lancet [Internet]. 2016 [cited 2017 Nov 27];388(10040):105–6. Available from: http://www.thelancet.com/journals/lancet/article/PIIS0140-6736(16)30194-5
13. Kirmayer L, Brass G, Guthrie G. Conclusion: Healing/invention/tradition. In: Kirmayer L, Valaskakis G, editors. Healing traditions: the mental health of Aboriginal peoples in Canada. Vancouver (BC): UBC Press; 2009. p. 440–72.

14. Kassam A. Encounters with the North: psychiatric consultation with Inuit youth. J Can Acad Child Adolesc Psychiatry [Internet]. 2006 [cited 2017 Nov 27];15(4): 174–8. Available from: https://www.ncbi.nlm.nih.gov/pmc/articles/PMC2277306/
15. Kral M. Postcolonial suicide among Inuit in Arctic Canada. Cult Med Psychiatry [Internet]. 2012 [cited 2017 Nov 27];36(2):306–25. Available from: http://www.ncbi.nlm.nih.gov/pubmed/22392639
16. Mehl-Madrona L. What traditional Indigenous Elders say about cross-cultural mental health training. Explore: J Sci Healing [Internet]. 2009 [cited 2017 Nov 27];5(1):20–9. Available from: http://www.ncbi.nlm.nih.gov/pubmed/19114260
17. Reading CL, Wien F. (2009). Health inequalities and social determinants of Aboriginal Peoples' health. Prince George (BC): National Collaborating Centre for Aboriginal Health.
18. Obed N. [no title]. Keynote speech presented at: Towards health and reconciliation. Annual University of Toronto Faculty of Medicine Indigenous Health Conference; 2016 May 26–27; Toronto, ON.
19. Day I. [no title]. Opening keynote speech presented at: Towards health and reconciliation. Annual University of Toronto Faculty of Medicine Indigenous Health Conference; 2016 May 26–27; Toronto, ON.
20. Blackstock C. Reconciliation means not saying sorry twice: remedying contemporary inequalities in First Nations children's health and wellbeing. Keynote speech presented at: Towards health and reconciliation. Annual University of Toronto Faculty of Medicine Indigenous Health Conference; 2016 May 26–27; Toronto, ON.
21. Littlechild W. [no title]. Keynote speech presented at: Towards health and reconciliation. Annual University of Toronto Faculty of Medicine Indigenous Health Conference; 2016 May 26–27; Toronto, ON.
22. Willison R, Fobister S Sr., Suzuki D, Mergler D. Panel presented at: Towards health and reconciliation. Annual University of Toronto Faculty of Medicine Indigenous Health Conference; 2016 May 26–27; Toronto, ON.
23. Chandler MJ, Lalonde CE. Cultural continuity as a moderator of suicide risk among Canada's First Nations. In: Kirmayer L, Valaskakis G, editors. Healing traditions: The mental health of Aboriginal peoples in Canada. Vancouver (BC): UBC Press; 2009. p. 221–48.
24. Young T, Chatwood S. Health care in the North: what Canada can learn from its circumpolar neighbours. CMAJ [Internet]. 2010 [cited 2017 Nov 27];183(2): 209–14. Available from: https://www.cmaj.ca/content/183/2/209
25. Kaspar V. The lifetime effect of residential school attendance on Indigenous health status. Am J Public Health [Internet]. 2014 [cited 2017 Nov 27];104(11):2184–90. Available from: http://www.ncbi.nlm.nih.gov/pubmed/24328622
26. Inuit Tapiriit Kanatami. National Inuit suicide prevention strategy [Internet]. Ottawa (ON): Inuit Tapiriit Kanatami; 2016 [cited 2017 Nov 27]. Available from:

http://www.itk.ca/wp-content/uploads/2016/07/ITK-National-Inuit-Suicide-Prevention-Strategy-2016.pdf

27. Kral M, Salusky I, Inuksuk P, Angutimarik L, Tulugardjuk N. Tunngajuq: Stress and resilience among Inuit youth in Nunavut, Canada. Transcult Psychiatry [Internet]. 2014 [cited 2017 Nov 27];51(5):673–92. Available from: http://www.ncbi.nlm.nih.gov/pubmed/24838171
28. Leske S, Harris MG, Charlson FJ, Ferrari AJ, Baxter AJ, Logan JM, Toombs M, Whiteford H. Systematic review of interventions for Indigenous adults with mental and substance use disorders in Australia, Canada, New Zealand and the United States. Aust NZ J Psychiatry [Internet]. 2016 [cited 2017 Nov 27];50(11):1040–54. Available from: http://www.ncbi.nlm.nih.gov/pubmed/27514405
29. Minore B, Boone M, Katt M, Kinch P, Birch S. Addressing the realities of health care in northern Aboriginal communities through participatory action research. J Interprof Care [Internet]. 2004 [cited 2017 Nov 27];18(4):360–8. Available from: http://www.ncbi.nlm.nih.gov/pubmed/15801551
30. Niezen R. Suicide as a way of belonging: causes and consequences of cluster suicides in Aboriginal communities. In: Kirmayer L, Valaskakis G, editors. Healing traditions: the mental health of Aboriginal peoples in Canada. Vancouver (BC): UBC Press; 2009. p. 178–95.
31. Métis Nation of Ontario [Internet]. Ottawa (ON): Métis Nation of Ontario; 2017. Mental health and addictions in the Métis Nation of Ontario fact sheet; 2017 [cited 2017 Nov 27]. Available from: http://www.metisnation.org
32. Petrasek MacDonald J, Cunsolo Willox A, Ford J, Shiwak I, Wood M. Protective factors for mental health and well-being in a changing climate: perspectives from Inuit youth in Nunatsiavut, Labrador. Soc Sci Med [Internet]. 2015 [cited 2017 Nov 27];14(1):133–41. Available from: http://www.ncbi.nlm.nih.gov/pubmed/26275362
33. Redvers J, Bjerregaard P, Eriksen H, Fanian S, Healey G, Hiratsuka V, Jong M, Larsen CV, Linton J, Pollock N, Silviken A, Stoor P, Chatwood S. A scoping review of Indigenous suicide prevention in circumpolar regions. Int J Circumpolar Health [Internet]. 2015 [cited 2017 Nov 27];74(1):27509. Available from: https://www.ncbi.nlm.nih.gov/pmc/articles/PMC4981753/
34. Restoule B, Hopkins C, Robinson J, Wiebe P. First Nations mental wellness: mobilizing change through partnership and collaboration. Can J Community Ment Health [Internet]. 2015 [cited 2017 Nov 27]; 34(4):89–109. Available from: http://www.cjcmh.com/doi/abs/10.7870/cjcmh-2015-014
35. Shankar J, Ip E, Khalema E, Couture J, Tan S, Zulla RT, Lam G. Education as a social determinant of health: issues facing Indigenous and visible minority students in postsecondary education in Western Canada. Int J Environ Res Public Health [Internet]. 2013 [cited 2017 Nov 27];10(9):3908–29. Available from: http://www.ncbi.nlm.nih.gov/pubmed/23989527

36. Tanner A. The origins of northern aboriginal social pathologies and the Quebec Cree healing movement. In: Kirmayer L, Valaskakis G, editors. Healing traditions: the mental health of Aboriginal peoples in Canada. Vancouver (BC): UBC Press; 2009. p. 249–71.
37. Wieman C. Six nations mental health services: a model of care for aboriginal communities. In: Kirmayer L, Valaskakis G, editors. Healing traditions: the mental health of Aboriginal peoples in Canada. Vancouver (BC): UBC Press; 2009. p. 401–18.
38. Williamson A, Andersen M, Redman S, Dadds M, D'Este C, Daniels J, Eades S, Raphael B. Measuring mental health in Indigenous young people: a review of the literature from 1998–2008. Clin Child Psychol Psychiatry [Internet]. 2014 [cited 2017 Nov 27];19(2):260–72. Available from: http://www.ncbi.nlm.nih.gov/pubmed/23737609
39. Zinck K, Marmion S. Global focus, local acts: providing mental health services to Indigenous people. Arch Psychiatr Nurs [Internet]. 2011 [cited 2017 Nov 27];25(5):311–9. Available from: http://www.ncbi.nlm.nih.gov/pubmed/21978799
40. Mathieu-Léger L, Kassam A. A First Nations community grappling with suicide crisis: "We're crying out for help." Guardian [Internet]. 2016 Apr 16 [cited 2017 Nov 27]. Available from: http://www.theguardian.com/world/2016/apr/16/canada-first-nations-suicide-crisis-attawapiskat-history
41. First Nations Child and Family Caring Society of Canada [Internet]. Ottawa (ON): First Nations Child and Family Caring Society of Canada; 2016. Jordan's principle; [updated 2021 Jan; cited 25 Nov 2017]. Available from: https://fncaringsociety.com/jordans-principle
42. Canadian Mental Health Association [Internet]. Toronto (ON): Canadian Mental Health Association; 2009. Rural and northern community issues in mental health; 2009 [cited 2017 Nov 27]. Available from: https://ontario.cmha.ca/documents/rural-and-northern-community-issues-in-mental-health/
43. Paltiel C, Foote V. Canada's rings of fire [Internet]. Mining Stories Productions, producers. Doha (QA): Al Jazeera Media Network. 2015 Jul 29 [cited 2017 Nov 27]. Video: 47:15 mins. Available from: http://www.aljazeera.com/programmes/witness/2015/07/rings-fire-150729124056943.html
44. Kandola K. Mental health in circumpolar Canada [Internet]. Yellowknife (NT): Canadian Society for Circumpolar Health; [2013?] [cited 2017 Nov 27]. Available from: https://a14c0b8b-8b55-4dca-8c23-8c3e0782aa2a.filesusr.com/ugd/a36a20_1415fc9fdd58456295e5b9db5ede7cb6.pdf
45. Jetty R. Understanding Inuit culture: an imperative for mental health care. Lecture presented at: University of Ottawa Culture and Psychiatry Seminar Series; 2017; Ottawa, ON.
46. Jiwa A, Kelly L, Pierre-Hansen N. Healing the community to heal the individual: literature review of aboriginal community-based alcohol and substance abuse

programs. Can Fam Physician [Internet]. 2008 Jul [cited 2017 Nov 27];54(7): 1000–1000.e7. Available from: http://www.ncbi.nlm.nih.gov/pubmed/18625824

47. Mental Health Commission of Canada. Changing directions, changing lives: the mental health strategy for Canada [Internet]. Calgary (AB): Mental Health Commission of Canada; 2012 [cited 2017 Nov 27]. Available from: https://www.mentalhealthcommission.ca/sites/default/files/MHStrategy_Strategy_ENG.pdf
48. Mental Health Commission of Canada. Working with First Nations, Inuit and Métis. In: Guidelines for recovery-oriented practice [Internet]. Ottawa (ON): Mental Health Commission of Canada; 2015 [cited 2017 Nov 27]. p. 66–77. Available from: http://www.mentalhealthcommission.ca/sites/default/files/MHCC_RecoveryGuidelines_ENG_0.pdf
49. Kirmayer J, Fung K, Rousseau C, Lo H, Menzies P, Guzder J, Ganesan S, Andermann L, McKenzie K. Guidelines for training in cultural psychiatry. Can J of Psychiatry [Internet]. 2011[cited 2017 Nov 27];57(3):1–17. Available from: http://www.multiculturalmentalhealth.ca/wp-content/uploads/2013/10/2012_CPA_Training-in-Cultural-PsychiatryEN.pdf
50. Strasser R, Hogenbirk JC, Minore B, Marsh DC, Berry S, Mccready WG, Graves L. Transforming health professional education through social accountability: Canada's Northern Ontario School of Medicine. Med Teach. 2013 [cited 2017 Nov 27];35(6):490–6. doi: 10.3109/0142159X.2013.774334
51. Canadian Federation of Medical Students [Internet]. Ottawa (ON): Canadian Federation of Medical Students; 2017 [cited 26 Nov 2017]. Available from: http://www.cfms.org
52. Eacott A. Racism, lack of resources "barriers" for Indigenous medical students. ABC News [Internet]. 2015 Sep 24 [cited 26 Nov 2017]. Available from: http://www.abc.net.au/news/2015-09-24/racism-a-barrier-for-indigenous-medical-students-being-doctors/6802730
53. University of Northern British Columbia [Internet] Prince George (BC): University of Northern British Columbia; 2017. Northern Medical Program; 2017 [cited 25 Nov 2017]. Available from: http://www.unbc.ca/northern-medical-program
54. Northern Ontario School of Medicine [Internet]. Thunder Bay (ON): Northern Ontario School of Medicine; 2017 [cited 26 Nov 2017]. Available from: http://www.nosm.ca
55. Gibson K, Coulson H, Miles R, Kakekakekung C, Daniels E, O'Donnell S. Conversations on telemental health: listening to remote and rural First Nations communities. Rural Remote Health [Internet]. 2011 [cited 26 Nov 2017];11:1656. Available from: http://www.rrh.org.au/journal/article/1656
56. Gibson K, O'Donnell S, Coulson H, Kakepetum-Schultz T. Mental health professionals' perspectives of telemental health with remote and rural First Nations communities. J Telemed Telecare [Internet]. 2011 [cited 26 Nov 2017];17(5):263–7. Available from: http://www.ncbi.nlm.nih.gov/pubmed/21824967

57. Monthuy-Blanc J, Bouchard S, Maïano C, Séguin M. Factors influencing mental health providers' intention to use telepsychotherapy in First Nations communities. Transcult Psychiatry [Internet]. 2013 [cited 26 Nov 2017];50(2):323–43. Available from: http://www.ncbi.nlm.nih.gov/pubmed/23666941
58. Health Canada, Assembly of First Nations. First Nations mental wellness continuum framework. Ottawa (ON): Minister of Health; 2015 Jan [cited 26 Nov 2017]. Available from: http://www.thunderbirdpf.org/wp-content/uploads/2015/01/24-14-1273-FN-Mental-Wellness-Framework-EN05_low.pdf
59. Kirmayer L, Guzder J, Rousseau C. Cultural consultation: encountering the other in mental health care. 1st ed. New York (NY): Springer-Verlag; 2014.
60. Inuit Tapiriit Kanatami [Internet]. Ottawa (ON): Inuit Tapiriit Kanatami; 2016. Inuktitut Magazine, issue 119; 2016 [cited 2017 Nov 27]. Available from: http://www.itk.ca/inuktitut-issue-119/
61. Portico Network [Internet]. Toronto (ON): Centre for Addiction and Mental Health; 2013. Trauma-informed care; 2013 [cited 2017 Nov 27]. Available from: http://www.porticonetwork.ca/treatments/approaches-to-care/trauma-informed-care
62. Fanian S, Young S, Mantla M, Daniels A, Chatwood S. Evaluation of the Kts'iìhtła ("We Light the Fire") project: building resiliency and connections through strengths-based creative arts programming for Indigenous youth. Int J Circumpolar Health [Internet]. 2015 [cited 2017 Nov 27];74(1):27672. Available from: http://www.ncbi.nlm.nih.gov/pmc/articles/PMC4532698/
63. Rowan M, Poole N, Shea B, Gone JP, Mykota D, Farag M, Hopkins C, Hall L, Mushquash C, Dell C. Cultural interventions to treat addictions in Indigenous populations: findings from a scoping study. Subst Abuse Treat Prev Policy [Internet]. 2014 [cited 2017 Nov 27];9(1):34. Available from: http://www.ncbi.nlm.nih.gov/pubmed/25179797
64. Yukon Hospital Corporation [Internet]. Whitehorse (YT): Yukon Hospital Corporation; 2017. First Nations health programs; 2017 [cited 2017 Nov 27]. Available from: https://yukonhospitals.ca/whitehorse-general-hospital/programs-and-services/first-nations-health-programs

12 Climate Change and Health: Remote Northern Community Health Service Provision in a Rapidly Changing Climate

ASHLEE CUNSOLO, EMILY MACLEOD, INEZ SHIWAK, MICHELE WOOD, THE INUIT MENTAL HEALTH ADAPTATION TO CLIMATE CHANGE TEAM*, AND SHERILEE HARPER

Living and Working at the Forefront of Climate Change Impacts on Health

Research has indicated that the Inuit throughout Inuit Nunangat (Inuit homelands) have been at the forefront of climate change impacts in Canada, and globally, experiencing some of the fastest rates of warming and sea ice loss on record (1–8). These changes are directly impacting health (9), as well as negatively affecting several determinants of health, including weather- and ice-related morbidity and mortality from unsafe travel conditions (10–16); disruptions to food and water security and increased foodborne and waterborne diseases (17–26); negative mental health outcomes, including strong emotional reactions, loss of place and sense of identity, increased drug and alcohol usage, and ecological grief and anxiety (27–31); and cultural continuity (3,5,6,32–35). The speed and severity of the changes, coupled with existing challenges in remote health service provision, are creating new challenges to health and wellness for Inuit and disrupting cultural systems of maintaining health that have existed for centuries. These changes and health impacts are experienced within the context of the already-present health disparities stemming from the legacies of colonization, forced acculturation, and systematic marginalization – contexts that have contributed to lower life expectancy, higher prevalence of

* The Inuit Mental Health Adaptation to Climate Change (IMHACC) authorship team: Anthony Andersen and Noah Nochasak, Nain Inuit Community Government; Wayne Piercy and Juliana Flowers, Hopedale Inuit Community Government; Diane Gear and Greg Jacque, Postville Inuit Community Government; Herb Jacque and Myrtle Groves, Makkovik Inuit Community Government; Charlotte Wolfrey and Marilyn Baikie, Rigolet Inuit Community Government.

chronic disease, higher incidence rates of infectious disease, and higher rates of substance usage, suicide, and addiction compared to the Canadian average (3,5,30).

At the forefront of responding to climate-related health impacts are health professionals. Yet health systems in Inuit Nunangat are often overstretched and face many challenges in service provision. These challenges stem from many factors, including communities situated in remote locations, reliant on weather-dependent modes of transportation to deliver health supplies; financial and human resource challenges, including regular access to doctors, dentists, and psychologists; decreased access to health-sustaining resources and services more readily available in less remote settings; high turnover of health professionals, often leading to disruptions in the continuity and quality of care; and an identified need for increased culturally based or culturally appropriate health programming (32,36–40).

Although health professionals are beginning to experience climate change impacts on these already-present challenges, less is known about the extent and nature of climatic pressures or stressors that will be placed on these health systems (3,32,36). Responding to this gap, this chapter examines the impacts and implications of climate change on remote health systems, services, and providers in the Nunatsiavut region of Labrador, Canada, to understand the linkages between climate change and remote health service provision, identify potential vulnerabilities of health systems within the context of a rapidly changing North, and consider opportunities for health systems to adapt in the region.

Nunatsiavut: "Our Beautiful Land"

Formed in 2005 from the Labrador Inuit Land Claims Agreement, the Labrador Inuit Land Claims Area of Nunatsiavut is located on the northeast coast of Labrador, Canada. Along with the Inuvialuit Settlement Region, Nunavut, and Nunavik, Nunatsiavut is one of Canada's four settled Inuit Land Claim Areas that make up Inuit Nunangat. Inuttitut for "Our Beautiful Land," Nunatsiavut is the homeland of the Northern Labrador Inuit, many of whom live in the communities of Nain (population 1125), Hopedale (population 574), Postville (population 177), Makkovik (population 377), and Rigolet (population 305) (see Figures 12.1 and 12.2). Similar to other Indigenous communities in Canada, Nunatsiavut has a young and growing population, with approximately 36 per cent of residents under the age of 25 (41).

All five of the communities in Nunatsiavut are remote and accessible only by boat and ferry in the summer, snowmobile over ice during the winter months, and planes year-round. There are no roads in or out of any of the communities,

Figure 12.1 The five Inuit communities located within the Labrador Inuit Land Claims Areas, Canada

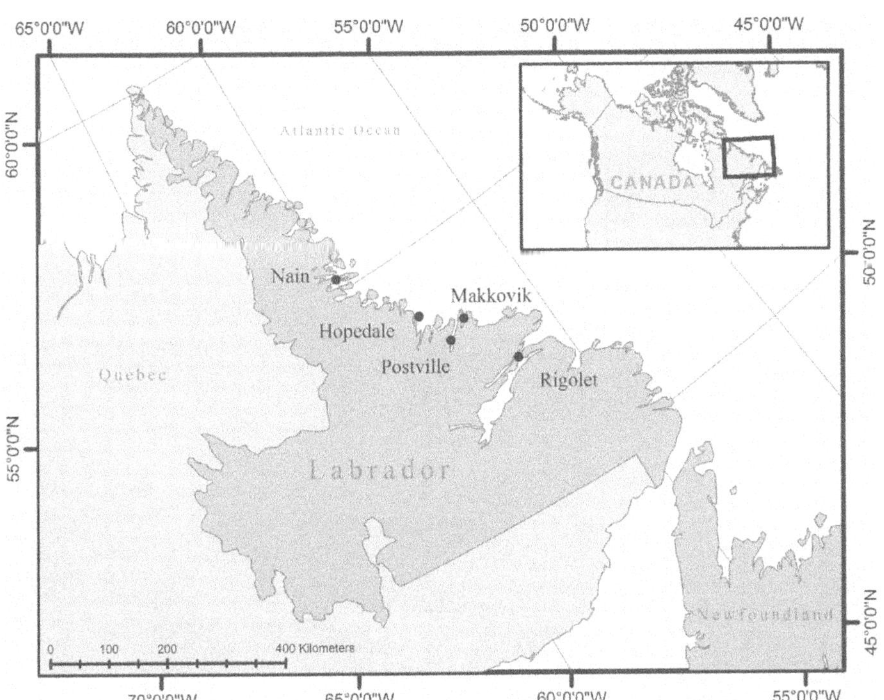

Figure source: Ashlee Cunsolo

and all modes of transportation are dependent on weather, snow, and ice conditions.

Although communities in the region experienced Settler contact from the late seventeenth century onwards and were subjected to assimilationist policies from the federal government in the nineteenth and twentieth centuries (42), Nunatsiavut Inuit have maintained a deep and vibrant connection to the land and to land-based cultural activities. Indeed, many residents of Nunatsiavut continue to live a semi-subsistence lifestyle and rely on hunting, fishing, trapping, foraging, and berry picking for food, nutrition, and wellness. The majority of residents also depend on the land for sociocultural connections and physical, emotional, mental, and spiritual health and well-being. The land is considered essential to Inuit culture and wellness (27,29,30).

Figure 12.2 Images from in and around Nunatsiavut communities

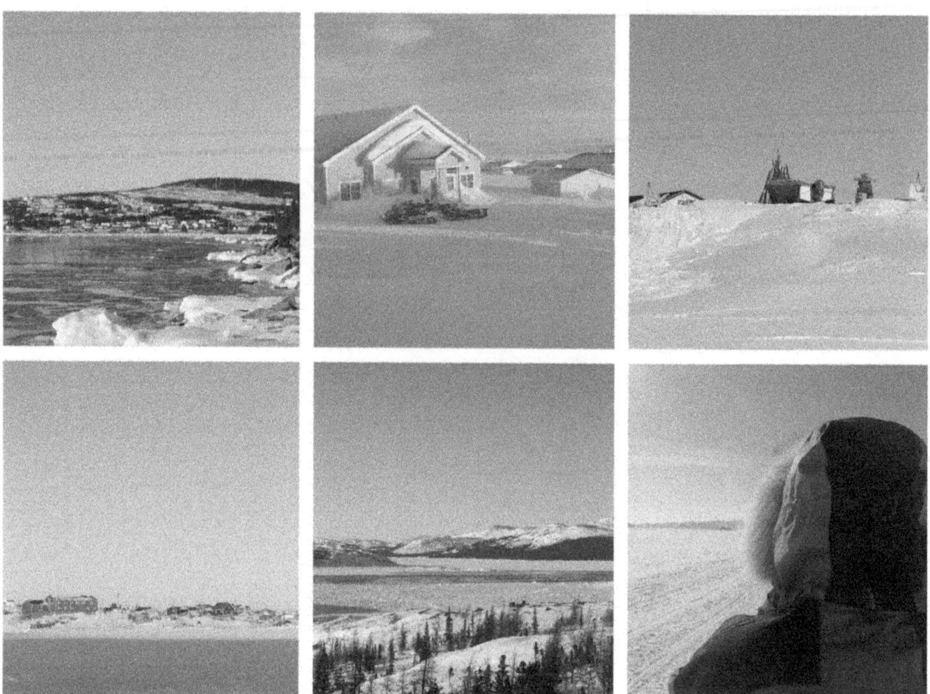

Left to right, top to bottom: Rigolet, Nunatsiavut, from the boardwalk; the Department of Health and Social Development building in Makkovik; an inuksuk with wood drying in Postville; Hopedale from the sea ice; open water just north of Nain; heading out on the land north of Nain

Photo source: Ashlee Cunsolo

In recent years, climate change and resulting shifts in environment, plants, and animals, have become an increasing concern for Inuit in Nunatsiavut. Research indicates changes in the timing of ice formation in the fall months and ice breakup in the spring months (later freeze-up and earlier breakup); a decrease in ice stability, thickness, and coverage; alterations in precipitation levels, including snow; increased frequency and severity of storms; and changes in animal migrations and plant growth patterns. A growing body of research indicates that all of these changes are already impacting Inuit health and well-being in the region (5–7,16,21,27,29, 31,32,43,44).

Like Inuit across Canada, Nunatsiavut residents experience higher incidences of acute and chronic diseases and substance abuse, addictions, and suicide. To support Inuit health, a variety of services are offered in the region through the Labrador-Grenfell Health (LGH) Authority at the provincial level, and regional services are provided through the Nunatsiavut Department of Health and Social Development (DHSD), including community health nursing, public health services, and addictions support. While there are no residential physicians in the Nunatsiavut region, each community has at least one full-time residential primary care nurse funded by LGH, as well as a public health nurse and community health workers funded by DHSD. Together, these health professionals offer a diverse range of health services, including emergency care and treatment and management of chronic illnesses and acute conditions. They also provide a variety of public health services and health advocacy. For serious or emergency conditions, clients are flown out of the community to receive care in a larger centre, usually Happy Valley-Goose Bay, Labrador, but for more serious cases, clients are treated in St. John's, Newfoundland. The majority of acute mental health issues are generally treated in Happy Valley-Goose Bay, including services for addictions recovery, suicide attempts or ideation, and treatment for dissociative, mood, and anxiety disorders (although these services are still quite limited compared to those available in larger or more urban centres). Once back in the community, clients are supported by nurses through ongoing counselling, monitoring, and medication management. The DHSD also supports culturally based programs focused on health promotion and healing, including Indigenous healing programs for residential school survivors, land-based and cultural programming that promotes wellness and mental resilience, and Inuit-relevant health education and promotion.

Listening to and Learning from Northern Labrador: Data Collection and Analysis

Data for our case study were drawn from a multi-year community-based research project run by the Rigolet Inuit Community Government and working in partnership with the Inuit community governments of Nain, Hopedale, Postville, and Makkovik. This project was community based and community led, following a participatory research process (9,28,45–47) and supporting the principles outlined in the National Inuit Strategy on Research (48): advancing Inuit governance in research; enhancing the ethical conduct of research; aligning funding with Inuit research priorities; ensuring Inuit access, ownership, and control over data and information; and building

Figure 12.3 Demographic and professional breakdown of interview participants in study of impact of climate change on health in Nunatsiavut communities

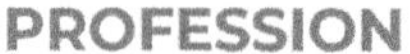

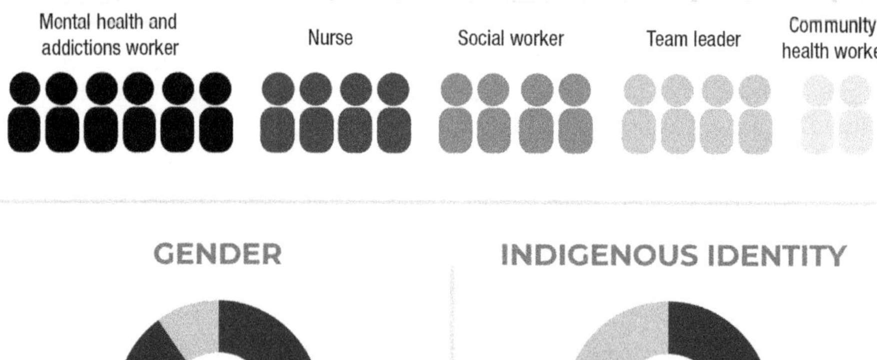

GENDER

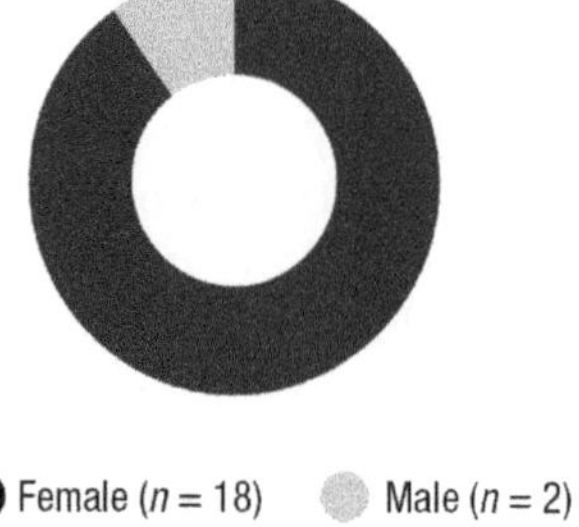

INDIGENOUS IDENTITY

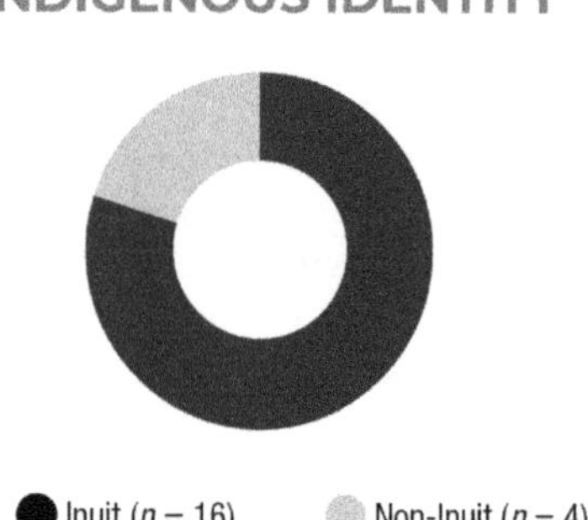

Figure source: Alex Sawatzky

capacity in Inuit Nunangat research. Data for this chapter were drawn from 14 in-depth conversational interviews (49) with a total of 20 DHSD health professionals (some interviews were conducted in pairs or small groups) (see Figure 12.3).

Qualitative data analysis was conducted using an immersive constant comparative method (50), which involved ongoing comparison of data between and within the interviews. Analysis was conducted through three main iterative steps: reflective memoing, group identification of emerging trends and themes, and collective creation of codes (Figure 12.4).

All subthemes and codes were continually discussed with key stakeholders and community members through results-sharing and verification meetings and open houses within the region for approval, authenticity, accuracy, and precise representation of the local and cultural context from which they emerged.

Figure 12.4 Iterative qualitative data analysis process used to characterize the linkages between climate change and remote health service provision and consider opportunities for adaptation

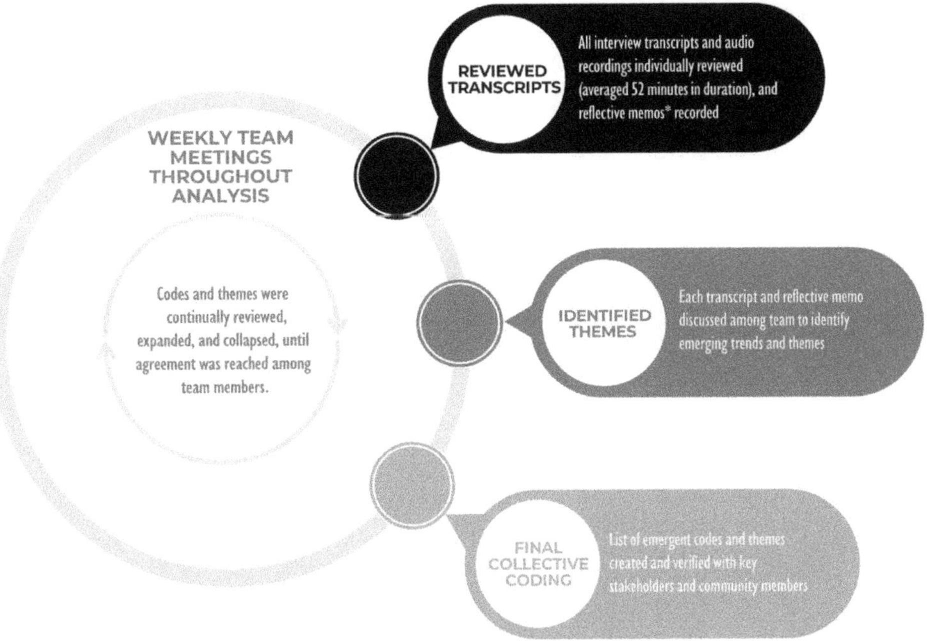

* Reflective memos included key quotations, questions for further consideration, general comments and reflections, links to other interviews, and key emerging themes and ideas.

Figure source: Alex Sawatzky

"It's Already Impacting Us:" Results and Discussion

Through the interviews conducted, all health professionals indicated that climate change – including long-term increases in surface air temperature, unstable ice conditions, diminishing ice coverage, and increased frequency and intensity of storms – was a growing concern for their communities, which also corroborates other work in the region (2,27–30,32,51,52). For people who are directly tied to and reliant on the land, even subtle changes to weather, snow, ice, plants, and animals can have significant impacts on health and health care systems. Indeed, those interviewed articulated that when environmental and climatic conditions that support wellness – including stability of weather and environment, and connection to place-based identities and histories – start shifting, there can be serious impacts on all facets of health, including impacts to individual and community wellness and strain on health care systems and resources (Table 12.1).

Table 12.1 Observed weather, climatic, and environmental changes in Nunatsiavut, and the related impacts on health and health care systems as experienced by research participants

Observed weather, climatic, and environmental changes in Nunatsiavut	Identified health impacts in Nunatsiavut	Impacts to health care system in Nunatsiavut
Declining ice coverage, stability, thickness, and extent	• Increased rates of injury and death from unsafe travel routes • Disruptions to hunting and fishing grounds, leading to increased food insecurity and potential nutritional deficiencies • Impacts to mental health, through loss of access to the land and land-based activities, emotional reactions to changes (fear, anxiety, stress, distress), and disruptions to food security and cultural continuity	• Increased client numbers and client care needs at the health care clinics • Higher expenses for increased medical supplies and needed health resources • Increased demand for mental health, counselling, and wellness services • Increased need for health resources to support increased client demands • Increased burnout in health professionals from job demands and inability to refresh on the land because of changes
Fluctuating weather patterns and increased storms	• Increased rates of injury and death from unpredictable travel conditions, accidents, and strandings • Increased gastrointestinal illnesses from runoffs from storms • Increased mental trauma from unsafe and unpredictable travel conditions, declining access to hunting and trapping opportunities, and disruptions to intergenerational knowledge transmission	• Increased client numbers and client care needs at the health care clinics • Higher expenses for increased medical supplies and needed health resources • Disruptions to fly-in health services and personnel or emergency medevac • Disruptions to health resource (medicine, supplies) delivery and access • Increased demand for mental health, counselling, and wellness services • Increased burnout in health professionals from job demands and inability to refresh on the land because of changes

Warming surface air temperatures and seasonal averages	• Increased foodborne, waterborne, and vectorborne diseases as changing temperatures create new environments for diseases • Increased asthma, respiratory challenges, and allergies • Increased incidences of sunburn • Increased incidences of heat-related distress • Increased mental stress from changing conditions and concerns about cultural continuity and traditional knowledge transmission	• Increased client numbers and client care needs • Higher expenses for increased medical supplies and needed health resources • Potential increases in need for diabetic support services
Shifts in wildlife and vegetation patterns	• Disruptions to food security and food sovereignty, as people find it increasingly difficult to hunt for wild food and forage for berries and edible plants • Increased reliance on store-bought food, leading to nutritional deficiencies, with potential implications for obesity and diabetes rates	• Increased client numbers and client care needs • Higher expenses for medical supplies and needed health resources • Potential increases in needs for nutritional, diabetic, and obesity-related support services • Increased demand for mental health, counselling, and wellness services

Figure 12.5 Pathways through which climate change is impacting remote health systems in Nunatsiavut, Labrador, Canada

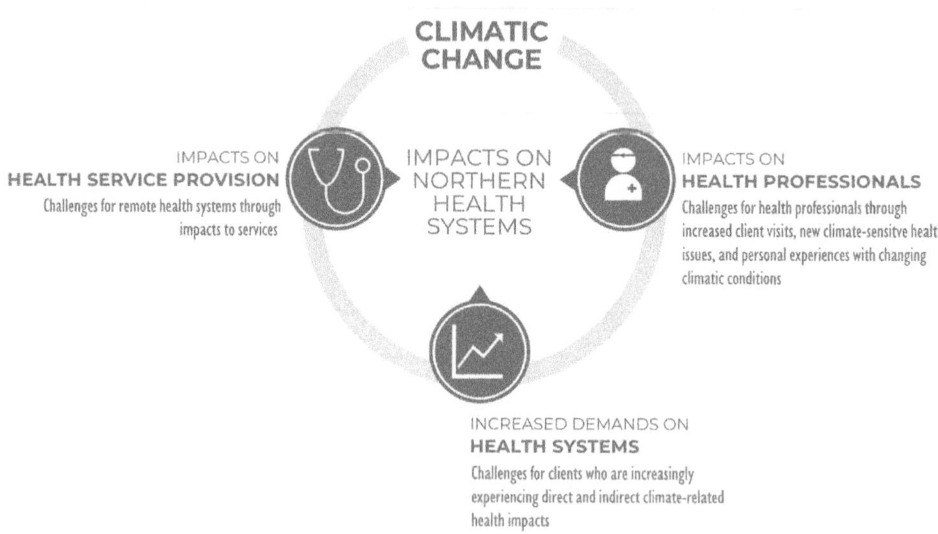

Figure source: Alex Sawatzky

Consistent with current literature in the region (2,6,27–32,51,52), as well as in other parts of the world (53,54), health professionals interviewed for this research indicated that climate change was becoming an increasing stressor on remote health systems through three main pathways: (1) challenges to remote health systems through impacts to services; (2) challenges for health professionals through increased client visits, new climate-sensitive health issues, and personal experiences with changing climatic and environmental conditions; and (3) challenges to clients who are increasingly experiencing direct and indirect climate-related health impacts (Figure 12.5).

Climate Change Impacts on Northern Health Service Provision

Health professionals explained that the observed changing climatic conditions leading to declining and unstable sea ice and unpredictable weather patterns were further contributing to the challenges of remote health care provision. Fluctuations in weather and ice quality can impact travel to and from the communities, and disrupt flight schedules in and out of the community, including for medical supplies or medical evacuation flights. These disruptions lead to health service provision becoming increasingly interrupted, fragmented, or limited, increasing or amplifying vulnerabilities in the health care system. For instance, participants reported that the non-residential health specialist visits were becoming more frequently delayed, cut short, or cancelled because of changes in climate conditions. These disruptions affect the overall quality of and access to health resources and may contribute to lack of trust among community members in non-residential health professionals. As one mental health and addictions worker stated, clients know when these non-residential health professionals are "watching the weather":

> You have to be very dedicated to what you're doing because [the clients] can feel it, and they know when you don't want to be there; they know when you're in a hurry to get out because of the weather ... we need community people trained to do those things on their own, without having to depend on somebody from outside, or depend on the weather.

Health professionals were also concerned about the ongoing and increasing climate-related disruptions to land-based programming (healing camps, skills-teaching trips, youth-Elder sharing experiences), which are often foundational strategies for supporting community wellness. With increasing changes to ice patterns, timing, extent, and stability, as well as unpredictability in weather, travelling safely on the land is not always possible and can be costly. As one health professional explained, "The ice is not safe sometimes, and the weather is very unpredictable, and money is a factor too." These programs are essential for providing culturally appropriate health services within the region, as Inuit remain closely tied to and reliant on the land for sustenance, livelihoods, and wellness. As another participant stated,

> I think I would have to say that the land – going out on the land – is everything to us. It's our heart and our soul. Going out on the land is a form of spirituality. And if you can't get there, then you almost feel like your spirit is dying. And then when you get out again, then you feel so much better when you come back, and I think it energizes you more and just frees your spirit more by being out on the land.

This recognition of the importance of the land to health, and understanding the land as an essential component of all aspects of Inuit health, resonates with research from across the North (10,27,29,30,32,55–57). Understanding the importance of the land-health interface for wellness, communities across the North are creating land-based programs as health-sustaining resources and supporting the revitalization of the connection between people and land for health (58–63). Yet depending solely on these land-based programs for health resilience is becoming an increasing challenge because of unstable, unreliable, and often unreadable weather, snow, and ice patterns and conditions.

Climate Change Is Impacting Health Professionals

Being a health care provider in small, remote communities presents many place-specific challenges for Nunatsiavut health professionals, including a limited number of regionally employed health professionals and the lack of access to health-sustaining resources that may be available or accessible in other places. The health professionals in the communities become the main care providers for all health issues, and often their day jobs turn into being on call (formally or informally) 24 hours a day, 7 days a week. Health professionals also indicated that the limited availability and accessibility of medical providers such as physicians, psychologists, and pharmacists has led to challenges regarding added responsibilities from extended scopes of practice. These working conditions and the relative isolation of being a health professional within these communities has made recruitment to the area difficult, and many positions remain unfilled. These conditions led to some interviewees sharing that they experience high levels of stress or burnout, because of being overstretched and overworked, and not being able to "get away" from the job. These experiences of limited resources, high turnover of staff, and burnout are common in the circumpolar North and resonate with existing literature (32,36–40,61,64,65), including chapter 8 by Møller in this volume.

Health professionals in Nunatsiavut explained that these challenges are exacerbated by climate change. As permanent residents of the communities in which they work and the majority self-identifying as Inuit, health care providers experience climate and environmental change impacts both professionally and personally: professionally, because they are supporting increasing numbers of clients who are experiencing health-related issues from disruptions to land access; and personally, because they, themselves, are no longer able to get out on the land to refresh and recharge. A health professional explained the effects of changing weather and ice patterns on her staff:

> People are more agitated and they just can't relax because they're just not getting off on the land. So, we see that in our programming, and even with our staff I see it … People who want to go off on the weekend or something like that, they can't get away and that affects their work.

To further elaborate, a community health worker described the feelings she experiences when she is able to "go off" and how it positively affects her state of mind:

> Well, for me personally, going out on the land is my saviour, I think, it's my healer … I grew up doing that, and I loved that, and I continued to do that as I got older … the minute I leave … I could feel the weight of the world fall off me, and I'm a totally whole different person. I'm really happy and everything, you know, everything is so different to me. I could feel everything fall away and I know I'm gonna be okay, even though it's just for a weekend. If I can't do that, then I get pretty moody.

Without reliable weather conditions for clients and health professionals to travel on the land safely and regularly, or to have access to weather-reliant health resources, health professionals indicated that they felt multiple levels of climate-related and place-based stress on their personal and professional lives. This manifested in feelings such as depression, anger, sadness, frustration, fear, distress, boredom, loneliness, agitation, and a sense of being "stuck" or "trapped" – climate change-related feelings for which they are simultaneously supporting their clients (see below), adding further to their personal and professional exhaustion. This further compounds the already-present challenges of providing health care in remote settings, magnifying stress and burnout rates, and impacting overall job satisfaction and the mental health of health care service providers (61–63,65).

Climate Change Is Increasing Demands on Health Systems

Health professionals indicated that their clients' health care needs were complex, requiring holistic approaches to community and mental health that are based in Inuit culture and tradition (Table 12.2). Similar to their personal experiences with the physical, mental, and emotional implications from a changing climate and subsequent land access, health professionals also expressed concerns about the impacts of climate change on their clients, from disruptions to land-based activities leading to depression and anxiety, to lack of access to health resources and supports (both within and outside the community) because of effects on weather-related services.

In addition, many who were interviewed expressed concerns that climate change would become an increasing stressor on other health-related issues, particularly mental health; indeed, many interviewees linked the disruptions of access to land-based activities as further compounding the mental health and addictions issues found in these remote communities:

> I can meet [clients] on the road, and we talk about hunting and what they done and where they went, and they'll talk about that … So, it affects them because it's a way of providing for their family, and if that's not there [because of climate change], then, I mean, look at other alternatives, and sometimes that's not there. So, you know, it makes a difference to their mental health because then they're thinking, oh, they're not providing for their family.

A community health nurse also linked changes in weather patterns and ice conditions to the triggering of depressive feelings, such as loneliness:

> When you're just stuck like that, there's a lot of despair, there's a lot of down feelings, you just want to go and that's the only way that you can go. So, people are always very anxious about getting the first ice and they can't wait for it to freeze up and then you know, a couple of months later, it's gone. And then you've got the whole rest of the year and then you're feeling stuck again … It's very lonely,

Table 12.2 Reported challenges for remote health care provision, providers, and clients, and additional challenges and impacts related to climate change in Nunatsiavut

Challenges	Climate change impacts
HEALTH CARE PROVISION	
• Lack of regular access to health resources • High staff turnover • Limited availability of health services and professionals in the region • Lack of understanding from outside workers or decision makers of local context and cultural needs	• Disruptions to travel and flights, impacting client transport, health professional visits, and needed medical supplies • Visiting health professionals may cancel or cut short visits and cancel appointments • Disruptions to land-based healing programs, which are essential to health and wellness
HEALTH PROFESSIONALS	
• Limited number of regionally employed staff leads to strong pressures on workers and high stress and burnout rates • Most health care providers have an expanded scope of practice, being one of only a few health care workers	• *Professional impacts:* greater client demands because of physical and mental health stressors from disruption to land access • *Personal impacts:* inability to get off on the land to refresh or recharge because of fluctuations in weather, snow, and ice
HEALTH CARE CLIENTS	
• Complex health needs stemming from intergenerational trauma, poverty, and lack of access to resources • Higher rates of acute and chronic diseases, addictions, and suicide than the non-Inuit Canadian population	• Increased emotional responses, including stress, anxiety, distress, depression, and sadness from disruptions to land-based activities and land access • Increased "empty time" leads to potential for greater substance abuse and suicide ideation

> because people are used to being on the land. When you're living in a small, isolated place and for the most part your whole livelihood revolves around the land and the ocean and that's changing, what do you do? What can you do?

This loneliness expressed by clients is not in terms of the desire or need for more contact with others, physically and socially, but rather the desire to feel a connection spiritually. This loneliness was identified as stemming from spiritual isolation as a result of not being able to access the land and the resulting impacts to place-based connections, identities, heritage, and health. If people are unable to access the land regularly because of changing climatic and environmental conditions (which compound already-existing socio-economic and health disparities) and increased place-based health stressors, the health professionals interviewed were concerned that health outcomes – particularly mental health outcomes, including increased substance usage and suicide ideation – were going to worsen in the coming years.

This decreased land access is also placing ever-greater strain on clients and thus on health professionals and remote health systems. Health professionals throughout this research continually expressed concern that many of these climate-change-related feelings may contribute to, or become an additional stressor for, other health challenges in the community, including addictions, acute and chronic physical and mental health conditions, and potentially even impact suicide ideation (2,27–30,32,51). These findings resonate with and support previous research conducted in the region examining the pathways through which climate change impacts mental health (2,27–30,32,51), as well as research from a circumpolar and a global context supporting this (10,31,33,66–77).

Climate Change and Northern Health Systems' Challenges: From Impacts to Adaptation

This research illustrates that climate change and its impacts on northern health systems is not experienced in isolation, and the effects are experienced through a complex web of health disparities, including the enduring legacies of colonialism and forced assimilation, and changing place-based identities and cultures.

It is clear that climate change is exacerbating and amplifying inequities in health care access and, as a result, is an increasing stressor to the health sector in many remote communities. Within this context, many Indigenous communities, such as Labrador Inuit, and their related health systems exist at the forefront of these changes and are already experiencing serious impacts throughout all parts of health care access and delivery. Building from this research, as well as relevant literature in the field, we have synthesized recommendations for mitigating climate-related health stressors in remote communities – recommendations that resonate with other research calling for changes in health care governance, service delivery, workforce development, educational awareness, infrastructure, and financial support (36,78–81) (Table 12.3).

How remote health systems respond, manage, and adapt to the stressors of climate change will be a defining issue in remote contexts in the coming years (81). Remote health service providers, health professionals, researchers, and decision makers have the opportunity and the responsibility to prepare for and meet this challenge through interdisciplinary research, health advocacy and leadership, and government action (36).

Table 12.3 Climate-related health challenges and identified recommendations and mobilization strategies to support health care systems' adaptation, health professionals, and remote communities

Climate-related health challenges	Identified recommendations	Potential mobilization strategies
Declining ice stability, thickness, and extent and snow conditions lead to disruptions in travel frequency and stability.	More resources for on-the-land programming to support wellness	• Land-based programs that are flexible and adaptable to deal with fluctuations in conditions • Increased funding for needed equipment to travel safely and effectively on the land (snowmobiles, boats, gas, food, ammunition, supplies, SPOT transmitters) • Emphasis on supporting youth, middle-age males, and Elders to support culturally relevant wellness activities
Fluctuations of weather, snow, and ice conditions and patterns are causing more people to be "stuck" in communities, with more "empty time."	Implement alternative strategies for engaging people in culturally relevant activities in the community to support wellness	• Creation of and funding for in-community programming to learn Inuit cultural skills, such as sewing with fur and animal skin, snowshoe making, carving, art, traditional cooking, fur preparation • More emphasis on language skills and training to reclaim Inuttitut language • More culturally based youth mentorship programs, connecting youth with positive adult role models to learn traditional knowledge and cultural skills
Research on climate-sensitive health impacts and outcomes is new and emerging; health professionals in remote settings do not often have access to research or resources on these topics.	Additional support and educational opportunities for health care providers (78,79,81–85)	• Creation of educational training materials to educate health professionals on health impacts of climate change • Additional support for health professionals to engage in professional development and collaborative brainstorming with colleagues on strategies to support community health • More relief staff to provide health care workers with breaks and time on the land • Support at local and regional levels for health professionals experiencing burnout and climate-related stressors

(*Continued*)

Table 12.3 (continued)

Climate-related health challenges	Identified recommendations	Potential mobilization strategies
Health professionals are over-burdened and staff time is overstretched; climate change is putting increasing pressures on the health care system and its workers, leaving little time for health care leadership and advocacy.	Increased participation of health professionals in leadership and advocacy roles, particularly in rural and remote regions (78–80,84)	• Encourage and support health care workers to become more involved with communities, researchers, and decision makers on climate-health research and policy • Encourage and support health professionals to become strong health advocates by providing professional development and training opportunities • Support health professionals interested in conducting climate-health research, or participating in research projects, by providing incentives • Provide needed tools to health care workers to further educate clients and communities on climate-sensitive health impacts
Access to funding to support remote health care system adaptation is limited, yet remote health care systems and providers in the North are on the frontlines of climate change and pressures to adapt are already present; little is known, however, about the extent of climate change impacts on remote health care systems.	More research and funding support at multiple levels of government to support remote health care system adaptation (36,81,83)	• Support multi-level and multi-sectoral research on climate-related impacts to remote health care, including risks and responses, distribution and frequency of impacts, and mitigation and adaptation strategies • Ensure research is conducted at the primary, secondary, and tertiary levels, with cohesive partnerships through all levels

ACKNOWLEDGMENTS

Our sincerest gratitude to all the research participants in Nain, Hopedale, Postville, Makkovik, and Rigolet, Nunatsiavut. Without you, this research would not have been possible, and we appreciate the time and wisdom you shared with the research team. In particular, thank you to Charlotte Wolfrey, Jack Shiwak, and the Rigolet Inuit Community Government for supporting, hosting, and leading this research. Thank you also to Alex Sawatzky for creating the diagrams and visuals in this article, and to Nia King for manuscript and referencing formatting and support. This research was supported through funding from Health Canada, Canadian Institutes of Health Research, Cape Breton University, and the Nunatsiavut Government Department of Health and Social Development.

REFERENCES

1. Intergovernmental Panel on Climate Change. Climate change 2013: the physical science basis – contribution of Working Group I to the fifth assessment report of the Intergovernmental Panel on Climate Change. Stocker T, Qin D, Plattner G, Tignor M, Allen S, Borschung J, Nauels A, Xia Y, Bex V, Midgley PM, editors. Cambridge (GB): Cambridge University Press; 2013.
2. Way RG, Viau AE. Natural and forced air temperature variability in the Labrador region of Canada during the past century. Theor Appl Climatol. 2015;121(3–4): 413–24.
3. Ford JD, Cunsolo Willox A, Chatwood S, Furgal C, Harper S, Mauro I, Pearce T. Adapting to the effects of climate change on Inuit health. Am J Public Health. 2014;104(S3):e9–17.
4. Ford JD, Labbé J, Flynn M, Araos M. Readiness for climate change adaptation in the Arctic: a case study from Nunavut, Canada. Clim Change. 2017;145(1–2): 85–100.
5. Inuit Tapiriit Kanatami. Inuit priorities for Canada's climate strategy: A Canadian Inuit vision for our common future in our homelands [Internet]. Ottawa (ON): Inuit Tapiriit Kanatami; 2016 [cited 2019 Dec 1]. Available from: https://www.itk.ca/wp-content/uploads/2016/09/ITK_Climate-Change-Report_English.pdf
6. Meredith M, Sommerkorn M, Cassota S, Derksen C, Eyaykin A, Hollowed A, Kofinas G, Mackintosh A, Melbourne-Thomas J, Muelbert MMC, Ottersen G, Pritchard H, Schuur EAG. Polar regions. In: Portner H-O, Roberts D, Masson-Delmotte V, Zhai P, Tignor M, Poloczanska E, Mintenbeck K, Alegría A, Nicolai M, Okem A, Petzold J, Rama B, Weyer NM, editors. IPCC special report on the ocean and cryosphere in a changing climate. Geneva (CH): Intergovernmental Panel on Climate Change; 2019. p. 203–320.
7. Inuit Tapiriit Kanatami. National Inuit climate change strategy [Internet]. Ottawa (ON): Inuit Tapiriit Kanatami; 2019 [cited 2019 Dec 1]. Available from: https://www.itk.ca/wp-content/uploads/2019/06/ITK_Climate-Change-Strategy_English.pdf
8. Ford JD, Couture N, Bell T, Clark DG. Climate change and Canada's north coast: research trends, progress, and future directions. Environ Rev. 2018;26:82–92.
9. Ford JD, Sherman M, Berrang-Ford L, Llanos A, Carcamo C, Harper S, Lwasa S, Namanya D, Marcello T, Maillet M, Edge V. Preparing for the health impacts

of climate change in Indigenous communities: the role of community-based adaptation. Glob Environ Chang. 2018;49:129–39.

10. Durkalec A, Furgal C, Skinner MW, Sheldon T. Climate change influences on environment as a determinant of Indigenous health: relationships to place, sea ice, and health in an Inuit community. Soc Sci Med. 2015;136–137:17–26.
11. Durkalec A, Furgal C, Skinner MW, Sheldon T. Investigating environmental determinants of injury and trauma in the Canadian North. Int J Environ Res Public Health. 2014;11(2):1536–48.
12. Clark DG, Ford JD. Emergency response in a rapidly changing arctic. Can Med Assoc J. 2017;189(4):E135–6.
13. Young SK, Tabish TB, Pollock NJ, Young TK. Backcountry travel emergencies in Arctic Canada: a pilot study in public health surveillance. Int J Environ Res Public Health. 2016;13(3):276.
14. Ford J, Clark D. Preparing for the impacts of climate change along Canada's Arctic coast: the importance of search and rescue. Mar Policy. 2019;108:103662.
15. Clark DG, Ford JD, Tabish T. What role can unmanned aerial vehicles play in emergency response in the Arctic? A case study from Canada. PLoS One. 2018;13(12):e0205299.
16. Ford JD, Clark D, Pearce T, Berrang-Ford L, Copland L, Dawson J, New MG, Harper S. Changing access to ice, land and water in Arctic communities. Nat Clim Chang. 2019;9(4):335–9.
17. Harper SL, Edge VL, Schuster-Wallace CJ, Berke O, McEwen SA. Weather, water quality and infectious gastrointestinal illness in two Inuit communities in Nunatsiavut, Canada: potential implications for climate change. Ecohealth. 2011;8(1):93–108.
18. Bakaic M, Medeiros AS. Vulnerability of northern water supply lakes to changing climate and demand. Arct Sci. 2017;3(1):1–16.
19. Medeiros AS, Wood P, Wesche SD, Bakaic M, Peters JF. Water security for northern peoples: review of threats to Arctic freshwater systems in Nunavut, Canada. Reg Environ Chang. 2017;17(3):635–47.
20. Wright CJ, Sargeant JM, Edge VL, Ford JD, Farahbakhsh K, Rigolet Inuit Community Government, Shiwak I, Flowers C; IHACC Research Team, Harper SL. Water quality and health in northern Canada: stored drinking water and acute gastrointestinal illness in Labrador Inuit. Environ Sci Pollut Res Int. 2018;25(33):32975–87.
21. Kenny T-A, Fillion M, Simpkin S, Wesche SD, Chan HM. Caribou (*Rangifer tarandus*) and Inuit nutrition security in Canada. Ecohealth. 2018;15(3):590–607.
22. Rosol R, Powell-Hellyer S, Chan HM. Impacts of decline harvest of country food on nutrient intake among Inuit in Arctic Canada: impact of climate change and possible adaptation plan. Int J Circumpolar Health. 2016;75(1):31127.
23. Berner J, Brubaker M, Revitch B, Kreummel E, Tcheripanoff M, Bell J. Adaptation in Arctic circumpolar communities: food and water security in a changing climate. Int J Circumpolar Health. 2016;75(1):33820.

24. Lam S, Dodd W, Skinner K, Papadopoulos A, Zivot C, Ford J, Garcia PJ, IHACC Research Team, Harper SL. Community-based monitoring of Indigenous food security in a changing climate: global trends and future directions. Environ Res Lett. 2019;14:073002.
25. Ford JD, Clark D, Naylor A. Food insecurity in Nunavut: are we going from bad to worse? Can Med Assoc J. 2019;191(20):E550–1.
26. Harper SL, Berrang-Ford L, Carcamo C, Cunsolo A, Edge VL, Ford JD, Llanos A, Lwasa S, Namanya DB. The Indigenous climate-food-health nexus. In: Reyes Mason L, Rigg J, editors. People and climate change: vulnerability, adaptation, and social justice. Oxford (GB): Oxford University Press; 2019. p. 184–212.
27. Cunsolo Willox A, Harper SL, Edge VL, Landman K, Houle K, Ford JD, Rigolet Inuit Community Government. The land enriches the soul: On climatic and environmental change, affect, and emotional health and well-being in Rigolet, Nunatsiavut, Canada. Emot Sp Soc. 2013;6(1):14–24.
28. Harper S, Edge VL, Cunsolo Willox A, Rigolet Inuit Community Government. Changing climate, changing health, changing stories profile: using an ecohealth approach to explore impacts of climate change on Inuit health. Ecohealth. 2012;9(1):89–101.
29. Cunsolo Willox A, Harper SL, Ford JD, Edge VL, Landman K, Houle K, Edge V, Rigolet Inuit Community Government. Climate change and mental health: an exploratory case study from Rigolet, Nunatsiavut, Canada. Clim Change. 2013;121(2):255–70.
30. Cunsolo Willox A, Harper SL, Ford JD, Landman K, Houle K, Edge VL, Rigolet Inuit Community Government. "From this place and of this place:" climate change, sense of place, and health in Nunatsiavut, Canada. Soc Sci Med. 2012;75(3):538–47.
31. Cunsolo A, Ellis NR. Ecological grief as a mental health response to climate change-related loss. Nat Clim Chang. 2018;8:275–81.
32. Harper SL, Edge VL, Ford J, Cunsolo Willox A, Wood M, IHACC Research Team, Rigolet Inuit Community Government, McEwen SA. Climate-sensitive health priorities in Nunatsiavut, Canada. BMC Public Health. 2015;15:605.
33. Cunsolo Willox A, Stephenson E, Allen J, Bourque F, Drossos A, Elgarøy S, Kral MJ, Mauro I, Moses J, Pearce T, Petrasek MacDonald J, Wexler L. Examining relationships between climate change and mental health in the circumpolar North. Reg Environ Chang. 2015;15(1):169–82.
34. Cunsolo A, Shiwak I, Wood M, The IlikKuset-Ilingannet Team. "You need to be a well-rounded cultural person": youth mentorship programs for cultural preservation, promotion, and sustainability in the Nunatsiavut region of Labrador. In: Fondahl G, Wilson G, editors. Northern sustainabilities: understanding and addressing change in the circumpolar world. Cham (CH): Springer Polar Sciences; 2017. p. 285–303.

35. Abram N, Gattuso J-P, Prakash A, Cheng L, Chidichimo MP, Crate S, Enomoto H, Garschagen M, Gruber N, Harper S, Holland E, Kudela RM, Rice J, Steffen K, Von Schuckmann K. Framing and context of the report. In: Portner H-O, Roberts DC, Masson-Delmotte V, Zhai P, Tignor M, Poloczanska E, Mintenbeck K, Alegría A, Nicolai M, Okem A, Petzold J, Rama B, Weyer NM, editors. IPCC special report on the ocean and cryosphere in a changing climate. Geneva (CH): Intergovernmental Panel on Climate Change; 2019. p. 73–129.
36. Ford JD, Berrang-Ford L, King M, Furgal C. Vulnerability of Aboriginal health systems in Canada to climate change. Glob Environ Chang. 2010;20(4):668–80.
37. Chatwood S, Young K. A new approach to health research in Canada's North. Can J Public Health. 2010;101(1):25–7.
38. Minore B, Boone M, Katt M, Kinch P, Birch S. Addressing the realties of health care in northern Aboriginal communities through participatory action research. J Interprof Care. 2004;18(4):360–8.
39. Young TK, Chatwood S. Health care in the North: what Canada can learn from its circumpolar neighbours. Can Med Assoc J. 2011;183(2):209–14.
40. Wexler L, Graves K. The importance of culturally-responsive training for building a behavioral health workforce in Alaska Native villages: a case study from Northwest Alaska. J Rural Ment Heal. 2008;33(3):209–14.
41. Statistics Canada. Census profile, 2016 census, Newfoundland and Labrador. Ottawa (ON): Statistics Canada; 2016.
42. Natcher D, Felt L, Procter A. Settlement, subsistence, and change among the Labrador Inuit: the Nunatsiavummiut experience. Winnipeg (MB): University of Manitoba Press; 2012.
43. Pearce T, Ford J, Cunsolo Willox A, Smit B. Inuit Traditional ecological knowledge (TEK), subsistence hunting and adaptation to climate change in the Canadian Arctic. Arctic. 2015;68(2):233–45.
44. Archer L, Ford JD, Pearce T, Kowal S, Gough WA, Allurut M. Longitudinal assessment of climate vulnerability: a case study from the Canadian Arctic. Sustain Sci. 2017;12(1):15–29.
45. Castleden H, Morgan VS, Lamb C. "I spent the first year drinking tea": exploring Canadian university researchers' perspectives on community-based participatory research involving Indigenous peoples. Can Geogr. 2012;56(2):160–79.
46. Pearce TD, Ford JD, Laidler GJ, Smit B, Duerden F, Allarut M, Andrachuk M, Baryluk S, Dialla A, Elee P, Goose A, Ikummaq T, Joamie E, Kataoyak F, Loring E, Meakin S, Nickels S, Shappa K, Shirley J, Wandelet J. Community collaboration and climate change research in the Canadian Arctic. Polar Res. 2009;28(1):10–27.
47. Ford JD, Stephenson E, Cunsolo Willox A, Edge V, Farahbakhsh K, Furgal C, Harper S, Chatwood S, Mauro I, Pearce T, Austin S, Bunce A, Bussalleu A, Diaz J, Finner K, Gordon A, Huet C, Kitching K, Lardeau M-P, McDowell G, McDonald E, Nakoneczny L, Sherman M. Community-based adaptation research in the Canadian Arctic. Wiley Interdiscip Rev Clim Chang. 2016;7(2):175–91.

48. Inuit Tapiriit Kanatami. National Inuit strategy on research. Ottawa (ON): Inuit Tapiriit Kanatami; 2018.
49. Steinar K, Brinkmann S. InterViews: Learning the craft of qualitative research interviewing. Thousand Oaks (CA): Sage; 2009.
50. Miles M, Huberman A. Qualitative data analysis: An expanded sourcebook. Thousand Oaks (CA): Sage; 1994.
51. Petrasek MacDonald J, Harper SL, Cunsolo Willox A, Edge VL, Rigolet Inuit Community Government. A necessary voice: Climate change and lived experiences of youth in Rigolet, Nunatsiavut, Canada. Glob Environ Chang. 2013;23(1):360–71.
52. Sawatzky A, Cunsolo A, Jones-Bitton A, Middleton J, Harper SL. Responding to climate and environmental change impacts on human health via integrated surveillance in the circumpolar North: a systematic realist review. Int J Environ Res Public Health. 2018;15:2706.
53. Costello A, Abbas M, Allen A, Ball S, Bell S, Bellamy R, Friel S, Groce N, Johnson A, Kett M, Lee M, Levy C, Maslin M, McCoy D, McGuire B, Montgomery H, Napier D, Pagel C, Patel J, de Oliveira JA, Redclift N, Rees H, Rogger D, Scott J, Stephenson J, Twigg J, Wolff J, Patterson C. Managing the health effects of climate change. Lancet. 2009;373(9676):1693–733.
54. Watts N, Adger WN, Agnolucci P, Blackstock J, Byass P, Cai W, Chaytor S, Colbourn T, Collins M, Cooper A, Cox PM, Depledge J, Drummond P, Ekins P, Galaz V, Grace D, Graham H, Grubb M, Haines A, Hamilton I, Hunter A, Jiang X, Li M, Kelman I, Liang L, Lott M, Lowe R, Luo Y, Mace G, Maslin M, Nilsson M, Oreszczyn T, Pye S, Quinn T, Svensdotter M, Venevsky S, Warner K, Xu B, Yang J, Yin Y, Yu C, Zhang Q, Gong P, Montgomery H, Costello A. Health and climate change: policy responses to protect public health. Lancet. 2015;386(10006):1861–914.
55. Petrasek MacDonald J, Cunsolo Willox A, Ford JD, Shiwak I, Wood M; IMHACC Team; Rigolet Inuit Community Government. Protective factors for mental health and well-being in a changing climate: perspectives from Inuit youth in Nunatsiavut, Labrador. Soc Sci Med. 2015;141:133–41.
56. Blakney S. Connections to the land: The politics of health and wellbeing in Arviat, Nunavut. Winnipeg (MB): University of Manitoba; 2009.
57. Petrasek MacDonald J, Ford JD, Cunsolo Willox A, Ross NA. A review of protective factors and causal mechanisms that enhance the mental health of Indigenous Circumpolar youth. Int J Circumpolar Health. 2013;72(1):21775.
58. Alfred T. The Akwesasne cultural restoration program: a Mohawk approach to land-based education. Decolonization Indig Educ Soc. 2014;3(3):134–44.
59. Freeland Ballantyne E. Dechinta Bush University: mobilizing a knowledge economy of reciprocity, resurgence and decolonization. Decolonization Indig Educ Soc. 2014;3(3):67–85.
60. Radu I, House LM, Pashagumskum E. Land, life, and knowledge in Chisasibi: intergenerational healing in the bush. Decolonization Indig Educ Soc. 2014;3(3):86–105.

61. Harper SL, Edge VL, Schuster-Wallace CJ, Ar-Rushdi M, McEwen SA. Improving Aboriginal health data capture: evidence from a health registry evaluation. Epidemiol Infect. 2011;139(11):1774–83.
62. Gibson O, Lisy K, Davy C, Aromataris E, Kite E, Lockwood C, Riitano D, McBride K, Brown A. Enablers and barriers to the implementation of primary health care interventions for Indigenous people with chronic diseases: a systematic review. Implement Sci. 2015;10:71.
63. O'Sullivan TL, Amaratunga CA, Hardt J, Dow D, Phillips KP, Corneil W. Are we ready? Evidence of support mechanisms for Canadian health care workers in multi-jurisdictional emergency planning. Can J Public Health. 2007;98(5):358–63.
64. Young T, Tabish T, Young SK, Healey G. Patient transportation in Canada's northern territories: patterns, costs, and providers' perspectives. Rural Remote Health. 2019;19:5113.
65. McDonnell L, Lavoie JG, Healy G, Wong S, Goulet S, Clark W. Non-clinical determinants of medevacs in Nunavut: perspectives from northern health service providers and decision-makers. Int J Circumpolar Health. 2019;78(1):1571384.
66. Berry H. Pearl in the oyster: climate change as a mental health opportunity. Australas Psychiatry. 2009;17(6):453–6.
67. Albrecht G, Sartore GM, Connor L, Higginbotham N, Freeman S, Kelly B, Stain H, Tonna A, Pollard G. Solastalgia: the distress caused by environmental change. Australas Psychiatry. 2007;15(S1):S95–8.
68. Dodd W, Scott P, Howard C, Scott C, Rose C, Cunsolo A, Orbinski J. Lived experience of a record wildfire season in the Northwest Territories, Canada. Can J Public Health. 2018;109:327–37.
69. Ellis NR, Albrecht GA. Climate change threats to family farmers' sense of place and mental wellbeing: a case study from the western Australian wheatbelt. Soc Sci Med. 2017;175:161–8.
70. Berry HL, Waite TD, Dear KBG, Capon AG, Murray V. The case for systems thinking about climate change and mental health. Nat Clim Chang. 2018;8(4):282–90.
71. Berry HL, Bowen K, Kjellstrom T. Climate change and mental health: a causal pathways framework. Int J Public Health. 2010;55(2):123–32.
72. Swim JK, Stern PC, Doherty TJ, Clayton S, Reser JP, Weber EU, Gifford R, Howard GS. Psychology's contributions to understanding and addressing global climate change. Am Psychol. 2011;66(4):241–50.
73. Sartore GM, Kelly B, Stain H, Albrecht G, Higginbotham N. Control, uncertainty, and expectations for the future: a qualitative study of the impact of drought on a rural Australian community. Rural Remote Health. 2008;8(3):950.
74. Rigby CW, Rosen A, Berry HL, Hart CR. If the land's sick, we're sick: the impact of prolonged drought on the social and emotional well-being of Aboriginal communities in rural New South Wales. Aust J Rural Health. 2011;19(5):249–54.
75. Doherty TJ, Clayton S. The psychological impacts of global climate change. Am Psychol. 2011;66(4):265–76.

76. Berry HL, Hogan A, Owen J, Rickwood D, Fragar L. Climate change and farmers' mental health: Risks and responses. Asia-Pacific J Public Heal. 2011;23(2):119S-132S.
77. Berry HL, Butler JR, Burgess CP, King UG, Tsey K, Cadet-James YL, Rigby CW, Raphael B. Mind, body, spirit: Co-benefits for mental health from climate change adaptation and caring for country in remote Aboriginal Australian communities. N S W Public Health Bull. 2010;21(5–6):139–45.
78. Austin SE, Ford JD, Berrang-Ford L, Biesbroek R, Ross NA. Enabling local public health adaptation to climate change. Soc Sci Med. 2019;220:236–44.
79. Sibbald BBJ. Physicians' roles on the front line of climate change. Can Med Assoc J. 2013;185(3):195.
80. Barlow G. Nurses feel impact of climate change. Aust Nurs J. 2008;15(10):24–6.
81. Blashki G, Armstrong G, Berry HL, Weaver HJ, Hanna EG, Bi P, Harley D, Spickett JT. Preparing health services for climate change in Australia. Asia-Pacific J Public Heal. 2011;23(2):133S – 43.
82. Green EIH, Blashki G, Berry HL, Harley D, Horton G, Hall G. Preparing Australian medical students for climate change. Aust Fam Physician. 2009;38(9):726–9.
83. McMichael AJ, Neira M, Bertollini R, Campbell-Lendrum D, Hales S. Climate change: a time of need and opportunity for the health sector. Lancet. 2009;374(9707):2123–5.
84. Purcell R, McGirr J. Preparing rural general practitioners and health services for climate change and extreme weather. Aust J Rural Health. 2014;22(1):8–14.
85. Blashki G, Abelsohn A, Woollard R, Arya N, Parkes MW, Kendal P, Bell E, Bell RW. General practitioners' responses to global climate change – lessons from clinical experience and the clinical method. Asia Pac Fam Med. 2012;11(6).

13 Suicide Prevention: A Sociocultural Approach to Understanding Suicide among Inuit – Issues and Prevention Strategies

JOSEPHINE TAN

I am an academic, a clinician, and a researcher who works in the area of cultural clinical psychology. My interest in Indigenous mental health was sparked when I started working with First Nations residential school survivors in 1996 as part of my clinical practice. My research on Inuit suicide prevention began in 2003 when I joined a mental health task force that was linked to a multi-site research centre. The task force members were a mix of Inuit and non-Inuit individuals from Nunavut who worked in the area of suicide prevention. I learned about Inuit, their history and culture, and the mental health issues that exist in Nunavut, as well as some of the history of those problems, from working with the task force members and from collaborating with the Nunavut Kamatsiaqtut Help Line (NKHL) on projects relating to suicide prevention. Our work together has continued to this day and has generated conference and workshop presentations and publications. I have visited Iqaluit as part of my work with the NKHL. With each visit, I come to know more people and my appreciation of the history, culture, and lived realities of Inuit continue to grow.

Over the years of working with the NKHL, I have witnessed the evolution of suicide prevention work in Nunavut. In 2017, I was invited to be part of a Canadian Institutes of Health Research knowledge exchange workshop involving key stakeholders, researchers, community leaders, and policymakers and decision makers from various levels of governments. The aim of the workshop was to discuss research evidence on the topic of suicide among Inuit and the applicability of the research findings to Nunavut. By then, Nunavut had developed its own Suicide Prevention Strategy. I am impressed with the details and comprehensiveness of the strategy and its recommendations, which take into consideration the unique realities of Inuit lifestyle and society. However, although information about the Strategy is available on websites and in reports, little information can be found in academic literature. In writing this chapter, I hope to bring together information from peer-reviewed and grey literature to highlight the link between colonization, the disruption of Inuit society, and suicide among Inuit today; the suicide prevention strategies that have been proposed and adopted by Inuit for Inuit; and the current status of suicide prevention in Nunavut.

Introduction

Inuit represent 4.2 per cent of the Indigenous peoples in Canada and 0.2 per cent of the entire population in the country (1). About 73.1 per cent of Inuit live in communities located across the northern regions of Canada. A large proportion of Inuit (45.4 per cent) live in Nunavut, and 85.4 per cent of Nunavut residents are Inuit. The suicide rate for Inuit has been increasing over the years, with male youth being the group at greatest risk (2). The most recent national statistics covering 2011 to 2016 indicated the suicide rate among Inuit to be nine times the rate for non-Indigenous individuals, but when comparing young females ages 15 to 24, the rate increased dramatically among Inuit to 33 times the rate for non-Indigenous people (3). Several attempts have been made to address the problem, such as the establishment of the NKHL (4); the Isaksimagit Inuusirmi Katujjiqaatigiit Embrace Life Council (5), which provides programs and community-based training to promote the value of life; and the Nunavut Suicide Prevention Strategic Plan (6) to guide suicide prevention efforts in the territory. In 2013, the suicide rate in Nunavut reached a high of 13.5 times the national rate. The chief coroner of Nunavut called for an inquest (7), which was held in September 2015. Subsequent to the inquest, the premier of Nunavut declared suicide to be a "crisis" in the territory (8 para10).

Factors that may increase Inuit youth's risk for suicide attempts include being male (9–11), knowing someone who attempted or died by suicide, solvent abuse, parental drug or alcohol problem (11), alcohol and/or marijuana use, and history of physical violence and sexual abuse (12). A large-scale study on Inuit in Nunavut who died by suicide between the years of 2003 to 2006 indicated a greater likelihood of having experienced child abuse and having a family history of clinical depression or of family members who died by suicide (13). As well, people who died by suicide were more likely to have had personal difficulties with clinical depression and alcohol or cannabis dependence within the previous six months of their death, to have higher levels of impulsivity and aggressive behaviours, and to have been diagnosed with personality disorders such as borderline personality disorder or antisocial personality disorder. Similar to reports on the general population, these findings reveal a relationship between suicide and psychopathology, substance use, and early childhood adversity (14–18).

A comprehensive understanding of suicide among Indigenous peoples must consider historical and sociocultural context, in particular the colonial history and the consequent devastation of Indigenous people's culture and societies that contribute to the high rates of suicide among Inuit today. The call for using a contextual approach is increasingly being echoed by researchers (e.g., 19,20) and Inuit themselves (21). This chapter begins with a literature review of the historical, sociopolitical, cultural, and structural factors associated with suicide among Inuit, followed by the implications for developing suicide prevention strategies that are culturally appropriate and informed by the lived experiences of Inuit.

Brief Overview of the Colonial History

Contact between Inuit and non-Inuit or Qallunaat (the Inuktitut term for non-Inuit people) goes back to the sixteenth century (22). More substantial contact took place in the nineteenth and twentieth centuries between Inuit and Caucasian whalers. Historically, Inuit lived with extended families and on the land; they migrated to follow animals as part of their hunting pattern (23). Social roles of men and women were defined, kinship was very important, and marriages were often arranged (24).

When the Canadian government took control of the Canadian Arctic between the 1940s and 1960s (21), Inuit were forced into fixed settlements, some Inuit communities were relocated to regions that were of considerable distance from their place of origin (25), and many children were separated from their parents and sent to residential schools (22,26). As well, tuberculosis, which was a national concern at that time, affected Indigenous communities to a far greater degree than the non-Indigenous society (27). Many Inuit who had contracted the illness were sent to southern sanitoria for treatment and separated from their family for several years (28). For more details on the colonial history, see Crawford (29) and Kral and Idlout (22). The policies and practices of the Canadian government had far-reaching impacts because they led to rapid social transformation in all areas of Inuit life, especially on family and social relationships (22,30). The transformation unravelled Inuit social structure, which led to high psychological distress and contributed to the high rates of suicide, as discussed in this chapter.

A significant amount of research has examined the specific ways in which government policies and actions have led to adversities experienced by Inuit. These adverse outcomes can be broadly classified into changes in lifestyle, intergenerational trauma specifically tied to the residential school system, breakdown in relationships and intergenerational segregation, cultural discontinuity, and structural and societal difficulties. The rest of the chapter will look at each of these outcomes, followed by a discussion of their implications for suicide prevention efforts. Recent developments in the area of Inuit suicide prevention strategies will also be discussed.

Changes in Lifestyle

When Inuit were forced by the Canadian government into fixed settlements, they had to abandon their traditional land-based lifestyle. Their subsistence economy was replaced by a wage economy that involved working in industries such as mining and in government civil service. However, there were barriers to Inuit employment, including lack of jobs that matched the individual's skill and the required level of formal education (31,32).

The drastic and rapid changes to Inuit economic structures and lifestyles were detrimental because the traditional subsistence style of living had not only afforded Inuit several benefits but also contributed to the stability of their social organization. For example, harvesting of traditional foods (e.g., seals, whales, caribou, and various fish and fowl) reinforced cultural identity and helped to develop and strengthen the relational and social ties among individuals, families, and communities (33). Inuit viewed, and many still view, traditional or "country" foods to have healing properties, seeing an integral link among food, blood, and mental well-being (34–36); their positive view has been supported by scientific evidence that points to the nutritional benefits of Inuit traditional food (37–39). Engagement in traditional activities also allowed Inuit men to fulfil their social responsibilities as hunters and providers (33). When the government killed Inuit sled dogs in the 1950s and 1960s, it not only took away from Inuit their means of transportation; it also deprived the men of the opportunity to hunt, provide for their families, and be productive (40–41).

Equally important, connection with the land is essential to Inuit health. The land is linked to Inuit personal and cultural history, and its vista provides Inuit with a sense of harmony and rejuvenation. Furthermore, activities on the land facilitate teaching where younger learn from older individuals, increase resilience, contribute to the development of skills and self-esteem, and promote relationships among individuals and families within and across generations (34). Forced relocation into permanent settlements in many cases removed the resources that were critical to Inuit personal, family, and community health (25).

The housing built by the government when Inuit moved into settlements did not address their needs; for example, they were too small for Inuit families and led to overcrowding, there was no indoor space to prepare seal meat, and the construction materials were inadequate for the northern climate. Furthermore, the costs of purchasing the housing units and paying for utilities were often beyond the financial means of Inuit (42).

The housing problems continue to this day. In 2017, the Standing Senate Committee on Indigenous Peoples released a report (43), which indicated that Inuit still lack appropriate and affordable housing and linked inadequate housing and overcrowding to ill health, lack of employment, and poor socio-economic and development outcomes. Other reports have also linked housing issues with health problems (44), low academic achievement, depression, substance use, domestic violence (45), and homelessness (46). The Canadian government is attempting to address the housing problems by including investments in housing for Inuit in its federal budget (47).

Residential School and Intergenerational Trauma

The residential school system, part of the colonial endeavour, was designed by the Canadian government to assimilate Indigenous peoples, including Inuit, into mainstream society by breaking the bonds that children had with their family and culture (48–50). Many children who attended residential school were abused psychologically, physically, and/or sexually (48) resulting in complex psychological trauma, use of maladaptive coping behaviours (e.g., alcohol and substance use), and increased risk of revictimization (51). The cycle of trauma was repeated over subsequent generations when the former students raised their own children because they had not learned about nurturing relationships or positive parenting skills because of the lack of appropriate role models in the residential schools (52).

Traditionally, Inuit parenting consists of modelling by the parents and imitation by children (34). Child abuse and neglect are not part of traditional Inuit culture. However, in contemporary times, a high percentage of respondents of the 2007–2008 Inuit Health Survey (53) indicated having experienced severe childhood sexual abuse (41 per cent) and severe childhood physical abuse (31 per cent). Furthermore, 29 per cent of respondents disclosed that they had made at least one suicide attempt in their lifetime. Comparisons between Inuit individuals who had died by suicide and those who were still living revealed that the suicide group was more likely to have experienced child abuse (13). Relatedly, another study showed that having a stable family environment differentiated Inuit who had never attempted suicide from those who had attempted suicide or died by suicide (54). Not surprisingly, links have been made between the adverse effects of residential school attendance, psychological distress, and suicide (55,56). Moreover, researchers who analysed the data from the 2002/2003 Manitoba First Nation Regional Longitudinal Adult Health Survey also found an association between suicide behaviour and having attended residential school or having a parent or grandparent who had attended residential school (56). Another group of researchers who analysed the 2008–10 First Nations Regional Health Survey reported that the odds of having suicidal ideation and attempts among individuals who had one familial generation of residential school history were higher than among those who had no familial history of residential school attendance, and that the odds of suicide attempts were higher among persons with two generations than persons with one generation of residential school family history (57). Collectively, these findings underscore the adverse intergenerational effects of the residential school system.

Relationship Breakdown and Intergenerational Segregation

Colonization and continued colonialism have had (and continue to have) a very marked and deleterious effect on Inuit family and relationships (34). In many communities, forced settlement led to decreased economic cooperation among kin networks, and for those who attended residential school, relational ties were often broken between child and family, leading to intergenerational segregation and conflict (22). In these cases, children often came to rely on peers instead of parents for support (58), and some of the young people entered into romantic and sexual relations with no guidance or role models (22).

Distress and suicide among Inuit often appear to be linked to relationship difficulties within the family or with romantic partners (58,59) and to feelings of anger and loneliness (60). Relationship problems and loneliness/boredom are the two leading reasons for Inuit reaching out for help outside their families, such as when using the NKHL (61). Some Inuit who have attempted suicide have noted that just before they made the attempt, they had feelings of depression, anger, boredom, or being tired of life, as well as thoughts of relationship conflicts or breakups (53).

The rapid cultural, social, and economic changes in Inuit society also contribute to the problem of intergenerational segregation in another way. The experiences of older Inuit and Elders are linked more to traditional ways of learning and being; in contrast, many Inuit youth receive formal education in schools that are often cast in a Euro-Canadian mould and taught by non-Inuit teachers (62), and are also exposed to a greater degree to non-Inuit culture (34). In some cases, older individuals might feel marginalized and ineffective because of the rapid transition from a subsistence economy that involved hunting to a wage and market economy that requires dealing with hierarchical authority and bureaucracy (34). Some youth might feel caught between two worlds – their own lifestyle and the one presented in mass media (19) or even in the schools (62,63). In all, older Inuit are more likely to identify with their traditional culture while some of the younger generations might not fully identify with either traditional Inuit or mainstream culture, thereby leading to an intergenerational divergence in interests and lived experiences. The importance of intergenerational connectedness is underscored by research that shows close relationships with parents, being connected to the family, the extended family, and adopted kin relational systems, as well as mentorship from older generations, to be factors that promote mental health and well-being among Indigenous circumpolar youth (64) and Inuit youth specifically (65; see also Healey et al., chapter 5 in this volume).

Cultural Discontinuity

Intergenerational segregation has meant fewer opportunities for parents and grandparents to mentor youth and pass on traditional Inuit values and teachings (58,66). Traditional teachings and knowledge can promote healthy self-image and positive identity (67). A study with two Inuit communities revealed a link between well-being and happiness and family, talking, and Inuit cultural values and traditional practices. Unhappiness was linked to an absence of these factors (19).

Intergenerational segregation does not reflect a refusal to interact on the part of either younger or older Inuit, but rather a gap in knowing how to reach out and communicate with each other. Kral (58) found that youth did not know how to approach the Elders, and some Elders feared that talking about suicide with youth would encourage suicidality (68). Another difficulty in discussing suicide is the lack of appropriate terminology for suicide in Inuit languages that can be used without appearing to blame those who died by suicide (68).

Structural and Societal Difficulties

The 2014 report by Inuit Tapiriit Kanatami (ITK) (66) identified 11 social determinants of Inuit health that are informed by those defined by the World Health Organization (69). Within these, a number of challenges identified were associated with employment, education, poverty, high costs of living, crowded housing and poor ventilation, homelessness, personal safety issues (interpersonal violence, children witnessing violence, substance and alcohol abuse), low access to health care, poor food security, climate change, and environmental contaminants, as well as the decline of the traditional culture and use of Inuit languages. All these factors reflect adverse living conditions that are considerably substandard when compared to Canadian mainstream society and that contribute to socio-economic distress and poor health in Inuit communities. An examination of each of these social determinants is beyond the scope of this chapter; see ITK (66) for details. However, the report supports the position that sociopolitical, historical, and environmental factors are highly relevant to our understanding of suicide among Inuit and that improving access to basic necessities and addressing inequity should be part of suicide prevention initiatives.

Thus it is prudent to stress that, as noted by ITK, "traditional values such as sharing, respect for elders and cooperation remain central to Inuit community life" and "Inuit communities [and individuals] are among the most culturally resilient in North America" (70 para1). A majority (60 per cent) of Inuit are able to converse in Inuktitut, and traditional practices such as harvesting and preparing country foods (e.g., seal, caribou, and narwhal) are still being followed (70). It is important to understand the factors that promote resilience and to use the information to inform suicide prevention initiatives. Unfortunately, only a few researchers (71,72; see also Healey et al. this volume, chapter 5) have paid attention to the strength of Inuit individuals, families, and communities or the factors that promote resilience among Inuit. Inuit Elders have identified a number of traditional values (e.g., patience, perseverance, love, and caring) and effective coping behaviours (e.g., talking to others, being active in nature, learning traditional skills) to be important to the development of resilience (73). Future research could use the information as a springboard to create more knowledge on the specific resilience factors that can protect against suicide.

Implications for Suicide Prevention Strategies

As discussed above, colonization and continued colonialism of Inuit by Qallunaat have resulted in cultural disruption for Inuit society with very significant consequences for the health of the individual, the family unit, and communities. The repercussions are transmitted across generations. Clearly, suicide prevention efforts for Inuit need to be sensitive to the cultural and contextual needs of the people. Indeed, the report by the Inungni Sapujjijiit Task Force on Suicide Prevention and Community Healing (74) indicated that participants in Inuit committee meetings have expressed the need for suicide prevention training by Inuit for Inuit, instead of adopting training programs from mainstream Canadian society or those that have been developed for other Indigenous groups, because they often do not hold cultural resonance for Inuit. The authors of the report also noted that employees from the south often do not understand Inuit culture and traditions or respect Inuit ways of dealing with issues. The Inuit Mental Wellness Framework calls for a holistic approach that includes Inuit traditional knowledge and practices (75).

Some research shows that suicide prevention interventions for Indigenous communities that are developed and carried out by Indigenous peoples themselves lead to positive outcomes (59,76). These interventions tend to include traditional cultural values and practices that serve as a protective factor against suicide among Indigenous peoples (77). Similarly, preliminary but promising results have been obtained when suicide prevention initiatives are guided by Inuit themselves. While it is not known exactly which factors are responsible for the success of home-grown suicide prevention initiatives, research with two communities, which had developed and implemented their own suicide prevention efforts, showed a decrease in the rates of suicide (22). In both instances, there was open communication among community members and among the youth themselves where concerns about suicides were expressed, and tangible suicide prevention strategies were identified and implemented. In one community, closet rods that were commonly used in youth suicides were removed. In the other community, the youth opened a youth centre.

They developed a crisis help line, received training to operate it, organized activities where youth and Elders could get together, and provided opportunities for youth to engage in and learn traditional practices and the Inuktitut language. When the centre closed down for lack of funding, the number of suicides increased. Several years later, the centre reopened after securing funding and the number of suicides decreased (22).

Developing suicide interventions that are simultaneously evidence based and culturally sensitive is not easy. Inuit and Western conceptualizations of mental health and approaches to addressing mental difficulties are very different. Western models generally focus on individual factors where treatment is guided by evidence derived from Western scientific health paradigms and delivered by trained mental health professionals within the context of Western mental health interventions. In contrast, Inuit often connect health and mental health to the land, family, culture, and traditional food and practices (19,34; see also Healey et al. this volume, chapter 5), similar to other Indigenous peoples (20; see also Mushquash et al. this volume, chapter 15). These results imply that suicide prevention may be best served by strengthening traditional values and practices, as well as relational ties, in addition to non-Inuit adopting decolonizing measures, which could take various forms, such as gaining familiarity with Canadian colonial history, Inuit culture, and their world views; and working towards social and economic equality for Inuit individuals and communities (20).

The disparities in perspectives are aptly captured by Wexler and Gone (20), who contrasted the assumptions about suicide from Western and Indigenous viewpoints. They noted that Western views on suicide are that it is a personal choice carried out as an expression of individual psychological pain. Thus, suicide prevention is considered to be best carried out by trained mental health professionals operating within a formal mental health system, who can deliver targeted interventions to alleviate the psychological distress. In contrast, Indigenous views of suicide are that it is the result of historical oppression, social suffering, and longstanding disruptions to Indigenous culture, families, and communities, and that the act itself is an expression of shared social anguish. Therefore, suicidality is best addressed by those who understand the social context of the individual at risk; for example, trusted family, friends, and community members who can provide the necessary social support. In addition, suicide prevention would be undertaken at the community level through locally designed decolonization projects that increase cultural engagement and strengthen community activism, such as those that work towards the promotion of Indigenous sovereignty rights, language, culture, and knowledge.

Clearly, it is inappropriate to employ Western models of health and interventions within Inuit society if they conflict with Inuit cultural values, as that would perpetuate colonialism. Thus, the challenge lies in finding ways to use

Inuit cultural and traditional practices for suicide prevention, where appropriate, alongside Western interventions that are grounded in culturally safe evidence. One example of such attempt is reflected in the Nunavut Suicide Prevention Strategic Plan (78).

Following the 2015 inquest into the high suicide rates in Nunavut, the territory's Suicide Prevention Strategic Plan, 2011–2014 was re-adopted, and an action plan, Resiliency Within (78), was developed for the 2016–2017 year. The strategic plan is a formulation that integrates comprehensive efforts between government and community sectors. It has eight commitments that are intended to mobilize organizations and individuals to be part of suicide prevention strategies, ensure that Nunavummiut (Nunavut residents) have access to a wide range of mental health services, assist youth to increase their resilience to adversity, provide suicide prevention training to interested individuals, carry out research on suicidality, engage in public education and dialogues about suicide, foster safe and healthy development for the young, and support communities in the development of local solutions (78).

The suicide prevention efforts listed included in the Resiliency Within action plan reflect a combination of Western and Inuit cultural approaches. For instance, psychiatric and mental health and addictions services, a mobile trauma response team, a public awareness campaign, and research can be found listed alongside efforts that have specific Inuit traditional focus, such as a hunter education program, a youth mentorship program that builds life skills and provides opportunities for youth to interact with Elders, and cultural sensitivity training for frontline staff. Although spirituality has been identified as a protective factor against suicide in both non-Indigenous (79) and Indigenous groups (80,81), it is not included in the action plan. Evidence shows that the benefits conferred by spirituality are not necessarily universal. For instance, minority religious groups that feel isolated and unsupported by mainstream culture might not experience reduced risk of suicidality associated with their spirituality (82).

Implementation of the strategic plan requires resources that might be available in bigger communities such as Iqaluit, which has a population of over 7000 (83). Suicide prevention efforts for smaller communities, several of which have a population count of under 1000, might require somewhat different approaches. Moreover, some communities might prefer to develop their own strategies that fit with their own lived realities instead of adopting them from elsewhere (68). As indicated in the work by Kral and Idlout (22), it is more likely that community-developed efforts will be successful.

In 2016, ITK revealed the National Inuit Suicide Prevention Strategy (84,85). It identified six priority areas: creating social equity, creating cultural continuity, nurturing healthy Inuit children from birth, providing access to mental wellness services, healing unresolved trauma and grief, and mobilizing Inuit knowledge for resilience and suicide prevention. For each priority area, objectives and action plans are laid out that are Inuit specific and led by Inuit. Western-based approaches are incorporated primarily in the priority area of mental wellness. Built into the strategy is a mandate to evaluate its implementation and outcomes and to learn about and add to gaps in knowledge, promote promising practices, and link communities and regions for mutual learning. The authors of the national strategy explained that it is not designed to replace local and community suicide prevention efforts; rather it offers a means for the different stakeholders to understand, communicate, and cooperate with one another so that they can develop policies and specific roles among themselves and coordinate their initiatives towards shared goals (84).

Recently, ITK (86) provided an update on the progress made during the first two years of the National Inuit Suicide Prevention Strategy. It reported on the development and implementation of new programming and services designed to reduce risk factors, such as historical trauma, mental distress, substance use, sexual violence, and homelessness for at-risk youth, individuals, and families. At the same time, programming and services are also available to Inuit to strengthen protective factors, such as intergenerational learning, employment skills, improved housing, parenting supports, early childhood education, counsellor training, and gatherings of Elders and youth to talk about issues of deaths by suicide. Outcomes of these new programming and services have yet to be evaluated.

Conclusion

Death by suicide and suicide attempts among Inuit are strongly connected to colonization and continued colonial interventions by the Canadian government, which led to drastic changes in Inuit social organization and lifestyle. Assimilation efforts by the government included forced fixed settlement of families into inadequate living units, rapid transition from subsistence to wage economy without sufficient access to wage labour, and implementation of a residential school system that resulted in mental health difficulties and intergenerational segregation. All these activities have had a ripple effect laterally across different aspects of Inuit society and vertically across generations. Moreover, the move into fixed settlements was very rapid for Inuit and compounded difficulties in adapting to a new way of living. One of the outcomes of government interventions has been the heavy toll on Inuit health; particularly. suicide among young Inuit has been identified to be of pressing concern.

Given that suicidality is linked to the disruption of Inuit society and culture, consideration of cultural and sociohistorical factors is essential to any plan that proposes to reduce suicide rates. Indeed, some data suggest that when suicide prevention efforts are developed and implemented by Inuit communities themselves, the outcome is promising. The philosophy that suicide prevention initiatives need to be developed and controlled by Inuit and incorporate cultural aspects is adopted in contemporary and comprehensive Nunavut and national Inuit suicide prevention strategies. These strategies go beyond addressing the psychological or personal suicide risk factors; they incorporate other mental-health-related factors, such as early childhood health and social equity, among many others.

In conclusion, it is of utmost importance that Inuit control efforts focusing on suicide prevention and that researchers and clinicians who work in the area of suicide among Inuit be familiar with the historical and contemporary political, social, and cultural forces that impact suicidality. Understanding the effects of colonization and colonialism is critical. Future research needs to focus on resilience among Inuit, which can offer culturally appropriate information to guide suicide prevention efforts. However, there is a risk that such information, which is often derived from qualitative and ethnographic studies, might not make it into mainstream scientific journals, because these journals are still defined by Western research paradigms, which place a high value on quantitative studies (87). Thus, the way that research on Inuit suicide and suicide prevention is being carried out, disseminated, and used needs to move in the direction of including Inuit perspectives more fully. Finally, it is vital to keep in mind that while non-Inuit can contribute to issues related to Inuit health, the efforts that are led by Inuit are more likely to have relevance and resonance for Inuit.

REFERENCES

1. Statistics Canada. Aboriginal peoples in Canada: First Nations peoples, Métis, and Inuit. National Household Survey 2011 [Internet]. Ottawa (ON): Minister of Industry; 2013 [cited 2016 Oct 1]. Catalogue No. 99-011-X2011001. Available from: http://www.stratejuste.ca/uploads/3/1/8/4/31849453/aboriginal_release_nhs_briefs_sept_16.pdf
2. Suicide Prevention Strategy Working Group. Nunavut Suicide Prevention Strategy [Internet]. Iqaluit (NU): Suicide Prevention Strategy Working Group; 2010. [cited 2011 Dec 25]. Available from: http://www.naho.ca/documents/it/2010-10-26-Nunavut-Suicide-Prevention-Strategy-English.pdf
3. Kumar MB, Tjepkema M. Suicide among First Nations people, Métis and Inuit (2011–2016): findings from the 2011 Canadian census health and environment cohort (CanCHEC) [Internet]. Ottawa (ON): Minister of Industry; 2019 [cited 2020 Jan 7]. Available from https://www150.statcan.gc.ca/n1/pub/99-011-x/99-011-x2019001-eng.pdf

4. Tan JCH, Maranzan AK, Boone M, Vander Velde J, Levy S. Usage of the Nunavut Kamatsiaqtut Help Line: An analysis of 11 years of database [Internet]. Thunder Bay (ON): Centre of Excellence for Children and Adolescents with Special Needs; 2005 [cited 2010 Jul 9]. Available from: https://www.deslibris.ca/ID/223867
5. Isaksimagit Inuusirmi Katujjiqaatigiit Embrace Life Council [Internet]. Iqaluit (NU): Embrace Life Council; 2019. About Embrace Life Council; 2019 [cited 2019 Apr 14]. Available from http://inuusiq.com/about/overview/
6. Government of Nunavut, Nunavut Tunngavik Inc., Embrace Life Council, Royal Canadian Mounted Police. Nunavut Suicide Prevention Strategy October 2010 [Internet]. Iqaluit (NU): Nunavut Tunngavik; 2010. Available from: http://www.gov.nu.ca/sites/default/files/files/NSPS_final_English_Oct%202010(1).pdf
7. Eggertson L. Nunavut calls inquest into record number of suicides. CMAJ. 2014;186(3):E109–10.
8. Nunatsiaq News. Nunavut premier declares suicide a "crisis," names minister to file. Nunatsiaq News [Internet], 2015 Oct 23 [cited 2017 Feb 10]. Available from: http://www.nunatsiaqonline.ca/stories/article/65674nunavut_premier_declares_suicide_crisis_names_minister_to_file/
9. Bjerregaard P, Young TK, Dewailly E, Ebbesson, SOE. Indigenous health in the Arctic: an overview of the circumpolar Inuit population. Scand J Public Health. 2004;32:390–5.
10. Hicks, J, Bjerregaard, P, Berman, M. The transition from the historical Inuit suicide pattern to the present Inuit suicide pattern. In: White JP, Wingert S, Beavon D, Maxim P, editors. Vol. 4, Moving forward, making a difference [Internet]. Toronto (ON): Thompson Educational Publishing; 2007 [cited 2019 Apr 13]. p. 39–53. Available from https://ir.lib.uwo.ca/aprci/113
11. Kirmayer LJ, Malus M, Boothroyd LJ. Suicide attempts among Inuit youth: a community survey of prevalence and risk factors. Acta Psychiatry Scand. 1996;94(1):8–17.
12. Fraser SL, Geoffroy D, Chachamovich E, Kirmayer LJ. Changing rates of suicide ideation and attempts among Inuit youth: a gender-based analysis of risk and protective factors. Suicide Life Threat Behav. 2015;45(2):141–56.
13. Chachamovich E, Kirmayer LJ, Haggarty JM, Cargo M, McCormick R, Turecki G. Suicide among Inuit: results from a large, epidemiologically representative follow-back study in Nunavut. Can J Psychiatry. 2015;60(6):268–75.
14. Bohnert ASB, Roeder K, Ilgen MA. Unintentional overdose and suicide among substance users: a review of overlap and risk factors. Drug Alcohol Depend. 2010;110:183–92.
15. Cavanagh JTO, Carson AJ, Sharpe M, Lawrie SM. Psychological autopsy studies of suicide: a systematic review. Psychol Med. 2003;33:395–405.
16. Gvion Y, Apter A. Aggression, impulsivity, and suicide behavior: a review of the literature. Arch Suicide Res. 2011;15(2):93–112.

17. Maniglio R. The role of child sexual abuse in the etiology of suicide and non-suicidal self-injury. Acta Psychiatry Scand. 2011;124(1):30–41.
18. Schneider B, Wetterling T, Sargk D, Schneider F, Schnabel A, Maurer K, Fritze J. Axis I disorders and personality disorders as risk factors for suicide. Eur Arch Psychiatry Clin Neurosci. 2006;256(1):17–27.
19. Kral MJ, Idlout L, Minore JB, Dyck RJ, Kirmayer LJ. Unikkaartuit: Meanings of well-being, unhappiness, health, and community change among Inuit in Nunavut, Canada. Am J Community Psychol. 2011;48(3–4):426–38.
20. Wexler LM, Gone JP. Culturally responsive suicide prevention in indigenous communities: unexamined assumptions and new possibilities. Am J Public Health. 2012;102(5):800–6.
21. Morris M, Crook, C. Structural and cultural factors in suicide prevention: the contrast between mainstream and Inuit approaches to understanding and preventing suicide. J Soc Work Pract. 2015;29(3):321–38.
22. Kral MJ, Idlout L. Indigenous best practices. Community-based suicide prevention in Nunavut, Canada. In: White J, Marsh I, Kral MJ, Morris J, editors. Critical suicidology: transforming suicide research and prevention for the 21st century. Vancouver (BC): UBC Press; 2016. p. 229–243.
23. Damas, D. Arctic migrants/Arctic villagers: the transformation of Inuit settlement in the central Arctic. Montreal (QC): McGill-Queen's University Press; 2002.
24. McElroy A. Canadian Arctic modernization and change in female Inuit role identification. Am Ethnol. 1975;2(4):662–86.
25. Tester FJ, Kulchyski P. Tammarniit (mistakes): Inuit relocations in the Eastern Arctic, 1939–63. Vancouver (BC): UBC Press; 1994.
26. King D. A brief report of the federal government of Canada's residential school system for Inuit. Ottawa (ON): Aboriginal Healing Foundation; 2006.
27. Tester FJ, McNicol P, Irniq P. Writing for our lives: The language of homesickness, self-esteem and the Inuit TB "epidemic." Etudes Inuit. 2001:25(1/2);121–40.
28. Wherret GJ. The miracle of the empty beds. Toronto (ON): University of Toronto Press; 1977.
29. Crawford A. "The trauma experienced by generations past having an effect in their descendants": narrative and historical trauma among Inuit in Nunavut, Canada. Transcult Psychiatry. 2014;51(3):339–69.
30. Kral M. The return of the sun: suicide and reclamation among Inuit of Arctic Canada. New York (NY): Oxford University Press; 2019.
31. Bonesteel S. Canada's relationship with Inuit: a history of policy and program development (report prepared for Indian and Northern Affairs Canada) [Internet]. Ottawa (ON): Minister of Public Works and Government Services Canada; 2006 [cited 2015 May 3]. Available from: http://www.aadnc-aandc.gc.ca/DAM/DAM-INTER-HQ/STAGING/texte-text/inuit-book_1100100016901_eng.pdf
32. Senécal, S. Employment, industry and occupations of Inuit in Canada, 1981–2001. Ottawa (ON): Indian and Northern Affairs Canada; 2007.

33. Richmond CAM. The social determinants of Inuit health: a focus on social support in the Canadian arctic. Int J Circumpolar Health. 2009:68(5):471–87.
34. Kirmayer LJ, Fletcher C, Watt R. Locating the ecocentric self: Inuit concepts of mental health and illness. In: Kirmayer LJ, Valaskakis, GG, editors. Healing traditions: the mental health of Aboriginal peoples in Canada. Vancouver (BC): University of British Columbia Press; 2008. p. 289–314.
35. Borré, K. Seal blood, Inuit blood, and diet: a biocultural model of physiology and cultural identity. Med Anthropol Q. 1991;5(1):48–62.
36. Laugrand F, Uhttuvak I, Therrien, M. Interviewing Inuit Elders, Volume 5: perspectives on traditional health. Iqaluit (NU): Nunavut Arctic College; 2001.
37. Gagné D, Blanchet R, Lauzière J, Vaissière E, Vézina C, Ayotte P, Déry S, Turgeon O'Brien H. Traditional food consumption is associated with higher nutrient intakes in Inuit children attending childcare centres in Nunavik. Int J Circumpolar Health. 2012;71(1):18401.
38. Hu XF, Kenny TA, Chan HM. Country food diet pattern is associated with lower risk of coronary heart disease. J Acad Nutr Diet. 2018;118(7):1237–48.
39. Sheehy T, Kolahdooz F, Roache C, Sharma S. Traditional food consumption is associated with better diet quality and adequacy among Inuit adults in Nunavut, Canada. Int J Food Sci Nutr. 2015;66(4):445–51.
40. Qikiqtani Inuit Association. Qikiqtani Truth Commission: thematic reports and special studies, 1950–1975. Qimmiliriniq: Inuit sled dogs in Qikiqtaaluk. Iqaluit (NU): Inhabit Media Inc.; 2013.
41. Inuit Tuttarvingat of NAHO, executive director. How are we as men? [television series episode; Internet]. In: Qanuqtuurniq – Finding the balance [edited DVD transcript]. Iqaluit (NU): Inuit Communications; 2009 [cited 2019 Apr 14]. Available at http://archives.algomau.ca/main/sites/default/files/2012-25_004_033_002.pdf
42. Duffy RQ. The road to Nunavut: the progress of the eastern Arctic Inuit since the Second World War. Montreal (QC): McGill-Queen's University Press; 1988.
43. Standing Senate Committee on Aboriginal Peoples. We can do better: Housing in Inuit Nunangat [Internet]. Ottawa (ON): Senate Canada; 2017 [cited 2020 January 8]. Available from https://sencanada.ca/content/sen/committee/421/APPA/Reports/Housing_e.pdf
44. Project HOPE. Housing and health. An overview of the literature. Health Affairs health policy brief [Internet]. Bethesda (MD): Project HOPE – The People-to-People Foundation, Inc.; 2018 Jun 7 [cited 2021 Mar 8]. Available from https://www.healthaffairs.org/do/10.1377/hpb20180313.396577/full/HPB_2018_RWJF_01_W.pdf
45. Inuit Tapiriit Kanatami. Backgrounder on Inuit and housing: for discussion at Housing Sectoral Meeting, November 24 and 25th in Ottawa [Internet]. Ottawa (ON): Inuit Tapiriit Kanatami; 2004 Nov 1 [cited 2019 Apr 14]. Available from: http://www.cca.qc.ca/charrette/2008/texts/ITK_BgPaper_e.pdf

46. Christensen J, Arnfjord S, Carraher S, Hedwig T. Homelessness across Alaska, the Canadian North and Greenland: a review of the literature on a developing social phenomenon in the circumpolar north. Arctic. 2017;70(4);349–64.
47. Inuit Tapiriit Kanatami. Inuit Nunangat housing strategy [Internet]. Ottawa (ON): Inuit Tapiriit Kanatami; 2019 [cited 2020 Jan 8]. Available from: http://www.itk.ca/wp-content/uploads/2019/04/2019-Inuit-Nunangat-Housing-Strategy-English.pdf
48. Milloy JS. A national crime: the Canadian government and the residential school system, 1879–1986. Winnipeg (MB): University of Manitoba Press; 1999.
49. The Legacy of Hope Foundation. Inuit and the residential school system [Internet]. Ottawa (ON): Legacy of Hope Foundation; 2013 [cited 2019 Apr 14]. Available from http://weweresofaraway.ca/wp-content/uploads/2013/04/Inuit-and-the-RSS.pdf
50. Truth and Reconciliation Commission of Canada. Canada's residential schools: the Inuit and northern experience – the final report of the Truth and Reconciliation Commission of Canada, Volume 2 [Internet]. Montreal (PQ): McGill-Queen's University Press, 2015 [cited 2019 Apr 14]. https://www.jstor.org/stable/j.ctt19rm9tm
51. Söchting I, Corrado R, Cohen IM, Ley RG, Brasfield C. Traumatic pasts in Canadian Aboriginal people: further support for a complex trauma conceptualization? BC Medical Journal. 2007;49(6):320–6.
52. Menzies P. Intergenerational trauma from a mental health perspective. Native Soc Work J. 2010;7:63–85.
53. Galloway T, Saudny H. Inuit health survey, 2007–2008. Nunavut community and personal wellness [Internet]. Ste-Anne-de-Bellevue (QC): Centre for Indigenous Peoples' Nutrition and Environment; 2012 [cited 2016 Dec 18]. Available from: http://www.tunngavik.com/files/2012/09/IHS_NUNAVUT-FV-V11_FINAL_AUG-15_2012.pdf
54. Beaudoin V, Seguin M, Chawky N, Affleck W, Chachamovich E, Turecki G. Protective factors in the Inuit population of Nunavut: a comparative study of people who died by suicide, people who attempted suicide, and people who never attempted suicide. Int J Environ Res Public Health. 2018;15(1):144.
55. Bombay A, Matheson K, Anisman H. The impact of stressors on second generation Indian residential school survivors. Transcult Psychiatry. 2011;48(4):367–91.
56. Elias B, Mignone J, Hall M, Hong SP, Hart L, Sareen J. Trauma and suicide behaviour histories among a Canadian indigenous population: an empirical exploration of the potential role of Canada's residential school system. Soc Sci Med. 2012;74(10):1560–9.
57. McQuaid R, Bombay A, McInnis O, Humeny C, Matheson K, Anisman H. Suicide ideation and attempts among First Nations peoples living on-reserve in Canada: the intergenerational and cumulative effects of Indian residential schools. Can J Psychiatry. 2017;62(6):422–30. doi: 10.1177/0706743717702075

58. Kral MJ. Postcolonial suicide among Inuit in Arctic Canada. Cult Med Psychiatry. 2012;36(2):306–25.
59. Kral MJ, Idlout L. Community wellness and social action in the Canadian Arctic: collective agency as subjective well-being. In: Kirmayer, LJ, Valaskakis, GG, editors. Healing traditions: the mental health of Aboriginal peoples in Canada. Vancouver (BC): UBC Press; 2009. p. 315–34.
60. Kral MJ, Idlout L, Minore JB, Dyck RJ, Kirmayer LJ. Unikkaartuit: meanings and experiences of suicide among Inuit in Nunavut, Canada. Int J Indig Health. 2014;10(1):55–67.
61. Tan JCH, Maranzan AK, Boone M, Vander Velde J, Levy S. Caller characteristics, call contents, and types of assistance provided by caller sex and age group in a Canadian Inuit crisis line in Nunavut, 1991–2001. Suicide Life Threat Behav. 2012;42(2):210–16.
62. Bentham M. The changing tides of education in Nunavut: a non-Inuit perspective of Inuit Qaujimajatuqangit [master's thesis on the Internet]. Toronto (ON): Ontario Institute for Studies in Education, University of Toronto; 2017 [cited 2019 Jul 20]. 114 p. Available from: http://www.researchgate.net/publication/316673255_The_Changing_Tides_of_Education_in_Nunavut_A_Non-Inuit_Perspective_of_Inuit_Qaujimajatuqangit
63. Møller H. "Double culturedness": the "capital" of Inuit nurses. Int J Circumpolar Health. 2013;72:21266.
64. MacDonald JP, Ford JD, Willox AC, Ross NA. A review of protective factors and causal mechanisms that enhance the mental health of Indigenous circumpolar youth. Int J Circumpolar Health. 2013;72(1):21775.
65. Tagalik, S. Inunnguiniq, caring for children the Inuit way [Internet]. Ottawa (ON): National Collaborating Centre for Aboriginal Health; 2009–2010 [cited 2019 Jul 20]. Available from: http://inuuqatigiit.ca/wp-content/uploads/2015/01/Inuit-caring-EN-web.pdf
66. Inuit Tapiriit Kanatami. Social determinants of Inuit health in Canada [Internet]. Ottawa (ON): Inuit Tapiriit Kanatami; 2014 [cited 2016 Sept 28]. Available from: http://www.itk.ca/wp-content/uploads/2016/07/ITK_Social_Determinants_Report.pdf
67. King M, Smith A, Gracey M. Indigenous health part 2: the underlying causes of the health gap. Lancet. 2009;374:76–85.
68. Tan JCH, Borg C, Levy L, Levy S, Tierney J. Report on the workshop on suicide contagion among Inuit youth aged 12–19. 2015. Available on request from the chapter author.
69. World Health Organization [Internet]. Geneva (CH): World Health Organization; 2019. Social determinants of health; 2019 [cited 2019 Jul 20]. Available from: http://www.who.int/social_determinants/en/
70. Inuit Tapiriit Kanatami [Internet]. Ottawa (ON): Inuit Tapiriit Kanatami; 2020. About Canadian Inuit; 2020 [cited 2020 Jan 7]. Available from https://www.itk.ca/about-canadian-inuit/

71. Kirmayer LJ, Dandeneau S, Marshall E, Phillips MK, Williamson KJ. Rethinking resilience from Indigenous perspectives. Can J Psychiatry. 2011;56(2):84–91.
72. Kral MJ, Salusky I, Inuksuk P, Angutimarik L, Tulugardjuk N. Tunngajuq: Stress and resilience among Inuit youth in Nunavut, Canada. Transcult Psychiatry. 2014;51(5):673–92.
73. Korhonen M. Suicide prevention. Inuit traditional practices that encouraged resilience and coping [Internet]. Ottawa (ON): National Aboriginal Health Organization; 2006 [cited 2016 Jan 7]. Available from: http://www.naho.ca/documents/it/2006_Suicide_Prevention-Elders.pdf
74. Inungni Sapujjijiit Task Force on Suicide Prevention and Community Healing. Our words must come back to us [Internet]. Iqaluit (NU): Nunavut Department of Health and Social Services; 2003 [cited 2019 Apr 14]. Available from: http://pubs.aina.ucalgary.ca/health/61941E.pdf
75. Alianait Inuit-specific Mental Wellness Task Group. Alianait Inuit mental wellness action plan [Internet]. Ottawa (ON): Inuit Tapiriit Kanatami; 2007 [cited 2019 Apr 14]. Available from: http://www.itk.ca/wp-content/uploads/2009/12/Alianait-Inuit-Mental-Wellness-Action-Plan-2009.pdf
76. Masecar D. What is working, what is hopeful: supporting community-based suicide prevention strategies within Indigenous communities [Internet]. Ottawa (ON): First Nations Inuit Health Branch, Health Canada; 2006 [cited 2017 Mar 7]. Available from: http://www.douglas.qc.ca/uploads/File/what-is-working-report.pdf
77. Chandler MJ, Lalonde CE. Cultural continuity as a hedge against suicide in Canada's First Nations. Transcult Psychiatry. 1998;35(2):193–219.
78. Government of Nunavut, Nunavut Tunngavik Incorporated, Royal Canadian Mounted Police V-Division, Embrace Life Council. Resiliency within. an action plan for suicide prevention in Nunavut 2016/2017 [Internet]. Nunavut: The Government of Nunavut, Nunavut Tunngavik Incorporated, Royal Canadian Mounted Police V-Division, Embrace Life Council; 2016 Mar [cited 2016 Sep 28]. Available from: http://www.gov.nu.ca/sites/default/files/resiliency_within_eng.pdf
79. Wu A, Wang JY, Jia CX. Religion and completed suicide: A meta-analysis. PLoS One. 2015;10(6):e0131715.
80. Fleming J, Ledogar RJ. Resilience and Indigenous spirituality: a literature review. Pimatisiwin. 2008;6(2): 47–64.
81. Hatala AR. Spirituality and Aboriginal mental health: an examination of the relationship between Aboriginal spirituality and mental health. Adv Mind-Body Med. 2008;23(1):6–12.
82. Lawrence RE, Oquendo MA, Stanley B. Religion and suicide risk: a systematic review. Arch Suicide Res. 2016;20:1–21.
83. Nunavut Bureau of Statistics. Population estimates July 1, 2015 [Internet]. Iqaluit (NU): Government of Nunavut; 2016 [cited 2017 Feb 10]. Available from: http://www.stats.gov.nu.ca/Publications/Popest/Population/Population%20Estimates%20Report,%20July%201,%202015.pdf

84. Inuit Tapiriit Kanatami. National Inuit suicide prevention strategy [Internet]. Ottawa (ON): Inuit Tapiriit Kanatami; 2016 [cited 2016 Dec 18]. Available from: http://www.itk.ca/wp-content/uploads/2016/07/ITK-National-Inuit-Suicide-Prevention-Strategy-2016.pdf
85. Cullen C. Inuit-led suicide prevention strategy to focus on mental wellness, social equity. CBC News [Internet]. 2016 Jul 27 [cited 2017 Feb 10]. Available from: http://www.cbc.ca/news/politics/inuit-led-suicide-prevention-strategy-1.3696914
86. Inuit Tapiriit Kanatami. National Inuit suicide prevention strategy: year two [Internet]. Ottawa (ON): Inuit Tapiriit Kanatami; 2019 [cited 2019 Apr 14]. Available from: http://www.itk.ca/national-inuit-suicide-prevention-strategy-year-two/
87. Hjelmeland H. A critical look at current suicide research. In: White J, Marsh I, Kral MJ, Morris J, editors. Critical suicidology: transforming suicide research and prevention for the 21st century. Vancouver (BC): UBC Press; 2016. p. 31–55.

SECTION III

New Directions – Innovation, Collaboration, and Resilience

REBECCA SCHIFF

As the previous sections and chapters in the volume illustrate, northerners experience numerous unique challenges in their health and health care. Dimensions of health and wellness in the North are impacted by uniquely northern contexts and experiences, including the social and ecological determinants of health that are distinct to or felt more acutely in the North, as well as the distinct interaction and interplay among these determinants. Northerners are also challenged by geographic, climatic, and other issues that create significant limitations in health care access and delivery, limitations that are felt even more acutely than in southern and more accessible rural communities.

What is missing from this picture is a reflection on the incredible resilience that northerners have demonstrated and the innovation they have inspired in the face of social, economic, political, and environmental change and challenges. Many of the chapters in Sections I and II of this volume have reflected on this resilience and on some of the innovative changes to programs, policy, and health care practice in northern Canada. This section puts a specific focus on these changes and what is needed to achieve health equity for the North.

While the chapters in Section II presented proposals for many social policies and programs to affect change to the social determinants of northern health, this section focuses more specifically on changes needed in health care systems and more broadly in terms of health research and governance. We want to emphasize here that these solutions need to be place-based and contextually relevant: developed in the North, led by northerners, and created with particular attention to the unique characteristics and strengths of the North. In other words, northern health challenges should not and cannot be addressed by replicating models that have developed for the dense, highly populated regions of Canada. Section III presents a strong focus on decolonization, which we assert is critical to achieving health equity for the many Indigenous peoples who reside in the North, and who make up a significant proportion of the population of northern Canada. Decolonizing health care delivery, health research, health policy, and governance are given specific attention. This section also proposes changes to health care policy and practice in terms of improving access to timely and specialized care, culturally safe care, and care that extends beyond biomedical conceptualizations of health. Governance and political self-determination are longstanding issues for Indigenous and non-Indigenous residents of both the Provincial North and the territories. Therefore, the chapters in this section also consider changes to political systems, health care governance, and policy that might be critical to achieving health equity for the North.

The chapters in this section are meant to provide an overview of some of the key proposals for policy and practice change as they relate to northern health care practice and governance. The section begins with several chapters focused on specific changes needed to achieve health equity in the North. This focus occurs through an examination of adopting strength-based approaches to health and social programs, such as those focused on resilience (see Matheson et al., chapter 14), and then particular innovations in health care delivery (see Mushquash et al., chapter 15, and Spadoni et al., chapter 16). The first chapter in this section focuses on resilience: Matheson, Asokumar, Anisman, and Gordon provide important insight into the need for an emphasis on strengths-based approaches that build on the inherent resilience of northern youth and their communities. They also highlight some of the new ways in which resilience is being supported and fostered in northern Indigenous communities. The chapter by Mushquash, Drawson, and Toombs returns to a topic discussed in Section II by Kassam and builds on Kassam's suggestion that culturally relevant strategies are necessary. They elaborate on the determinants of mental health framework presented by Kassam and focus on the need for mental health and addictions care in northern Indigenous communities to be grounded in Indigenous conceptualization of health and wellness. The authors provide a basis to move towards Indigenous-designed frameworks for mental health and addictions supports and services, and some practical ways in which these frameworks are and can be implemented in northern contexts.

Continuing with a discussion of innovation for specific aspects of service delivery, Spadoni, Dampier, and Sevean examine telehealth/telemedicine, an increasingly popular approach to solving some of the geographic and human resource barriers to northern health care delivery. As health care practitioners, they provide unique reflection on their experiences with and the potentials for telehealth in northern contexts. The chapter provides a broad overview of telemedicine, as well as a case study of a relatively new and innovative Indigenous-led telemedicine program operating across northern Ontario. The authors contextualize the challenges and promise of telehealth and telemedicine for the future of northern health care.

The section then moves on to examine some key approaches to decolonizing health care delivery for Indigenous peoples in the North. First, chapter 17 by

Crawford, Waddell, and Lund examines cultural safety education and training for health care providers. The chapter takes a close look at some of the historical and current trauma produced through Inuit interactions with health care systems. The authors present the potential of cultural safety for improving health care experiences and health outcomes, as well as the lack of knowledge about this still new and emerging concept. The chapter also describes the outcomes and lessons learned through implementation of an innovative cultural safety training program for health care providers working with Inuit in Nunavut. Their conclusions point to the value of cultural safety training, as well as the need for a broader and more comprehensive response to cultural issues in northern health care systems.

The examination of decolonizing health care continues with chapter 18 by Peltier on traditional medicine and traditional healing. Peltier begins with a key consideration for any health care provision with northern communities: a discussion of northern Indigenous peoples' conceptualizations of health and well-being. These conceptualizations inform northern Indigenous approaches to healing, and Peltier describes a novel framework that models Indigenous approaches to healing at proximal, intermediate, and distal levels. The chapter also makes clear the importance of more holistic approaches to understanding health and wellness, and the potential relevance of dimensions language to move past the unidirectional and biomedically oriented implications of traditional health determinants theory. The chapter examines a new and novel approach to the complexity of using both biomedical and traditional healing approaches simultaneously. Peltier offers practical processes for "braiding" contemporary biomedical approaches with northern Indigenous healing and describes the necessity of such approaches for processes of decolonization.

Chapter 19 by Brunger and Chubbs considers an issue that is critical to ongoing knowledge creation and knowledge mobilization on northern health and health care issues. In particular, they consider the contemporary context of Canadian health research ethics review processes and the limitations of these current processes for northern communities. They also pay additional, specific attention to unique research review needs and considerations for northern and northern Indigenous communities. Northern Indigenous communities are often mistaken to be homogenous, and contemporary structures can fail to account for the diversity of opinion and experiences within isolated communities. Brunger and Chubbs describe new strategies to improve health research ethics review for the North, suggestions that attend to issues of authority and representation for diverse and complex communities.

Chapter 20, the final chapter in this section, by Lavoie, Kornelsen, and Boyer, considers the colonial nature of northern health policy, and the impact of southern – centric decision making in health care governance. They provide a broad overview of the frameworks informing health legislation and policy in northern Canada, as well as some of the complexities and innovations in northern Canadian health care delivery. This chapter includes a discussion on policy and legislation that is relevant to all Indigenous peoples in Canada; it highlights the failure of our legal, political, and health care systems to differentiate between northern and southern (as well as rural and urban) experiences. Their discussion illustrates the difficulty of northern policymaking when much policy development (and particularly that for Indigenous peoples) does not pay specific attention to the unique needs of northerners. They present new and innovative options for federal-level policy that are applicable to both southern and northern communities. This discussion is accompanied by a comparative analysis with health policy and governance in other circumpolar regions, an analysis that reveals potential areas for improvement to legislative and policy frameworks for health care in northern Canada. We hope that this, as the final chapter in this book, will direct the discussion to the southern-centric policies and systems that currently play a significant role in shaping northern health care and health outcomes. The chapter points to the possibilities for redesigning and reimagining federal and provincial or territorial policymaking and decision making in ways that privilege northern and northern Indigenous voices, and focus on equity in northern health governance.

14 Youth Resilience: Resilience among Indigenous Youth in Northern Canada

KIMBERLY MATHESON, AJANI ASOKUMAR, HYMIE ANISMAN, AND JANET GORDON

You have purpose. Your heart beats like our ancestors' drums. If you don't have reason, make one. We represent resilience. It flows throughout our bloodstream, like rain flows down the mountain. – Youth (1)

When we consider the wellness of Indigenous youth in northern regions of Canada, we typically think in terms of its absence. We note disproportionately high rates of depression, suicide, and substance use emanating from historical and current trauma; lower levels of educational attainment and employment prospects that foster lifestyles that undermine health (smoking, lack of physical activity); housing that is insufficient and inadequate, contributing to epidemic levels of respiratory illnesses, in particular tuberculosis; and the outrageous cost of nutritious foods and diminished skills to access traditional food sources, resulting in poor diets, obesity, and diabetes. Although these issues cannot be ignored, a singular focus on the gaps in health and wellness perpetuates a view of northern Indigenous populations as victims, rife with illness, and suffering as a result of historical and continuing systemic discrimination.

An alternative perspective that is being increasingly advocated is to recognize the factors that promote resilience and wellness, and to incorporate an understanding of the contradictions, complexity, and self-determination of the lives of Indigenous peoples as the driver for change (2). Indigenous peoples in Canada are empowering themselves to revive their cultural identities and reclaim their inherent rights to self-determination and autonomy as nations, a course of action that is grounded in strength.

It is in this light that we will discuss the resilience of Indigenous youth in northern regions of Canada. Resilience is not about an absence of challenges, and indeed the challenges faced by these youth are well documented. As a result of colonialist policies and practices, the resources that have traditionally fostered resilience among Indigenous youth, in particular connections to the land and to cultural identities (through relationships), have been systematically undermined.

Yet despite the challenges and disruptions in the lives of northern Indigenous youth, there is clear evidence of their capacity to persevere and thrive, even if scarred, in the face of such adversities (3–5). Many northern Indigenous youth are demonstrating the strengths needed to flourish, mobilize, and take on leadership roles to bring about a better future. The goal of this chapter is to integrate Indigenous and Western understandings of resilience to reflect on how northern Indigenous youth contend with distinct challenges, and the unique resources they draw upon that enable them to thrive. We place particular focus on how such resilience is derived from intergenerational relationships (including biological processes) and from youths' connection to the land in which their identities are embedded.

Although we are using the term *northern* Indigenous youth, such singularity is a misnomer. Northern Indigenous cultures vary extensively, reflecting variations of language, kinship lines, ceremonies and legends, and land-based practices. While existing literature provides insights into youth experiences across the North, we present in this chapter our own understandings, which are grounded in the First Nations communities in the territory of the Nishnawbe Aski Nation (NAN). NAN comprises 49 First Nations communities (population 45,000) spread over the northern two-thirds of Ontario known as the Arctic watershed. The majority of the communities are rural or remote, with access only by air or winter ice roads. They range in population from less than 50 to 2500 people, and about half the population in most communities is less than 25 years of age. These communities vary in language (Cree, Ojibway, Oji-Cree), spiritual beliefs and ceremonies, and even treaty area (Treaties 3 and 9 and the Ontario portion of Treaty 5).

Each of our own backgrounds also vary. Janet Gordon is originally from one of the most northern communities of NAN, Kasabonika Lake First Nation. She has three children who she raised with her husband. They now spend significant time in Lac Seul First Nation, which is a road-accessible community close to Sioux Lookout. Gordon is a nurse by training and is currently the chief operating officer of the Sioux Lookout First Nations Health Authority, which has responsibility for the community health resources for 33 First Nations in the Sioux Lookout zone of northwestern Ontario. Together with Kimberly Matheson, she is the co-lead of the Indigenous Youth Futures Partnership (IYFP), a community-led action research program that brings together Western academics from multiple disciplines with First Nations service organizations and communities in the NAN region to create the conditions for youth to thrive. A key aspect of the IYFP is to use a two-eyed seeing approach to understand the context of communities and to support the strategies they develop to promote youth resilience.

Matheson is a settler ally residing in rural Ottawa. She was trained as a social/health psychologist and has been conducting research assessing the intergenerational consequences of the Indian residential schools (IRSs) on the psychological wellness of descendants of survivors. Her research regarding the IRSs has been in collaboration with Hymie Anisman, whose parents were Holocaust survivors who emigrated from Poland following World War II to Montreal, where he grew up. Anisman is a behavioural neuroscientist whose research focuses on the environmental and biological factors that render individuals more resilient or vulnerable to stress-related pathologies. Ajani Asokumar's parents are refugees from Sri Lanka. She is completing her doctoral research regarding the importance of reconciling place identity for the wellness of immigrants transitioning to Canada, and is working with Matheson and Anisman.

In this chapter, we will begin with an overview of how resilience has been understood in relation to Indigenous populations. By grounding our understanding of resilience in a cultural and socioecological context, it becomes apparent that youth resilience is imbedded in relationships across generations, within families, and among peers. We will explore the role of relationships from a cultural, social, and biological perspective. Moreover, relationships with family and community and relationships with the land are inseparable within Indigenous culture. Thus, the importance of the land and connections to place in promoting resilience among northern Indigenous youth will be discussed. In our analysis, we have tried to be guided by the voices of Indigenous youth by quoting their views and through the presentation of the results of participatory research conducted with youth.

Understandings of Resilience

> We are the change. Remember the teachings. Remember our families' voices. Hope. Education. Courage. Relationships. Awe for the resiliency that students have shown. – Youth (6)

Simply stated, resilience is the capacity to use the personal, social, cultural, and environmental resources available to adapt successfully in the face of adversity (7,8). Understandings of resilience have evolved in terms of what is meant by adaptation, and, in particular, it has been suggested that it is not simply about maintaining or returning to baseline wellness following a challenge. Instead, it may entail a process of adjustment, transformation, and even growth (3,7,9). Typically, research conducted to identify the factors that promote resilience has placed particular emphasis on individual difference characteristics, such as personal hardiness, coping skills, and cognitive styles. While such attributes contribute to resilience among Indigenous youth (10), in the past decade, it has been increasingly recognized that the nature of the adversities encountered, the meaning of successful adaptation, and the protective factors that contribute to it are culturally contextualized (7,9,11–13). Research adopting socioecological frameworks for understanding resilience among Indigenous populations has highlighted connections to culture, language, spirituality, and the land (9,12,14–17). In addition, relationships across generations, within families, and within communities have emerged as playing a key role in the resilience of Indigenous peoples (12,14). In this regard, resilience emerges as a holistic and relational process involving the interplay of individual, social, cultural, and environmental factors (5).

Although the importance of relationships and connections to the land appear to be central to many Indigenous cultures and identities in Canada, how these elements are expressed and the meanings derived vary substantially (9). Particularly relevant to northern Indigenous peoples, it has been suggested that the meaning of resilience among the Inuit is reflected in the concept of *niriunniq*, which is an Inuktitut word for hope. Based on an analysis of the narratives of Inuit, Kirmayer and colleagues (4,9,18) suggested that "faced with adversity, people talk of hope and wait for it to reveal itself. For many, it is an elusive experience, but its potency as a life-giving force is never questioned. Being animists at heart, Inuit understand the world as shaped by powerful forces coming together – forces that really are beyond one person's control. Expressions such as *ajurnarmat* [cannot be helped] or *isumamminik* [on its own will], reflect the Inuit recognition of human limitations" (9 p88). Such expressions have their roots in the need to survive the harsh environmental conditions that northern peoples live with. This contrasts with other collective narratives of resilience that emphasize different features, such as collaboration among the Mi'kmaq, resistance among the Mohawk, or self-reliance among the Métis (9,18). Although these features of resilience may be common across cultures, variations in how central they are to the actions that enable resilience are likely grounded in the community experiences and values that define wellness and socialized understandings (often through language) and behaviours to cope with adversity. Thus, the meaning of resilience varies broadly from one community to another and from one geographical region to another.

Recognizing the culturally and environmentally based features that contribute to resilience, in recent years, considerable efforts have been made to engage in community-led collaborative processes to promote resilience among northern Indigenous youth. The collaborative process and focus on community narratives, in themselves, are seen to encourage the validation of Indigenous voices through the assertion of their identities and affirmation of the core values inherent to these identities that enable youth to face the challenges they encounter (9). In effect, the collaborative community-based processes involved in developing, implementing, and evaluating programs may contribute to collective resilience (19–22). Such approaches facilitate the revival of traditional practices that emerge from the narratives of Elders and Knowledge Keepers. These narratives often emphasize the importance of intergenerational relationships, the strengths that are infused into connections to the land, and how these factors combine to form the localized cultural identities that promote collective and individual resilience.

Intergenerational Resilience through Relationships

The love of her children. The love of her family, and the love of her grandchildren to be. This is my grandmother's legacy. What she's given me through intergenerational trauma. I'm able to stand here today, a strong Indigenous Gwitch'in woman. – Youth (23)

Intergenerational relationships, particularly between Elders and youth, are regarded as a robust protective process that ground youth in familial bonds and cultural identity (24). These relationships form the core of numerous interventions that encourage storytelling (25–27) and the passing on of traditional skills and practices (24), and are integral to many land-based healing programs (28,29). In addition, older individuals (parents, grandparents) may pass on positive coping strategies (e.g., humour), traditional values (e.g., the seven sacred teachings), and strength by sharing stories of their own responses to past adversities and how they grew from them (30–32).

As much as children and youth yearn for the protection, understanding, and support of parental caregivers, and they take advantage of opportunities to spend time with family (10,33), they often do not turn to their parents in times of need (4). Indeed, in a survey of Indigenous youth in northern Saskatchewan, only 20 per cent believed that adults in their community valued youth (34). Relatedly, it has been suggested that the *spontaneous enactment* of communication across generations appears largely absent for northern Indigenous youth today (4,33). Traditional opportunities for the intergenerational transmission of values, wisdom, practices, and the meaning of cultural identities were virtually eradicated by colonialist policies and practices. These included (grand) parental attendance at residential or day schools (disrupting traditional socialization behaviours, including language), forced relocation and confinement to restricted land bases, namely, reserves (diminishing the relevance of land-based knowledge, activities, and sustenance), and changes in social relationships within communities to mirror Euro-Christian practices (altering gender and kinship relations). Contributing to the attenuation of intergenerational relationships more recently has been the role of technology and social media. Without exception, in the fly-in communities in which we are working, internet gaming and social media are viewed as being at the root of youths' lack of interest in engaging in community activities and events (see also 35). In addition, cyberbullying is reported to be particularly devastating to the esteem of First Nations children and youth (36) and is further perceived to exacerbate community rifts among adults.

To meet the need for enhancing intergenerational relationships, strategies for promoting youth resilience and wellness have commonly focused on promoting parental involvement (10) and enabling youth to build more positive relationships with Elders and to hear their stories to document the strengths that emerge from these stories (37). As youth engage in their own efforts towards self-actualization and reshaping their futures, some seek the guidance of Elders (38), but others have expressed dismay at the entrenchment of Elders in the "old ways" and in their experiences of trauma. At the same time, youth wish that the Elders could provide them with a better understanding of who they are as Indigenous peoples (33). Limited research has assessed the mechanisms by which Elders' social participation and the strengthening of intergenerational relationships occur and how they contribute to youth, community, and family well-being (39).

Intergenerational Resilience through Biological Connections

> The resiliency of our people, though deeply disturbed by the processes of impoverishment, is like a spring of hope that is tapped into again and again. This hope is found inside the prophecy of the seven generations and somehow continues even though it is under the surface and not always visible, even to the ones who are affected by it. – Elders (40)

Consistent with the belief held by some Indigenous cultures that what happens today will affect the next seven generations, Western approaches to understanding the impacts of exposure to adversity are increasingly recognizing that experiential factors can affect subsequent generations through alterations of biological processes. Biomarkers are being identified that predict and diagnose various illnesses, including their interaction with risk and protective factors that contribute to resilience and health inequities between cultural groups. However, because of the infrequent participation of Indigenous and other marginalized groups in genetic research (41), little is known about how underlying biological processes operate across cultures. The lack of participation in such research is not surprising given the numerous instances in which Indigenous peoples have been experimented on without consent, lied to about the goals of research (42), and over-researched but at the same time remain invisible in research (2). Moreover, there is a concern that such research might be used to undermine the responsibility of colonial governments to acknowledge the causal role of history in relation to health inequities. Thus, it is recognized that environmental conditions and intergenerational trauma can influence biological processes that affect vulnerability or resilience in the face of adversity, but there is currently an absence of mutually beneficial research addressing these issues among Indigenous peoples in Canada.

This said, there are biological mechanisms that may be relevant to the intergenerational transmission of historical trauma, as well as to the factors that promote resilience. Historical trauma entails a process by which the negative consequences of multiple traumas experienced by a group are cumulative and are carried forward to influence the emotional, psychological, and physical well-being of subsequent generations. Several factors might contribute to the intergenerational effects of historical trauma, including dysfunctional parenting, communication processes, and disruption of social relationships and cultural norms that might otherwise serve as protective factors (43). Of particular relevance to the intergenerational transmission of the effects of historical trauma among Indigenous peoples may be epigenetic processes. Epigenetic research is built on the understanding that environmental conditions, social challenges, and even dietary factors can alter the expression of a great number of genes. Through various processes, the functioning of particular genes can be silenced or activated, which can promote multiple phenotypes (44). Thus, a history of trauma encountered by Indigenous peoples, including IRS experiences, may have altered gene expression, leading to either elevated vulnerability to psychological and physical illnesses or, conversely, to greater resilience. At one time it was assumed that epigenetic actions were infrequent, but it is now known that epigenetic changes are exceedingly common, some becoming fixed (permanent), whereas others are transient. Childhood abuse, for instance, was accompanied by a great many epigenetic marks beyond those evident among individuals who had not experienced early life abuse (45). In view of the numerous epigenetic changes that occur, it is difficult to determine the correspondence between specific changes and particular phenotypes. Moreover, finding such relationships does not imply causality (46).

Enthusiasm for this line of inquiry increased when it was understood that if epigenetic changes occurred in germline cells (sperm or ova), they could be passed on across generations (47). Studies in humans have been less conclusive than were the studies in rodents in demonstrating epigenetic changes across generations. Nevertheless, it seemed that some epigenetic modifications related to genes associated with cortisol (a stress hormone) were altered among children of survivors of the Holocaust (48). There are also indications of persisting epigenetic marks among individuals affected by the 1944–5 Dutch Hunger Winter (49), and the 1959–61 famine in China (50), which could be transmitted across generations (51).

Given the sensitivity to early life experiences, particular attention has been paid to this developmental period (52). While adverse childhood experiences appear to exacerbate stress sensitivities associated with epigenetic changes, it is also possible that positive early life experiences or "time to heal" can promote resilience. Epigenetic processes are not static, and providing nurturing environments can alter previously programmed epigenetic actions. For instance, raising rodents in an enriched environment attenuated the adverse transgenerational actions attributable to earlier maternal stressors (53), just as enrichment during the adolescent period could reverse the negative epigenetic consequences otherwise engendered by poor early life maternal care (54). In effect, the bell can be un-rung (46).

In short, typically, discussions of epigenetics have focused on the adverse outcomes created by various challenges, including historical trauma. But this may be too narrow a perspective. Natural selection involves advantageous gene mutations being passed on across generations, thereby enhancing resilience and increasing the fitness of successive generations. In a like fashion, certain epigenetic effects may persist across generations because they promote resilience, enhancing adaptations that facilitate health and survival (55). To be sure, data supporting this view are only now emerging (56) but suggest that, in conjunction with cultural, social, and interpersonal factors, biological processes might also contribute to the intergenerational connections that are foundational to youth resilience.

The Land: Place-Based Resilience

> My way of coping with overwhelming amounts of stress and sadness is to go out on our land to smell, feel, and listen to the waves of the water, the wind, and the creatures that inhabit them. – Youth (57)

Among Indigenous peoples, resilience and wellness are profoundly connected to the land (5,58,59). Such connections shape Indigenous peoples' understanding of who they are, their relationships to one another, and their sense of agency. Although northern Indigenous peoples were largely nomadic, there was a deep understanding of the territories in which they traditionally sought sustenance (fishing, hunting, gathering). At the heart of many northern Indigenous cultures, the land and specific places are infused with meaning that is expressed through language, stories, music, and art. Thus, the intergenerational resilience derived from the symbiotic relationship to the land often involves the integration of cultural identity with the features of specific places. In effect, attachment to the land not only reflects the distinctive physical aspects of a geographical location but also encompasses non-physical elements, such as the social, emotional, and spiritual aspects that provide the foundation of identity, social connectedness, and a sense of community and belonging (59,60).

Given the structural, cultural, and spiritual characteristics of the land and specific places, disruptions to such connections can impact health and well-being (61). The colonialist policies and actions imposed on northern peoples involving forced relocations and restriction of movements, and assimilationist policies associated with education, loss of language, health, and governance, have all contributed to the erosion of the knowledge of the land that was passed down through generations, including a holistic understanding of purpose and meaning (3). To this day, disconnection from the places in which their roots were formed is profoundly experienced by northern Indigenous youth, particularly as they are compelled to leave their remote or rural home communities to seek education and employment prospects in more urban settings. When the social and cultural relationships that are inherent to specific places are inaccessible, individuals feel "out of place" and negative impacts on well-being may emerge (62).

Environmental issues and climate change are having a further impact on the health and well-being of Indigenous peoples, especially in the North (63,64). For example, many First Nations communities in northern Ontario have been contending with critical environmental issues within their communities, including toxicity of local bodies of water and exposure to natural and human-made disasters, such as floods and forest fires. In addition, warming temperatures and changes in weather patterns and ice stability are altering access to resources critical to community survival (i.e., winter hunting grounds and hence traditional diet), shortening the time ice roads are open, and creating barriers for community members' participation in land-based practices, resulting in diminished cultural identity and well-being (65).

A growing body of research has demonstrated that disturbances to an individual's sense of place that are beyond their control can result in feelings of placelessness (61). For instance, Elders from two Anishinaabe communities in northern Ontario recounted decreased physical, mental, and emotional health after experiencing dispossession from the land (17). Elders described a diminished sense of place identity because of the inability to pass on traditional Indigenous knowledge to younger generations, reduced access to the land preventing its use for ceremonies and traditional practices, and the loss of language that is essential to express their connection with, and knowledge of, the land.

The connections to land and place have become an important consideration for understanding the physical and psychological wellness of Indigenous youth, particularly those from rural and remote northern communities. Land-based programs have been emerging across northern communities as a strategy for building youth resilience (66). Key features of these programs include developing traditional sustenance skills (e.g., hunting, trapping, food preparation), building relationships with peers and Elders, and solving problems and making decisions (67). To enable youth to embrace land-based or cultural practices, activities that are relevant to their modern lives are often intermingled with traditional activities, such as sports or expeditions (38,68). Other programs integrate traditional and modern identities by encouraging youth to reshape traditional ways by incorporating creative adaptations, for example, through music, dance, and art (69), or by including the use of technology, such as digital storytelling or sharing through social media (63,66,70). The objective of these programs is to build confidence, esteem, cultural connections, and positive relationships among youth, particularly those who are considered "at risk" (24,28,66). Strengthening social ties that are linked to the land may alleviate feelings of dislocation and homesickness among youth and may thus act as a source of resiliency (71).

Connection to the land goes hand in hand with the strength of intergenerational relationships. The majority of land-based programs encourage the participation of Elders, thereby promoting youths' connections across generations, including exposure to their own languages and to the teaching strategies that enable the sharing of knowledge that is transmitted nonverbally or through stories (29). In addition, some programs impart a sense of belonging and purpose among youth by integrating activities to meet collective needs, such as creating community freezers (24). In essence, relationships with the land and relationships with family and community are inseparable within Indigenous culture (24,66,70). The people and the land are one.

Conclusions

Emanating from a socioecological understanding that resilience is culturally shaped and that among northern Indigenous peoples, relationships across generations and connections to the land provide a basis for strengthening cultural identity, numerous programs to expose children and youth to such factors have been developed. Many of these programs have intuitive appeal and buy-in from communities and youth who are seeking opportunities to know who they are and to embrace a positive cultural identity. Many appear to incorporate protective factors that contribute to resiliency and wellness. At the same time, it was conveyed by an Elder in one of the NAN communities that these programs remain constrained by administrative burdens (e.g., rules associated with insurance concerns, age restrictions, accountability reports) and limited parental or family involvement (thereby minimizing continuity of intergenerational relationships). In addition, programs structured around organized activities and arranged opportunities for the sharing of knowledge differ from the normalized day-to-day social interactions across generations (from Elders to infants) that enable the passing on of teachings as part of a way of life (see also 72).

While systematic evaluation of the effectiveness of such programs is limited (12,73), in actuality, initiatives that focus on specific activities within the context of the broad range of adversities might set an unrealistic bar for success. Indeed, outcome measures are often very targeted and limited in scope and longevity of effects. For example, traditional language use (74) and cultural and land-based activities (75) were associated with greater wellness indicators, such as reduced smoking and more physical activity, among Indigenous youth. Others have evaluated self-reported resilience and enjoyment of the program (70), educational outcomes (15), and reduced substance use (58). To derive a richer, broad-based understanding of impacts, some evaluations assessed the narratives of program implementers (28,66) or the youth participants (4). All of these methodologies are critical to providing the culturally and locally contextualized meaning associated with resilience and wellness (3). At the same time, it has been suggested that because of the lack of "rigorous" research methods, or consistent operationalizations of resilience and measures of wellness outcomes, definitive conclusions regarding the causal importance of particular factors in promoting resilience among Indigenous youth cannot be derived (12).

In actuality, the accumulation of programs that address multiple, complex, and interacting elements over a sustained time and across generations is likely needed before anything but short-term incremental changes will be evident. Indigenous understandings of wellness are inherently holistic, with resilience emanating from the adaptive balance of protective and risk factors over time and place (72).

REFERENCES

1. Coady S. Street smarts [video on the Internet]. Toronto (ON): Project CREATeS; 2019 [cited 2019 Jul 1]. Video: 1:45 min. Available from: http://www.projectcreates.com/videos/street-smarts
2. Tuck E. Suspending damage: a letter to communities. Harvard Educ Rev. 2009 Sep 1;79(3):409–28.
3. Allen J, Hopper K, Wexler L, Kral M, Rasmus S, Nystad K. Mapping resilience pathways of indigenous youth in five circumpolar communities. Transcult Psychiatry. 2014 Oct;51(5):601–31.
4. Kral MJ, Salusky I, Inuksuk P, Angutimarik L, Tulugardjuk N. Tunngajuq: stress and resilience among Inuit youth in Nunavut, Canada. Transcult Psychiatry. 2014 Oct;51(5):673–92.
5. Liebenberg L, Ikeda J, Wood M. "It's just part of my culture": understanding language and land in the resilience processes of Aboriginal youth. In: Theron L, Liebenberg L, Ungar M, editors. Youth resilience and culture. Dordrecht (NL): Springer; 2015. p 105–16.
6. Indigenous Youth Futures Partnership [Internet]. Ottawa (ON): Indigenous Youth Futures Partnership; 2019. Youth forum on First Nations youth transitions to high school, Thunder Bay, Ontario; 2017 Nov [cited 2019 Jul 2]. Available from: http://www.indigenousyouthfutures.ca/first-nations-youth-transition-to-high-school-forum.html
7. Ungar M. Resilience across cultures. Brit J Soc Work. 2008 Feb 1;38(2):218–35.
8. Ungar M. Resilience, trauma, context, and culture. Trauma Viol Abuse. 2013 Jul;14(3):255–66.

9. Kirmayer LJ, Dandeneau S, Marshall E, Phillips MK, Williamson KJ. Rethinking resilience from indigenous perspectives. Can J Psychiatry. 2011 Feb;56(2):84–91.
10. Andersson N, Ledogar RJ. The CIET Aboriginal youth resilience studies: 14 years of capacity building and methods development in Canada. Pimatisiwin. 2008;6(2):65.
11. Isbister-Bear O, Hatala AR, Sjoblom E. Strengthening Âhkamêyimo among Indigenous youth: the social determinants of health, justice, and resilience in Canada's north. J Indig Wellbeing. 2017 Dec 20;2(3):76–89.
12. Toombs E, Kowatch KR, Mushquash CJ. Resilience in Canadian Indigenous youth: A scoping review. Int Child Adol Resil. 2016;4(1):4–32.
13. Walls ML, Whitbeck L, Armenta B. A cautionary tale: examining the interplay of culturally specific risk and resilience factors in indigenous communities. Clin Psychol Sci. 2016 Jul;4(4):732–43.
14. Du Hamel P. Aboriginal youth: risk and resilience. Native Soc Work J. 2003; 5:213–24.
15. Lafferty D. Dǫ Edàezhe: building resiliency among Aboriginal youth. Pimatisiwin. 2012;10(2):217–30.
16. Snowshoe A, Crooks CV, Tremblay PF, Hinson RE. Cultural connectedness and its relation to mental wellness for First Nations youth. J Prim Prev. 2017 Apr 1;38(1–2):67–86.
17. Tobias JK, Richmond CA. "That land means everything to us as Anishinaabe ...": environmental dispossession and resilience on the north shore of Lake Superior. Health Place. 2014 Sep;29:26–33.
18. Kirmayer LJ, Dandeneau S, Marshall E, Phillips MK, Williamson KJ. Toward an ecology of stories: Indigenous perspectives on resilience. In: Unger M, editor. The social ecology of resilience. New York (NY): Springer; 2012. p. 399–414.
19. Halsall T, Forneris T. Evaluation of a leadership program for First Nations, Métis, and Inuit youth: stories of positive youth development and community engagement. App Dev Sci. 2018 Apr 3;22(2):125–38.
20. Kovach M. Indigenous methodologies: characteristics, conversations, and contexts. Toronto (ON): University of Toronto Press; 2009.
21. Trout L, Wexler L, Moses J. Beyond two worlds: identity narratives and the aspirational futures of Alaska Native youth. Transcult Psychiatry. 2018;55(6):800–20.
22. Ulturgasheva O, Rasmus S, Morrow P. Collapsing the distance: Indigenous-youth engagement in a circumpolar study of youth resilience. Arctic Anthropol. 2015 Jan 1;52(1):60–70.
23. Firth-Hager J. Natihthun Gwiintl'oo Choo [A whole lot of love] [video on Internet]. Toronto (ON): Project CREATeS; 2019 [cited 2019 Jul 1]. Video: 3:05 min. Available from: http://www.projectcreates.com/videos/natihthun-gwiintloo-choo-a-whole-lot-of-love
24. Hackett C, Furgal C, Angnatok D, Sheldon T, Karpik S, Baikie D, Pamak C, Bell T. Going off, growing strong: building resilience of Indigenous youth. Can J Community Ment Health. 2016 Oct 24;35(2):79–82.

25. Cunsolo Willox A, Harper SL, Edge VL, "My Word": Storytelling and Digital Media Lab, Rigolet Inuit Community Government. Storytelling in a digital age: digital storytelling as an emerging narrative method for preserving and promoting Indigenous oral wisdom. Qual Res. 2013 Apr;13(2):127–47.
26. Project CREATeS [Internet]. Ottawa (ON): Project CREATeS; 2019. 2019 Jun [cited July 22, 2019]. Available from: http://www.projectcreates.com
27. Wexler L. Intergenerational dialogue exchange and action: introducing a community-based participatory approach to connect youth, adults, and Elders in an Alaskan Native community. Int J Qual Methods. 2011;10:248–64.
28. Radu I, House LL, Pashagumskum E. Land, life, and knowledge in Chisasibi: Intergenerational healing in the bush. Decolonization. Indigeneity Educ Soc. 2014 Jul 2;3(3):86–105.
29. Roué M. Healing the wounds of school by returning to the land: Cree Elders come to the rescue of a lost generation. Int Soc Sci J. 2006 Mar;58(187):15–24.
30. Hatala AR, Desjardins M, Bombay A. Reframing narratives of Aboriginal health inequity: exploring Cree Elder resilience and well-being in contexts of historical trauma. Qual Health Res. 2016 Dec;26(14):1911–27.
31. Matheson K, Bombay A, Dixon K, Anisman H. Intergenerational communication regarding Indian residential schools: implications for cultural identity, perceived discrimination, and depressive symptoms. Transcult Psychiatry. 2020 Apr;57(2):304–20.
32. Wexler L. Looking across three generations of Alaska Natives to explore how culture fosters indigenous resilience. Transcult Psychiatry. 2014 Feb;51(1):73–92.
33. Provincial Advocate for Children and Youth. Feathers of Hope report: a First Nations youth action plan [Internet]. Toronto (ON): Provincial Advocate for Children and Youth; 2014. Available from: https://ocaarchives.files.wordpress.com/2019/01/foh-report.pdf
34. Irvine J, Quinn B, Stockdale D. Northern Saskatchewan health indicators report 2011. La Ronge (SK): Athabasca Health Authority and Keewatin Yatthé and Mamawetan Churchill River Regional Health Authorities; 2011.
35. Bombay A, Matheson K, Anisman H. Youth personal wellness and after-school activities. In: First Nations Information Governance Centre, editor. First Nations regional health survey (RHS) phase 2 (2008/10): national report on adults, youth, and children living in First Nations communities. Ottawa (ON): First Nations Information Governance Centre. p. 340–57.
36. Matsumoto C, Bocking N. Our children and youth health report. Sioux Lookout (ON): Sioux Lookout First Nations Health Authority; 2018.
37. Wexler L, Moses J, Hopper K, Joule L, Garoutte J, LSC CIPA Team. Central role of relatedness in Alaska Native youth resilience: preliminary themes from one site of the circumpolar Indigenous pathways to adulthood (CIPA) study. Am J Community Psychol. 2013 Dec 1;52(3–4):393–405.

38. Sasakamoose J, Scerbe A, Wenaus I, Scandrett A. First Nation and Métis youth perspectives of health: an Indigenous qualitative inquiry. Qual Inq. 2016 Oct;22(8):636–50.
39. Viscogliosi C, Asselin H, Basile S, Couturier Y, Drolet MJ, Gagnon D, Torrie J, Levasseur M. A scoping review protocol on social participation of indigenous elders, intergenerational solidarity and their influence on individual and community wellness. BMJ Open. 2017 May 1;7(5):e015931.
40. Clarkson L, Morrissette V, Régallet G. Our responsibility to the seventh generation: Indigenous peoples and sustainable development [Internet]. Winnipeg (MB): International Institute for Sustainable Development; 1992 [cited 2019 Jul 1]. Available from: https://www.iisd.org/system/files/publications/seventh_gen.pdf
41. Gurdasani D, Barroso I, Zeggini E, Sandhu MS. Genomics of disease risk in globally diverse populations. Nat Rev Genet. 2019 Sep;20(9):520–35.
42. Yancey AK, Ortega AN, Kumanyika SK. Effective recruitment and retention of minority research participants. Annu Rev Public Health. 2006 Apr 21;27:1–28.
43. Bombay A, Matheson K, Anisman H. Psychological perspectives on intergenerational transmission of trauma. In: Blume A, editor. Social issues in living color: challenges and solutions from the perspective of ethnic minority psychology. Santa Barbara (CA): Praeger; 2017. p. 171–98.
44. Meaney MJ, Szyf M. Environmental programming of stress responses through DNA methylation: life at the interface between a dynamic environment and a fixed genome. Dialogues Clin Neurosci. 2005 Jun;7(2):103–23.
45. Suderman M, Borghol N, Pappas JJ, Pinto Pereira SM, Pembrey M, Hertzman C, Power C, Szyf M. Childhood abuse is associated with methylation of multiple loci in adult DNA. BMC Med Genomics. 2014 Mar 11;7:13.
46. Anisman H. Introduction to stress and health. London (GB): Sage; 2014.
47. Franklin TB, Russig H, Weiss IC, Gräff J, Linder N, Michalon A, Vizi S, Mansuy IM. Epigenetic transmission of the impact of early stress across generations. Bio Psychiatry. 2010 Sep 1;68(5):408–15.
48. Yehuda R, Daskalakis NP, Bierer LM, Bader HN, Klengel T, Holsboer F, Binder EB. Holocaust exposure induced intergenerational effects on FKBP5 methylation. Biol Psychiatry. 2016 Sep 1;80(5):372–80.
49. Heijmans BT, Tobi EW, Stein AD, Putter H, Blauw GJ, Susser ES, Slagboom PE, Lumey LH. Persistent epigenetic differences associated with prenatal exposure to famine in humans. Proc Natl Acad Sci USA. 2008 Nov 4;105(44):17046–9.
50. Li J, Liu S, Li S, Feng R, Na L, Chu X, Wu X, Niu Y, Sun Z, Han T, Deng H, Meng X, Xu H, Zhang Z, Qu Q, Zhang Q, Li Y, Sun C. Prenatal exposure to famine and the development of hyperglycemia and type 2 diabetes in adulthood across consecutive generations: a population-based cohort study of families in Suihua, China. Am J Clin Nutrition. 2016 Dec 7;105(1):221–7.
51. Tobi EW, Goeman JJ, Monajemi R, Gu H, Putter H, Zhang Y, Slieker RC, Stok AP, Thijssen PE, Müller F, van Zwet EW, Bock C, Meissner A, Lumey LH, Eline

Slagboom P, Heijmans BT. DNA methylation signatures link prenatal famine exposure to growth and metabolism. Nat Commun. 2014 Nov 26;5:5592.

52. Stenz L, Schechter DS, Serpa SR, Paoloni-Giacobino A. Intergenerational transmission of DNA methylation signatures associated with early life stress. Curr Genomics. 2018 Dec;19(8):665–75.
53. Gapp K, Bohacek J, Grossmann J, Brunner AM, Manuella F, Nanni P, Mansuy IM. Potential of environmental enrichment to prevent transgenerational effects of paternal trauma. Neuropsychopharmacol. 2016 Oct;41(11):2749–58.
54. Champagne FA, Meaney MJ. Transgenerational effects of social environment on variations in maternal care and behavioural response to novelty. Beh Neurosci. 2007 Dec;121(6):1353–63.
55. Tian FY, Marsit CJ. Environmentally induced epigenetic plasticity in development: epigenetic toxicity and epigenetic adaptation. Curr Epidemiol Rep. 2018 Dec;5(4):450–60.
56. Serpeloni F, Radtke KM, Hecker T, Sill J, Vukojevic V, Assis SG, Schauer M, Elbert T, Nätt D. Does prenatal stress shape postnatal resilience? An epigenome-wide study on violence and mental health in humans. Fron Gen. 2019 Apr 16; 10:269.
57. Calvin O. Children, my hope for the future [video on Internet]. Toronto (ON): Project CREATeS; 2019 [cited 2019 Jul 1]. Video: 1:53 mins. Available from: http://www.projectcreates.com/videos/children-my-hope-for-the-future
58. Dell CA, Seguin M, Hopkins C, Tempier R, Mehl-Madrona L, Dell D, Duncan R, Mosier K. From benzos to berries: treatment offered at an Aboriginal youth solvent abuse treatment centre relays the importance of culture. Can J Psychiatry. 2011 Feb;56(2):75–83.
59. Wilson K. Therapeutic landscapes and First Nations peoples: an exploration of culture, health and place. Health Place. 2003 Jun;9(2):83–93.
60. Qazimi S. Sense of place and place identity. Eur J Soc Sci Educ Res. 2014 May;1(1):306–10.
61. Williams A, Kitchen P. Sense of place and health in Hamilton, Ontario: a case study. Soc Indicators Res. 2012 Sep;108(2):257–76.
62. Atkinson S, Fuller S, Painter J. Well-being and place. Surrey (GB): Ashgate; 2012.
63. Cunsolo Willox A, Harper SL, Ford JD, Landman K, Houle K, Edge VL, Rigolet Inuit Community Government. "From this place and of this place:" climate change, sense of place, and health in Nunatsiavut, Canada. Soc Sci Med. 2012;75(3):538–47.
64. Sarkar A, Hanrahan M, Hudson A. Water insecurity in Canadian Indigenous communities: some inconvenient truths. Rural Remote Health. 2015 Oct 1; 15(4):3354.
65. Willox AC, Harper SL, Ford JD, Edge VL, Landman K, Houle K, Blake S, Wolfrey C. Climate change and mental health: an exploratory case study from Rigolet, Nunatsiavut, Canada. Climatic Change. 2013 Nov 1;121(2):255–70.

66. Walsh R, Danto D, Sommerfeld J. Land-based intervention: a qualitative study of the knowledge and practices associated with one approach to mental health in a Cree community. Int J Mental Health Addict. 2018:1–15.
67. Dobson C, Brazzoni R. Land based healing: Carrier First Nations' addiction recovery program. J Indig Wellbeing. 2016 Dec 16;2(2):9–17.
68. Gaudet JC. An Indigenous methodology for coming to know Milo Pimatisiwin as land-based initiatives for Indigenous youth. Ottawa (ON): University of Ottawa; 2016.
69. Fanian S, Young SK, Mantla M, Daniels A, Chatwood S. Evaluation of the Kts'iìhtła ("We Light the Fire") project: building resiliency and connections through strengths-based creative arts programming for Indigenous youth. Int J Circumpolar Health. 2015 Aug 10;74(1):27672.
70. Ritchie SD, Wabano MJ, Russell K, Enosse L, Young NL. Promoting resilience and wellbeing through an outdoor intervention designed for Aboriginal adolescents. Rural Remote Health. 2014 Mar 26;14:2523.
71. Chow K, Healey M. Place attachment and place identity: first-year undergraduates making the transition from home to university. J Env Psychol. 2008 Dec;28(4):362–72.
72. Hansen JG, Antsanen, R. Elders' teachings about resilience and its implications for education in Dene and Cree communities. Int Indig Policy J. 2016 Jan;7(1):2.
73. Redvers J, Bjerregaard P, Eriksen H, Fanian S, Healey G, Hiratsuka V, Jong M, Larsen CV, Linton J, Pollock N, Silviken A, Stoor P, Chatwood S. A scoping review of Indigenous suicide prevention in circumpolar regions. Int J Circumpolar Health. 2015 Jan 31;74(1):27509.
74. Whalen DH, Moss M, Baldwin D. Healing through language: positive physical health effects of indigenous language use. F1000Research. 2016 May 9;5.
75. Baillie CP, Galaviz KI, Emiry K, Bruner MW, Bruner BG, Lévesque L. Physical activity interventions to promote positive youth development among indigenous youth: a RE-AIM review. Translat Beh Med. 2016 Jul 21;7(1):43–51.

15 Innovation for Northern Mental Health and Addiction Services: Indigenous Frameworks

CHRISTOPHER MUSHQUASH, ALEXANDRA S. DRAWSON, AND ELAINE TOOMBS

Overview

Northern Canadians bears a disproportionate burden of health disparities, including higher rates of mental health difficulties and addiction, in comparison to other Canadians. In northwestern Ontario, for example, addiction to opioids and other substance misuse is a public health crisis that places tremendous burden on the social and economic fabric of communities. At the same time, however, there remains limited regional capacity both to clinically support and to engage in research with communities to develop local, effective, and sustainable approaches to wellness that are culturally and contextually appropriate. This chapter will review what is known about mental health and addiction in northern and remote Canada, and among Indigenous peoples, and discuss the importance of the recent Indigenous mental health and addiction policy document *Honouring Our Strengths: A Renewed Framework to Address Substance Use Issues Among First Nations People in Canada* and the First Nations Mental Wellness Continuum Framework. Both frameworks have relevance for all living in northern Canada given their focus on systems-level organization towards holistic conceptual models grounded in culture.

Margaret's Story

There was an old lady named Margaret. Once while she was going about her day, she happened to swallow a fly. We don't know why she swallowed a fly. But the fact remained. Margaret now had a fly problem. And fly problems, as we know, left unchecked, can turn into much worse problems. Margaret spent some time thinking about what she was going to do. She thought, *What takes care of flies?* Then it occurred to her: spiders eat flies! Margaret decided that she needed to find herself a spider to swallow to catch the fly.

As luck would have it, Margaret was successful in finding just the right spider. In fact, the task was not even really that difficult. Spiders are quite common, and it did not take her much time before she found a suitable one. And then Margaret went about swallowing the spider. That took a little more effort. Swallowing a spider was a little difficult to stomach but she managed. If there was one thing that Margaret was good at, it was doing what was needed when needed. Margaret was pleased with herself. She had solved her fly problem. However, it was not long before Margaret realized she had a new problem. She now had a spider problem. She could feel it wriggling inside her. Just as in the case of her fly problem, Margaret thought about what to do about the spider. Success! Birds eat spiders. She went about finding just the right bird.

It never occurred to Margaret how absurd it was to swallow a bird. All she knew was that she swallowed the bird to catch the spider that wriggled inside her. Now, if you are an experienced reader, you might know what happened to Margaret next. However, the interesting thing is that a series of events had been put into motion and now the story unfolds quite predictably. Margaret's bird problem needed to be solved so she swallowed a cat. Fancy that, to swallow a cat! She swallowed the cat to catch the bird and swallowed the bird to catch the spider and swallowed the spider to catch the fly. Nevertheless, we still do not know why she swallowed a fly. Margaret continued her efforts to solve her new emerging problems. She swallowed a dog. She swallowed a cow. Finally, she swallowed a horse. She swallowed the horse to catch the cow; she swallowed the cow to catch the dog; she swallowed the dog to catch the cat; she swallowed the cat to catch the bird; she swallowed the bird to catch the spider; she swallowed the spider to catch the fly. But we don't know why she swallowed the fly. Perhaps she'll die.

Introduction

Authors have many ways to introduce their audience to an academic chapter on mental health and addiction among people in northern Canada. For example, consistent with an academic tradition, this chapter could have begun by framing the scope of the issues of mental health and addiction among northerners, Indigenous peoples, broadly in Canada and then make noncontextualized comparisons of limited base rate data. This approach would include statistics demonstrating the significant health, mental health, and addiction issues faced by Indigenous and non-Indigenous people living in northern Canada. The chapter would provide an overview of the determinants of these difficulties, including an overview of such essential topics as residential schools, child welfare systems, the Indian Act, and ongoing funding disparities and the resultant crescendo of poverty, poor housing conditions, lack of clean drinking water, food insecurity, crumbling infrastructure, lack of access to education and health, and economic development disadvantage. However, although a chapter of this nature would summarize what is known, it would exclude, through its traditional academic focus, new developments in mental health and addiction in Canada.

Instead, we started with a story about an old lady named Margaret. Margaret's story serves as a metaphorical framework to illustrate the current approaches to addressing mental health and addiction difficulties in northern populations generally and in Indigenous communities specifically. Margaret applied multiple interventions, which aimed to treat symptoms that sprung from treatments of prior issues. As her own health care provider, she treated the presenting problem but did not address the cause of the problems. Within our current medical systems, we expect that when an individual – for example, Margaret presents with a mental health or addiction difficulty, we go about a familiar process that is supposed to involve referral to an appropriate care provider, assessment, diagnosis, treatment, and follow-up. One could also sprinkle waitlists at each stage in the care pathway that would reduce the likelihood of Margaret receiving timely evidence-based treatment. But is this common approach appropriate? Although conceptually it makes intuitive sense to proceed in this manner, the care pathway is rarely this linear, and we know that individuals often present with complexity in the form of comorbidity. By the time Margaret receives treatment for her presenting "horse problem," service providers often do not inquire about the cascading events that led to it. Her family history, her childhood experiences, and the additional structural or system-level issues that exacerbate her symptoms may never be discussed although they affect her ability to benefit from the prescribed treatment. In addition, the likelihood that the requisite mental health support is accessible to those requiring it in the North is very low.

Generally, there is a lack of sufficient evidence regarding both rates of mental disorders in and adequate treatment of Canadian Indigenous peoples (1), particularly for those living in northern regions. This lack of data creates difficulty and confusion at individual, community, provincial and territorial, and national levels. How can we effectively prevent and treat the disproportionate burden of mental health and addiction if we do not have access to simple base rates or have high-quality information about which treatment protocols and wider programming bring positive change? For example, population-level data, like the census collected by Statistics Canada, do not portray all health-specific data by region (2). Such data are typically available at a provincial or territorial level, but it remains challenging to determine regional differences within a province or territory. The lack of availability of these data reduce the feasibility and utility of analyses dedicated to examining specific populations and regions, such as Indigenous communities in the North.

Rural and northern regions bear a disproportionate burden of disease with respect to mental health and addiction and, at the same time, have limited or less consistent access to health services, particularly when it comes to specialist care (3). Difficulties with access are caused by a number of system-level issues, such as transportation/geography, lack of comprehensive services, recruitment and retention problems, and unequal access to the services that exist (4). Indigenous peoples in northern and remote Canada are significantly more likely to experience a variety of physical health, mental health, and addictions difficulties (5–7). Across a variety of settings, approximately 50 per cent of First Nations adults have been diagnosed with a mental disorder (8,9). While 60 per cent of the non–First Nations adult population rate their health as "excellent" or "very good," only 44.1 per cent of First Nations adults report the same. Similarly, approximately 30 per cent of non–First Nations adults appraise their psychological stress as "moderate" or "high," compared to almost 50 per cent of First Nations adults (9). First Nations people in Canada are five to seven times as likely to commit suicide as majority-population Canadians – however, this rate varies greatly from community to community and is contingent on social determinants of health (1). Northern families are more likely to experience housing instability, inconsistent access to mental health services, and poverty (10). The relative risk of unintentional injury requiring hospitalization for First Nations individuals living in northern communities was higher (19.4 per 1000 individuals) than for non–First Nations people living in northern (7.9 per 1000) and southern (6.5 per 1000) small communities (11). These regional differences have encouraged some to consider geographical location as a social determinant of Indigenous health in Canada (12).

Determinants of Health

Systemic disparities in social determinants of health contribute to these high rates of mental health difficulties and addictions within communities (5,13). As discussed by Schiff in this volume, and previously described by Reading and Wein, social determinants of Indigenous health can be considered on three levels: distal, intermediate, and proximal (14). Distal determinants exist at the widest level and include political and historical contexts, such as colonization, continued colonization, and the impact of these, while intermediate determinants can be considered community-wide factors that affect all members (14). Proximal determinants often vary at the individual level and are those determinants that directly affect any aspect of health, including employment status, education, overcrowding, and family violence (14). Most social determinants of health affect the presence, identification, and treatment of various health conditions in all regions of Canada. At all levels of health, specific factors remain particularly relevant for individuals living in northern Canada, and some are especially relevant for Indigenous populations. Consideration of both culture and context for Indigenous communities in the northern regions of Canada can further the understanding of how the health and well-being needs of the individuals living in these communities are met (see also Healey et al., this volume, chapter 5). The effect of these determinants in a northern context are discussed below.

Distal Determinants

COLONIZATION

Colonization is a significant determinant of health that continues to adversely affect Indigenous peoples and communities in Canada (15–18). Poor outcomes in communities (including poverty, lack of housing, limited access to health care) have been attributed to both direct and indirect effects of colonization and assimilation policies and attempts (14,19). Residential schools, an aspect of colonization and the distal determinants of health, also have a significant influence on the current state of Indigenous peoples in Canada (7). The effects of these institutions may have regional implications, given that the majority of residential schools were located in northern and western regions of Canada (7). In Phase 2 of the First Nations Regional Health Survey, 20 per cent of respondents had attended residential school, while approximately half reported that one of their parents (52.5 per cent) or one of their grandparents (46.2 per cent) had attended (20). Survivors of residential school report many negative health outcomes as a result, including loss of cultural identity, noted by 76.3 per cent of respondents (7). Unfortunately, the effects are not limited to the attendees; both second- and third-generation survivors of residential school report a variety of poorer mental health outcomes (21,22). In fact, in Phase 3 of the Regional Health Survey, 74.4 per cent of adult respondents reported direct or intergenerational effects of their parents' or grandparents' residential school attendance (23). Given the higher prevalence of residential schools in northern regions, it is possible that the health implications of these institutions disproportionally affect northern communities today.

Intermediate Determinants

CULTURE AND TRADITION AS PROTECTIVE FACTORS

Traditional and cultural activities are essential to the mental health and well-being of Indigenous peoples living in northern communities. Involvement results in enhanced self-reported balance (spiritual, mental, emotional, and physical) and sense of control in life, as well as reduced substance use and symptoms of depression (9). Culture as an intervention approach has been proposed for Indigenous well-being promotion, but the current scope of these interventions in northern communities is limited (3,4). Language serves as the vehicle by which culture is communicated; without a common language, social norms, symbols, and history may be lost (24). Through colonization and other attempts at assimilation, such as residential schools and the Sixties Scoop, the linguistic legacy of Indigenous peoples in Canada has been damaged; there are fewer fluent speakers of the approximately 60 existing Indigenous languages, and some Indigenous languages have become extinct (12,24–27). Speaking a traditional language is a protective factor against a variety of poor mental health outcomes, such as substance use, depression, anxiety, and suicide (6,8,12,28). Although the number of primary Indigenous language speakers has decreased (from 21.4 per cent in 2006 to 15.6 per cent in 2016), there was a 3.1 per cent increase of Indigenous people speaking an Indigenous language overall. In northern regions, particularly among Inuit populations, almost two-thirds of the population reported they could hold a conversation in an Indigenous language. Similar results have been found for First Nations in remote or northern regions, particularly for communities in which the majority population identified as Indigenous (27). Traditional language revitalization has been explored as one way to promote resilience in Indigenous communities (29).

HEALTH CARE

The current health care system, for Indigenous peoples in Canada, is considered an intermediate social determinant of health. Current efforts in Indigenous health prevention are focused on communicable disease as opposed to the chronic illnesses that are actually leading to high mortality in these communities (14). Access to care is also contributing to poor health outcomes, particularly for those Indigenous peoples who reside in rural or remote northern communities, which are infrequently visited by health professionals (with the exception of regular nursing staff) (1,14) and face recruitment and retention challenges, as discussed by Pong (physicians, chapter 7) and Møller (nurses, chapter 8) both in this volume.

INDIGENOUS CONCEPTUALIZATIONS OF HEALTH AND HEALING

Significant differences exist between mainstream and Indigenous conceptualizations of health and, thereby, of mental health. The primary contrast is that in mainstream conceptualizations, health often can be separated from the rest of our existence (30), whereas in many Indigenous views, health is the outcome of balance between several domains (30–32). From Indigenous perspectives, illness is viewed as a symptom or descriptor of one's existence, as opposed to as an isolated incident (30–32). This balance is often illustrated through the medicine wheel (30–32). The medicine wheel does not allow for the simplification of any physical or mental health disorder to a disparity in one discrete area or system of the body and, in fact, does not allow for illness to be conceptualized as only residing in the ill individual (30). Instead, the medicine wheel conceptualization of illness may reflect that disorder exists in the individual's relationships and community as well (30–32). When the health of Indigenous peoples is viewed through this lens, the influence of community-wide difficulties, such as residential school history, can be appreciated (33). This discrepancy is illustrated by the Anishinabek word *mino bmaddis*. This word directly translates to *being alive well*, but conceptually communicates one's health status and the balance of the four domains of the medicine wheel (30). The Anishinabek word for illness *aakozi* translates more accurately to *being out of balance*.

Mental health care for Indigenous peoples in Canada has routinely included mainly mainstream perspectives on healing. In the literature, there is now an increasing demand for and understanding of the benefits of traditional approaches to healing or the importance of considering an individual's Indigenous identity in the healing process. This is not to say that mainstream approaches to treatment of mental disorders and addictions are not useful when working with Indigenous peoples, but rather that they may not always be sufficient. Just as mainstream conceptualizations and explanations for illness are often not as holistic as Indigenous views, neither are mainstream approaches to healing (32). Some northern Ontario health care centres (e.g., the Thunder Bay Regional Health Sciences Centre and Sioux Lookout Meno Ya Win Health Centre) have recognized these integrative systems of knowledge and incorporated Indigenous patient navigators, while also providing access to traditional ceremonies, such as smudging, to better address Indigenous health and well-being (10).

Proximal Determinants

ADVERSE CHILDHOOD EXPERIENCES

Proximal determinants are factors that directly affect physical, emotional, mental, or spiritual health (14). Adverse childhood experiences represent an important proximal determinant of health worth considering in the context of Indigenous communities (14). In fact, in terms of effect size, few relationships between determinants and outcomes are seen in epidemiological research. The initial Adverse Childhood Experiences Study was undertaken by the Centers for Disease Control and the Kaiser Permanente Healthcare Consortium (34); it involved 13,494 participants who were asked to answer questions about their first 18 years of life. Three categories of trauma were measured: abuse, household challenges, and neglect. Each category included several specific types of trauma, for a total of 10 types of trauma. The abuse category included emotional abuse, physical abuse, and sexual abuse; the household challenges category included mother treated violently, household substance abuse, mental illness in the household, parental separation or divorce, and criminal household member; and the neglect category included emotional neglect and physical neglect. This research found that these adverse childhood experiences are related to a number of difficulties, including (but not limited to) increased risk for alcoholism and alcohol abuse, chronic obstructive pulmonary disease, depression, illicit drug use, heart disease, liver failure, intimate partner violence, smoking, suicide, poor academic achievement, obesity, and diabetes. Most importantly, adverse childhood experiences are related to these difficulties in a dose-response relationship. That is, the more adverse childhood experiences an individual is exposed to, the more likely they are to experience the difficulties listed. For example, a male child with an adverse childhood experiences (ACE) score of 6 (i.e., who had six of the above adverse childhood experiences), when compared to a male child with an ACE score of 0, has a 46-fold (4600 per cent) increase in the likelihood of becoming an injection drug user sometime later in life (35). As well, an ACE score of 7 or more increased the risk of suicide attempts 51-fold among children and adolescents (36).

Research has shown that exposure to trauma has the ability to disrupt the way that our brains grow; the manner in which we develop in social, emotional, and cognitive domains; how we manage stress; our likelihood of developing chronic health issues; and our life expectancy. Much of the focus on trauma is oriented toward treating trauma that has already happened, which is important as many in our communities have experienced and continue to experience trauma. Healing those who have experienced trauma must remain a priority, in all regions across Canada. However, we must also turn our attention to preventing trauma from occurring. Working collaboratively as communities and nations with our service providers across health and social services fields will assist us in achieving prevention. This requires significant commitments from multiple levels of government, sufficient funding, development of appropriate teams, evidence-based treatment approaches, systematic monitoring, and flexible, responsive service delivery through adaptable policy – all within appropriate Indigenous governance models considering geographic-specific needs. After all, appropriate and high-quality service planning requires appropriate and high-quality data that represent regional similarities and differences. Given the magnitude of effect sizes in the ACEs literature, further research with Canadian Indigenous communities, specifically those located in the North, can be dedicated to development and delivery of mental health systems and services. These systems and services must necessarily include strong prevention approaches as a means of reducing the number of people exposed to preventable adverse childhood experiences and thus stem the onset of the full range of serious health and mental health negative consequences.

RESILIENCE

Indigenous people have persevered despite many obstacles not encountered by other populations in Canada (32). Although they are at increased risk for mental health difficulties, Indigenous peoples have also displayed remarkable resilience. In Phase 2 of the First Nations Regional Health Survey, over 70 per cent of adult respondents reported feeling balanced in at least one of the four domains of the medicine wheel: physical, emotional, mental, or spiritual well-being (21). Similar to definitions of health and well-being existing as more broad and holistic, so too are ideas of resilience for many Indigenous peoples. In Indigenous conceptualizations, resilience may arise as the result of shared language and cultural traditions, an individual and community connection with the environment and land, and re-examination of the history of hardships that many Indigenous groups have survived (29). Exploring these notions can strengthen an identity rooted in culture and create a dissonance with the colonial-related difficulties Indigenous peoples have experienced (29). Given the contextual nature of strategies to promote resilience, useful strategies have been determined based on geographical regions. For example, some factors identified to be relevant to specific circumpolar regions have included promotion of traditional knowledges, increased communication within the community, and cultural revitalization (37). Within the North, fostering resilience has been used to support education and Indigenous learners (38). Elder suggestions of how best to incorporate resilience within educational systems were provided, through advocating respect for one's self, the land, other people, and the spiritual world (38).

Despite what is known about the difficulties and disparities Indigenous peoples face in health, mental health, and addiction, a lot remains to be optimistic about. In 2016, 4.9 per cent (1,673,785) of the total population of Canada were Aboriginal, and between 2006 and 2016, there was a 42.5 per cent increase in the number of Indigenous people in Canada (39), including population increases in northern regions, such as a 12.5 per cent increase in Nunavut. Not only is this population experiencing growth, but it is also a very young population, with 28 per cent ages 14 or under (compared to 16.5 per cent of the majority population) and only 6 per cent ages 65 or over (compared to 14.2 per cent of the majority population) (39). Furthermore, increasingly more Indigenous peoples are accessing and completing higher education than ever before (40). Being hopeful about the future is a central cultural lever of mental wellness. By appropriately investing in our young people, we create a future that is characterized by wellness for our communities.

Culture as Healing: Honouring Our Strengths

Honouring Our Strengths: A Renewed Framework to Address Substance Use Issues Among First Nations People in Canada (41), is a policy document that was intended to address substance use and addiction-related treatment issues among First Nations people in Canada. This document provided a framework to guide the design, coordination, and delivery of mental health services within all levels of health care, including community, regional, and national levels.

Honouring Our Strengths emphasized community and cultural strengths within addictions treatment and resulted in the creation of practical care guidelines, making it an important resource for treatment providers.

Honouring Our Strengths provided a comprehensive guide that aimed to revive and renew substance use treatment services for First Nations people. This framework has been used successfully within Indigenous communities in the North. Six elements of care were identified as priorities that would increase the utility, effectiveness, and cultural relevance of existing substance use treatments:

1. Community development, universal prevention, and health promotion
2. Early identification, brief intervention, and aftercare
3. Secondary-risk reduction
4. Active treatment
5. Specialized treatment
6. Care facilitation

These elements of care provide a systems-wide response to substance use treatment for First Nations populations and account for individual treatment needs within sub-populations. All elements are implemented using guiding principles, which include balance, spirit-centring, connection, and holistic focus (41).

To continuously guide the framework, including facilitating ongoing communication, collaboration, and commitment to the partnerships, the National Native Alcohol and Drug Abuse Program Renewal Leadership Team was created in 2010. This team ensures the continuing implementation of *Honouring Our Strengths*, including dissemination of knowledge throughout systems of care. Ongoing conversations ensure that addictions treatment remains a priority. Through such initiatives, the priorities reviewed in *Honouring Our Strength* have moved from policy recommendations to systematic implementation within all levels of health care.

Other directions of this project included the development of a model to provide a holistic description of mental wellness rooted in Indigenous conceptualizations of community, family, and culture. The First Nations Mental Wellness Continuum Framework was created to meet these needs and extend the *Honouring Our Strengths* initiative into a measurable framework that reflects holistic Indigenous well-being.

First Nations Mental Wellness Continuum Framework

The First Nations Mental Wellness Continuum Framework (FNMWCF) is a unique approach to the conceptualization and development of First Nations mental wellness. The FNMWCF was developed in collaboration with the Assembly of First Nations, National Native Addictions Partnership Foundation, the Native Mental Health Association, Health Canada's First Nations and Inuit Health Branch, and additional community partners (42).

Mental wellness was conceptualized in the FNMWCF as a balance of spiritual, emotional, mental, and physical well-being. Individual balance and wellness has been identified through measurable indicators of hope, belonging, meaning, and purpose:

- Having **Hope** for the future, from the embodiment of unique Indigenous values, a sense of identity, and belief in spirit, is a marker of spiritual wellness.
- A sense of **Belonging**, facilitated through connectedness with individual attitudes towards living, as well as family, community, and cultural relations, indicated emotional well-being. Family relationships were prioritized by relevance to the individual and those that are culturally defined rather than Westernized values of bloodlines.
- **Meaning** was described as an indicator of mental wellness. It was defined as an individual understanding within people's personal lives and those of their families.
- Physical well-being was identified by **Purpose** achieved through living one's life with wholeness, including activities associated with employment, family, education, culture, and community involvement.

Rather than focusing on symptom presentation and behavioural concerns existing within an individual, this framework incorporates broader determinants of health and wellness. Overall holistic well-being is the priority of the framework for all First Nations peoples, rather than the mere absence of illness or symptoms. Mental wellness is placed on a wheel, illustrating the holistic and interrelational approach to well-being. The wheel is centred using the Four Directions of Hope, Belonging, Meaning, and Purpose. Community (represented by Kinship, Clan, Elders, and Community) circles the Four Directions. This is followed by circles related to Populations, Specific Population Needs, Continuum of Essential Services, Supporting Elements, Partners in Implementation, Key Themes for Mental Wellness, and, finally, Culture as Foundation. Culture is placed last on the wheel, as the practice that circles all others, and ultimately embodies wellness. Culture is defined within this framework as related to Elders, Cultural Practitioners, Kinship Relationships, Language, Practices, Ceremonies, Knowledge, Land, and Values (42).

Applying the FNMWCF in a Northern Context

The FNMWCF was created to provide a guideline by which program and service providers could align their own policies and priorities. To promote optimal mental wellness, the framework recognized the necessity of collaboration, communication, and cultural knowledge within all service settings. Given the challenges of mental health service provision in northern communities, implementing an adaptable, collaborative model of Indigenous wellness was warranted (42).

The framework was designed and developed using Indigenous values of wellness; however, it can be implemented within mainstream services as well. Recognizing broader social determinants of health, such as socio-economic status, housing, and gender, and the influence of such factors within an individual expands the scope of mental health and well-being for all populations. Combinations of exposure to such determinants can change symptom presentation within individuals and can create unique challenges that are not recognized within typical mental health treatments.

The framework provided themes that related to the expressed needs of communities but also identified priorities for action within each concept. It has identified five key themes that aim to enhance First Nations mental wellness. These themes resulted from intensive conversations with First Nations communities, including community leadership, youth, and Elders:

1. Culture as foundation
2. Community development, ownership, and capacity building
3. Quality care system and competent service delivery
4. Collaboration with partners
5. Enhanced flexible funding

These priorities continue to be addressed within First Nations communities. The framework has been used to inform federal policy and has been implemented at community, regional, and national levels. Specific projects have supported community adaptations, knowledge generation, and shared community mentorship for the FNMWCF in northern communities. For example, Kwanlin Dun First Nation, located in Yukon, has applied the framework to crisis management training within its community and established specific measures of hope, belonging, meaning, and purpose. Shibogama First Nation council in northwestern Ontario developed and evaluated a land-based healing program for families. Elements of the model have been prioritized by substance use treatment centres in northern Manitoba, have assessed quality of life and service delivery strategies through eHealth service providers for northern Ontario residents, and have facilitated collaboration of Indigenous communities across Canada (43).

Conclusion

This chapter was a quick visit through a number of interrelated issues in Indigenous mental health, addiction, and wellness in northern communities. In summary, we would like to reorient you to the story about Margaret. If Margaret had swallowed a fly and the system responded, it would likely try to find the best evidence-based spider possible to help Margaret manage the fly problem. As well, she might be offered concurrent treatment for the spider through the bird program. As an example, imagine Margaret presenting to a family physician with symptoms of depression. She might be prescribed an antidepressant. Margaret may or may not experience relief from her depressive symptoms. If not, she might be prescribed some other medication. Perhaps a different SSRI, or SNRI, or MAOI, or tricyclic, or tetracyclic, or atypical antipsychotic, or maybe even an anticonvulsant. She might also be prescribed an anxiolytic or hypnotic to help with the sleep difficulties she experiences.

When we liken Margaret's fly problem to a specific diagnosis, we understand that she requires interventions that are culturally appropriate, timely, and effective. She requires interventions that address systemic issues that may hinder her prognosis, using interdisciplinary circles of care that illuminate diverse needs. For example, if she is diagnosed with a substance use disorder and seeks addictions treatment, she requires a program that not only addresses her substance use but does so in a way that best supports her individual needs. Several conditions need to be met for Margaret to be able to access, successfully complete, and reap the best outcomes from such a program. She must be able to meet the eligibility criteria, she needs to be able to access the program regardless of her financial situation and physical location, and the program must have proven effective. Programs that have proven effective for Indigenous peoples often integrate cultural, spiritual, social, and mental needs and are delivered by care providers who know what it means to provide culturally safe care and treatment (44). After Margaret has completed treatment, she may require program bridging and continuity of care within her community to addresses lingering issues relevant to her clinical needs. Perhaps she needs to connect with a social worker to discuss employment, accessibility supports, or housing. Perhaps she needs to meet with a therapist to address attachment, trauma, or emotional regulation concerns. These are larger "horse problems" that can be addressed after proper first-line treatment has been successfully administered.

Whatever Margaret's needs may be, a fly problem can be effectively addressed if care providers have a good understanding of social determinants of health and strength-based approaches that support the specific needs of Indigenous populations (45 p19). The *Honouring Our Strengths* framework (41 p19) discusses six elements of care related to effectively addressing fly problems. These are displayed in a tiered care treatment model and are as follows:

1. Community development, universal prevention, and health promotion approaches
2. Early identification, brief intervention, and aftercare programs
3. Secondary-risk reduction

4. Active treatment
5. Specialized treatment
6. Care facilitation and case management

If Margaret's fly problem is related to substance use, programs such as the Nimkee NupiGawagan Healing Centre's residential solvent use program for youth (46,47), the New Choices program for young mothers who use substances (48,49), or a Seeking Safety (50) program that addresses intergenerational trauma in conjunction with substance use could be treatment options that meet Margaret's needs. Fortunately, some programs exist in northern regions that can meet her needs, but unfortunately, many are not offered as first-line, primary treatments.

To improve services and supports for Indigenous people in mental health and addiction, we must explore our conceptual models and integrate everything known that explains the variance in mental health and addiction difficulties for those living in northern Canada. This will require new thinking that includes broad conceptualizations and culture-based approaches. Fortunately, Indigenous peoples have been leading the way through the development of frameworks such as *Honouring Our Strengths* (41) and the Mental Wellness Continuum Framework (42). These frameworks outline the need and importance of integrated and responsive systems that collaborate across the range of typical silos that contribute to disruptions in continuity of care. It is time for systems to come along with us, to help facilitate the wellness for which we strive.

REFERENCES

1. Al-Hamad A, O'Gorman L. Northern Ontario health care priorities: access to culturally appropriate care for physical and mental health [Internet]. Thunder Bay (ON): Northern Policy Institute; 2015 Jun [cited 2018 Jun 12]. Available from: https://www.northernpolicy.ca/upload/documents/publications/briefing-notes/paper-health-policy-4-english-15.06.22.pdf
2. CMHA Ontario. Rural and northern health issues: challenges and new opportunities [Internet]. Toronto (ON): CMHA Ontario; 2014 Oct 9 [cited 2018 Jun 20]. Available from: https://ontario.cmha.ca/news/rural-northern-health-issues-challenges-new-opportunities/
3. Adelson N. The embodiment of inequity: health disparities in Aboriginal Canada. Can J Public Health. 2005 Mar 1;96(Suppl 2):S45–S61.
4. Bellamy S, Hardy C. Anxiety disorders and Aboriginal peoples in Canada: the current state of knowledge and directions for future research. Prince George (BC): National Collaborating Centre for Aboriginal Health; 2015.

5. National Collaborating Centre for Aboriginal Health. An overview of Aboriginal health in Canada [Internet]. Prince George (BC): National Collaborating Centre for Aboriginal Health; 2013 [cited 2018 Jun 12]. Available from: http://www.nccah-ccnsa.ca/Publications/Lists/Publications/Attachments/101/abororiginal_health_web.pdf
6. Firestone M, Smylie J, Maracle S, McKnight C, Spiller M, O'Campo P. Mental health and substance use in an urban First Nations population in Hamilton, Ontario. Can J Public Health. 2015 Sep 1;106(6):e375–e381.
7. First Nations Information Governance Centre. First Nations regional health survey (RHS) 2008/10: National report on adults, youth and children living in First Nations communities [Internet]. Ottawa (ON): First Nations Information Governance Centre; 2012 Jun [cited 2018 Jun 12]. Available from: ttps://fnigc.ca/wp-content/uploads/2020/09/5eedd1ce8f5784a69126edda537dccfc_first_nations_regional_health_survey_rhs_2008-10_-_national_report_adult_2.pdf
8. Kielland N, Simeone T. Current issues in mental health in Canada: the mental health of First Nations and Inuit communities [Internet]. Ottawa (ON): Library of Parliament; 2014 Jan 6 [cited 2018 June 12]. Publication No. 2014-02-E. Available from: https://lop.parl.ca/staticfiles/PublicWebsite/Home/ResearchPublications/InBriefs/PDF/2014-02-e.pdf
9. Redvers N, Marianayagam J, Blondin BS. Improving access to Indigenous medicine for patients in hospital-based settings: a challenge for health systems in northern Canada. Int J Circumpolar Health. 2019 Jan 1;78(1):1577093.
10. Fantus D, Shah BR, Qiu F, Hux J, Rochon P. Injury in First Nations communities in Ontario. Can J Public Health. 2009 Jul 1;100(4):258–62.
11. Barker B, Goodman A, DeBeck K. Reclaiming Indigenous identities: culture as strength against suicide among Indigenous youth in Canada. Can J Public Health. 2017 Mar 1;108(2):e208–e210.
12. Statistics Canada. Education in Canada: Key results from the 2016 census [Internet]. Ottawa (ON): Statistics Canada; 2017 [cited 2018 May 29]. Available from: https://www150.statcan.gc.ca/n1/en/daily-quotidien/171129/dq171129a-eng.pdf?st=vFcm75uE
13. Reading C, Wein F. Health inequalities and social determinants of Aboriginal peoples' health [Internet]. Prince George (BC): National Collaborating Centre for Aboriginal Health; 2009. Available from: http://www.ccnsa-nccah.ca/docs/determinants/RPT-HealthInequalities-Reading-Wien-EN.pdf
14. Kelly-Scott K, Smith K. Aboriginal Peoples: fact sheet for Canada [Internet]. Ottawa (ON): Statistics Canada; 2011 [cited 2018 May 30]. Online Catalogue No. 89-656-X. Available from: https://www.statcan.gc.ca/pub/89-656-x/89-656-x2015001-eng.htm
15. Smythe C, Caverson R. Alcohol, other drugs and related harms in Ontario: a scan of the environment – a background document to support the development of an Ontario Drug Strategy [Internet]. Barrie (ON): Simcoe Muskoka District Health

Unit; 2008 [cited 2018 Mar 16]. Available from: https://smdhu.files.wordpress.com/2012/02/aod_scan1.pdf

16. Dell CA, Roberts G, Kilty J, Taylor K, Daschuk M, Hopkins C, Dell D. Researching prescription drug misuse among First Nations in Canada: Starting from a health promotion framework. Subst Abuse. 2012 Jan;6:23–31.
17. Czyzewski K. Colonialism as a broader social determinant of health. Int Indig J. 2011;2(1):5.
18. Allan B, Smylie J. First Peoples, second class treatment: the role of racism in the health and well-being of Indigenous peoples in Canada [Internet]. Toronto (ON): Wellesley Institute; 2015 [cited 2018 Mar 16]. Available from: https://www.sac-oac.ca/sites/default/files/resources/Report-First-Peoples-Second-Class-Treatment.pdf
19. Truth and Reconciliation Commission of Canada. Truth and Reconciliation Commission of Canada: Calls to action [Internet]. Winnipeg (MB): Truth and Reconciliation Commission of Canada; 2015 [cited 2018 March 22]. Available from: http://trc.ca/assets/pdf/Calls_to_Action_English2.pdf
20. Bombay A, Matheson K, Anisman H. The impact of stressors on second generation Indian residential school survivors. Transcultural psychiatry. 2011 Sep;48(4):367–91.
21. Bombay A, Matheson K, Anisman H. The intergenerational effects of Indian Residential Schools: Implications for the concept of historical trauma. Transcultural psychiatry. 2014 Jun;51(3):320–38.
22. First Nations Information Governance Centre. National report of the First Nations regional health survey – phase 3, volume one [Internet]. Ottawa (ON): First Nations Information Governance Centre; 2018 Mar [revised 2018 Jul; cited 2018 Jun 12]. Available from: https://fnigc.ca/wp-content/uploads/2020/09/713c8fd606a8eeb021debc927332938d_FNIGC-RHS-Phase-III-Report1-FINAL-VERSION-Dec.2018.pdf
23. National Collaborating Centre for Aboriginal Health. Culture and language as social determinants of First Nations, Inuit and Métis health [Internet]. Prince George (BC): National Collaborating Centre for Aboriginal Health; 2016 [cited 2018 Jun 29]. Available from: http://www.ccnsa-nccah.ca/docs/determinants/FS-CultureLanguage-SDOH-FNMI-EN.pdf
24. Statistics Canada. Aboriginal languages in Canada [Internet]. Ottawa (ON): Statistics Canada; 2012 [modified 2018 Jul 23; cited 2018 Mar 8]. Catalogue No. 98-314-X2011003. Available from: http://www12.statcan.gc.ca/census-recensement/2011/as-sa/98-314-x/98-314-x2011003_3-eng.cfm
25. Statistics Canada. 2011 national household survey – Aboriginal language knowledge [Internet]. Ottawa (ON): Statistics Canada. [cited 2018 Jun 12]. Available from: https://www150.statcan.gc.ca/n1/en/catalogue/99-011-X2011030
26. Statistics Canada. The Aboriginal languages of First Nations people, Métis and Inuit [Internet]. Ottawa (ON): Statistics Canada; 2017 Oct 15 [modified 2019

Apr 3; cited 2018 March 8]. Catalogue No. 98-304-X. Available from: https://www12.statcan.gc.ca/census-recensement/2016/as-sa/98-200-x/2016022/98-200-x2016022-eng.cfm

27. Bellamy S, Hardy C. Understanding depression in Aboriginal communities and families [Internet]. Prince George (BC): National Collaborating Centre for Aboriginal Health; 2015 [cited 2017 May 19]. Available from: http://www.ccnsa-nccah.ca/docs/emerging/RPT-UnderstandingDepression-Bellamy-Hardy-EN.pdf
28. Isbister-Bear O, Hatala AR, Sjoblom E. Strengthening Âhkamêyimo among Indigenous youth: the social determinants of health, justice, and resilience in Canada's north. J Indig Wellbeing. 2017;2(3):76–89.
29. Vukic A, Gregory D, Martin-Misener R, Etowa J. Aboriginal and Western conceptions of mental health and illness. Pimatisiwin: J Aborig and Ind Community Health. 2011;9(1):65–86.
30. Blackstock C. Rooting mental health in an Aboriginal world view [Internet]. Ottawa (ON): Provincial Centre of Excellence for Child and Youth Mental Health at CHEO; 2008 Oct [cited 2014 Jun 3]. Available from: https://iknow-oce.esolutionsgroup.ca/api/ServiceItem/GetDocument?clientId=A1B5AA8F-88A1-4688-83F8-FF0A5B083EF3&documentId=949655ad-d9df-4cb3-9323-9de3602220e7
31. Kirmayer LJ, Brass GM, Tait CL. The mental health of Aboriginal peoples: transformations of identity and community. Can J Psychiatry. 2000 Sep;45(7):607–16.
32. Chandler MJ, Lalonde C. Cultural continuity as a hedge against suicide in Canada's First Nations. Transcult Psychiatry. 1998 Jun;35(2):191–219.
33. Felitti VJ, Anda RF, Nordenberg D, Williamson DF, Spitz AM, Edwards V, Koss MP, Marks JS. Relationship of childhood abuse and household dysfunction to many of the leading causes of death in adults: the adverse childhood experiences (ACE) study. Am J Prev Med. 1998 Jun 1;56(6):774–86.
34. Stein MD, Conti MT, Kenney S, Anderson BJ, Flori JN, Risi MM, Bailey GL. Adverse childhood experience effects on opioid use initiation, injection drug use, and overdose among persons with opioid use disorder. Drug Alcohol Depend. 2017 Oct 1;179:325–9.
35. Dube SR, Anda RF, Felitti VJ, Chapman DP, Williamson DF, Giles WH. Childhood abuse, household dysfunction, and the risk of attempted suicide throughout the life span: findings from the adverse childhood experiences study. JAMA. 2001 Dec 26;286(24):3089–96.
36. MacDonald JP, Ford JD, Willox AC, Ross NA. A review of protective factors and causal mechanisms that enhance the mental health of Indigenous circumpolar youth. Int J Circumpolar Health [Internet]. 2013 [cited 2018 Jun 12];72(1):21775. doi: 10.3402/ijch.v72i0.21775
37. Hansen JG, Antsanen R. Elders' teachings about resilience and its implications for education in Dene and Cree communities. Int Indig Policy J. 2016;7(1):2.

38. Minore B, Katt M, Hill, ME. Planning without facts: Ontario's Aboriginal health information challenge. J Agromedicine. 2009 May 7;14(2):90–6.
39. Statistics Canada. Aboriginal people in Canada: key results from the 2016 census [Internet]. Ottawa (ON): Statistics Canada; 2017 [cited 2018 Jun 12]. Available from: https://www150.statcan.gc.ca/n1/daily-quotidien/171025/dq171025a-eng.htm
40. Statistics Canada. Education in Canada: key results from the 2016 census [Internet]. Ottawa (ON): Statistics Canada; 2017 [cited 2018 May 29]. Available from: https://www150.statcan.gc.ca/n1/en/daily-quotidien/171129/dq171129a-eng.pdf?st=vFcm75uE
41. Assembly of First Nations, National Native Addictions Partnership Foundation, Health Canada. Honouring our strengths: a renewed framework to address substance use issues among First Nations people in Canada [Internet]. Ottawa: Minister of Health; 2011 [cited 2018 Mar 22]. Available from https://thunderbirdpf.org/honouring-our-strengths-full-version-2
42. Assembly of First Nations, Health Canada. The First Nations mental wellness continuum framework [Internet]. Ottawa: Minister of Health; 2015 Jan [cited 2018 Mar 22]. Publication Number 140358. Available from: https://thunderbirdpf.org/wp-content/uploads/2015/01/24-14-1273-FN-Mental-Wellness-Framework-EN05_low.pdf
43. Assembly of First Nations. Mental wellness bulletin: what does wellness mean to you? [Internet]. Ottawa (ON): Assembly of First Nations; 2015 [cited 2018 Mar 22]. Available from: http://www.cssspnql.com/docs/default-source/default-document-library/afn-mental-health-bulletin-fall-2015.pdf
44. Campbell S, Schiff R, Møller H, Scharf D, Kozorys M. Housing insecurity and justice system involvement among women in the Thunder Bay region. Thunder Bay (ON): Elizabeth Fry Society and Northwestern Ontario and Lakehead University; 2019.
45. McKenzie HA, Dell CA, Fornssler B. Understanding addictions among Indigenous people through social determinants of health frameworks and strength-based approaches: a review of the research literature from 2013 to 2016. Curr Addict Rep. 2016;3(4):378–86
46. Denwan, G. Agency helps free Indigenous youth from addictions. CTV News [Internet]. 2019 Dec 11 [cited 2019 Dec 12]. Available from: https://london.ctvnews.ca/agency-helps-free-indigenous-youth-from-addictions-1.4726239
47. Dell CA, Seguin M, Hopkins C, Tempier R, Mehl-Madrona L, Dell D, Duncan R, Mosier K. From benzos to berries: treatment offered at an Aboriginal youth solvent abuse treatment centre relays the importance of culture. Can J Psychiatry. 2011;56(2):75–83.
48. Niccols A, Sword W. "New choices" for substance-using mothers and their children: preliminary evaluation. J Subst Use. 2005 Jan 1;10(4):239–51.

49. Niccols A, Dell CA, Clarke S. Treatment issues for Aboriginal mothers with substance use problems and their children. Int J Ment Health Addict. 2010;8(2):320–35.
50. Marsh TN, Coholic D, Cote-Meek S, Najavits LM. Blending Aboriginal and Western healing methods to treat intergenerational trauma with substance use disorder in Aboriginal peoples who live in northeastern Ontario, Canada. Harm Reduct J. 2015 Dec;12(1):14.

16 The Evolving Role of Telehealth: From Tackle Box Emergency Kits to Telemedicine

MICHELLE SPADONI, SALLY DAMPIER, AND PATRICIA SEVEAN

Most of the North was in a whiteout. On the phone, we [doctor and nurse] were trying to figure out how to treat a patient we believed had developed septicemia (a serious blood infection). The patient had received chemotherapy two weeks prior, so the timing made it possible. Chemotherapy not only targets cancer cells but kills some white blood cells that normally help fight infections. It is all part of treating cancer. Typically, we would have the patient come to the clinic, order tests to investigate, and start antibiotics to treat the infection. But our patient lived eight hours away, in a remote First Nation community that had neither a nursing station nor a pharmacy. The patient had been staying in a neighbouring community with a small hospital but had returned home with the news of a family member's passing ... Late in the day, the patient was finally airlifted to the neighbouring community hospital. Two weeks later, an Elder from the community accompanied the patient to the clinic as a support person and Knowledge Keeper, and she had a plan! She had brought a new fishing tackle box with her, she suggested the creation of a "tackle box emergency kit" containing antibiotics, medicated mouthwash, and nausea medication to be stored at the community health station and to be opened if a patient was ill from chemotherapy or when weather prohibited transfer out. She thought that as a community (patient and community working with our clinic team), we could manage post-chemotherapy side effects: mouth sores, early signs of infection, nausea, diarrhea, and so forth. The tackle box represented the pharmacy they did not have, and the phone was our connection as a community (patient, community, and clinic). The tackle box would travel back to the clinic with the patient on chemotherapy days to be refilled and sealed.

Our experience with *health at a distance* began in our practice lives as nurses in the mid-1990s with patients and families navigating cancer. The tackle box emergency kit was one step in our experiences of caring for people in a rural centre. It was part of our journey of figuring out how to support patients and their families from a distance, when geography and rural health care resources (or lack of resources) shaped in tangible and intangible ways our ability (or inability) to provide just-in-time expertise, which could potentially change the health and well-being outcomes for patients and their families in positive (or negative) ways. Imagine driving eight hours in adverse weather conditions to get to a medical appointment, sometimes on roads that are paved or are winter roads. But other times, people are caught in snowbound communities and can neither drive nor fly out: in −40°C weather, with a wind chill that makes it feel like −60°C, helicopters cannot takeoff because their blades freeze once they are on the ground. *Telehealth* (the term used at the time), what we now think more broadly of as *telemedicine*, was one innovation among many technological innovations that expanded the ways in which we thought about delivering and practising cancer care for rural people living in our clinic catchment area.

In this chapter, we will explore the evolution of rural and remote telemedicine as it transpired for us (northern urban practitioners) through the mid-1990s, in contrast to the present in Canada. The discussion centres on the story of the tackle box emergency kits. A scoping review focused on rural and remote telemedicine informs the discussion. The opportunity to write this chapter provided us a means to move beyond our insular practice space, where our thoughts and actions were often confined within the orbit of *managing*. It gave us a rare chance to look both back and forwards to understand how telemedicine was taking root and evolving around us. In the last decade, efforts to provide health care beyond the hospital doors and to care for people in community and their homes has moved forward rapidly. These changes have been shaped by social demands, funding, and legislative limitations and possibilities in relation to the scope of practice of health professionals, and, more importantly by technology, from mobile devices to wearable body technology. In the 1990s, other compelling issues were in play, particularly for Indigenous people. Outside our clinic doors, not visible to us then, was a powerful movement by First Nations communities in northwestern Ontario towards what today is described as *self-determination* (1,2). The ability to look back and forwards, moves the chapter discussion beyond telemedicine as access, travel time, cost, statistics, and information communication technologies and evolves it into a discussion about colonization and self-determination. In this chapter, we explore the evolution of telemedicine in rural and remote areas of Ontario and for First Nation, Métis, and Inuit communities. As well, we examine more closely the Keewaytinook Okimakanak eHealth Telemedicine Services (KOeTS) in Ontario. Finally, we explore prospective areas for health care telemedicine curriculum development suggested by Indigenous practitioners for health care providers who work with Indigenous communities.

Understanding the Evolution of Health Technologies – "Healing at a Distance"

The term *telemedicine* first emerged in the 1970s and literally meant "healing at a distance" (3 p8). Telemedicine is a clustering of information and communication technologies aimed to improve patient outcomes and increase access to care and medical information for all people, with the particular goal of decreasing the divide between urban and rural populations, high- and low-income people, and access to specialist and generalist practitioners (3). The term *telemedicine* is frequently used interchangeably with telehealth. However, the term *telehealth* is confined to "service delivery by physicians only" (3 p9), while telemedicine includes health care provision from an interprofessional perspective.

From its inception, telemedicine was viewed as a means to bridge the gap between remote communities and urban centres, a pathway to equity and access in underserviced areas, and way to improve access to services that otherwise may not be available to patients, families and health care professionals in their home communities (4,5). Telemedicine provides a space for interprofessional health care teams to attend holistically to chronic disease, delivering medical management and psychosocial programming for secondary chronic disease health issues, such as depression, anxiety, and stress management (4–7). It also provides access to physiotherapy, occupational therapy, and social work (to name a few) to assist with the cascade of life changes that may ensue, such as financial, family, or housing issues, and grants for assistive devices (4–7). Telemedicine is a medium for patient and family education; it has been found to enhance people's abilities to manage their own diseases and, to varying degrees, reduce hospital admissions (4,5,7). For example, tele-glaucoma management is shown to be equally as effective as in-office visits, and both patients and practitioners have found it to be expedient (8). Telemedicine is being used across disciplines, with a wide variety of technologies, and by people living in both rural and urban settings, thus shifting the spaces and places people receive care from hospital and physician office to community and in-home care (3,4,9).

Although researchers have found telemedicine to increase health-related knowledge, change health behaviours, and encourage psychosocial adaptation (7), it's not for everyone. Dogba and colleagues found that, for some people, internet health interactions can feel expansive and impersonal, and not everyone can adapt to technology (7). The effectiveness of telemedicine interventions may be related to issues of user acceptance and factors such as patient or practitioner technological literacy, internet viability, and affordability (7). Patients' ease with technology-driven health information has been linked to compositional factors like education, self-efficacy, and computer skills (7). Patient and family responses to telemedicine vary depending on factors such as the urgency of the care need, distance, weather, geography, costs, ease and availability of technology, sense of safety, and consistency of providers (5,7). These sorts of variances make it difficult to evaluate telemedicine programs and their cost-effectiveness (7). Despite these challenges, telemedicine is shifting the grounds of practice, the notion of who is directing health care, and patient–practitioner relationships, and the ways in which telemedicine is accessed and delivered in Ontario is expanding.

Ontario Telemedicine Experience

The Ontario Telemedicine Network (OTN) is a prime example of how health care is shifting from hospital settings to community and home. The OTN is a not-for-profit organization funded by the Ontario Ministry of Health and Long-Term Care. It is the largest telemedicine service provider in Canada and one of the largest in the world with 2026 OTN sites in Ontario (10). In addition, OTN has an agreement with Keewaytinook Okimakanak (KO) communities to provide eHealth programs that are owned, governed, and delivered by First Nation communities (2). A quarter of OTN sites are in northern Ontario ($n = 522$), and half of those are located in rural parts of the north ($n = 286$) (10 p473). OTN services include *eVisit* (a secure videoconference between telemedicine sites and a patient's device), *Big White Wall* (a mental health online peer support community), and *eVisit Primary Care*, which connects patients (frequently at home) to family physicians in their office through secure audio, video, or messaging (9). In 2017–18 OTN provided 896,529 patient consultations, saving $71.9 million in Northern Health Travel Grants and avoiding 270 million kilometres in patient travel time (9 p6).

OTN's eVisit service is used by 28,000 members, including 3400 room-based systems in hospitals and clinics, covering medical and surgical pre- and post-assessment, and chronic disease management (9 p7). eVisits are booked through the *OTNhub*; many sites are resourced with nursing staff and medical peripheral devices (i.e., handheld cameras and digital stethoscopes) (9 p7). Chronic disease management now includes the *home video visits* pilot, which started in fall 2017; in the first four months of the program, 425 physicians reported 1406 virtual encounters, ranging from home video visits for oral chemotherapy to mental health consultations (9 p7). *Telehomecare* is a digital chronic disease self-management program, which helped patients avoid 3151 hospital admissions in 2016–17; 96.8 percent of the patients serviced reported they would recommend the program to others (9 p13). The 2017–18 annual report indicates that OTN's *telestroke* program served 2207 patients, and 24 percent of people seen were identified as needing emergency room intervention in the form of clot-busting treatment (9 p15). Telestroke provides health care staff with 24/7 access to neurologists who are experts in stroke care, leveraging OTN's eVisit service and *CritiCall* (an on-call program) to enable real-time neurologist consultations (9). *EConsults* conducted 33,643 telederm and teleophthalmology visits that resulted in "78% referral avoidance" (9 p6). As well, $2.8 million was saved by using virtual critical care visits (9 p6). The total number of patient home video visits was 21,498, reducing hospital admissions through telehomecare between 60 and 80 percent (9 p12). *Mental health and addictions* visits are 62 percent of telemedicine visits in the province (10 p476). As well, OTN (9) partnered with Ontario Ministry of Community Safety and Correctional Services and Correctional Service of Canada to provide virtual clinical services to all correctional facilities through a "telemedicine first" policy. Delivering service to the province's 24 correctional facilities reduces the need to transfer inmates to hospitals or community doctors' offices (9). Although there has been significant growth and innovation in health care services by OTN, including the evolution of KOeTS, it is unclear if funding for OTN through the Ministry of Health and Long-Term Care will remain, given a recent cut that has seen 44 staff positions eliminated (11). It is unclear how these cuts will impact patients seeking care and health providers' ability to engage in OTN services. In northern Ontario, the KOeTS is well developed, extensive, and worth taking a closer look at because of its focus on the care of First Nation people in distant rural and remote communities.

Ontario Telemedicine and First Nations' Health Systems

The KOeTS was born out of a partnership between KO (a council of six northern and isolated First Nations) and OTN in 1998 (12). It began with federal funding targeted for telehealth services for First Nation communities. A partnership agreement was signed between KOeTS and OTN in 2009. The KOeTS is considered the most comprehensive First Nations–operated regional telemedicine system in Canada, (12) currently servicing 26 remote northern First Nations communities. Orpah McKenzie (KOeTS manager) noted that, in 2016–17, 5630 requests made for KOeTS clinical services and 2984 of them were met (12 p10). The services that were delivered varied, including those in the areas of mental health and addictions, general surgery, general practitioner, endocrinology, and family visits (12). Over 30 new telemedicine systems were established with northern Indigenous communities in 2017–18 through the partnership of OTN and KOeTS (9 p19). Additionally, in 2017–18, a new model using secure desktop computers with videoconferencing devices (web cameras and echo-cancelling speakers) was introduced to northern First Nation communities that had adequate internet services; it is thought to be simpler and more confidential then existing systems (9).

KOeTS Experience

In 2017, Orpah McKenzie spoke at the Saskatchewan Indigenous Communities Telehealth Forum about the history and evolution of telemedicine in northern Ontario (12). The benefits of KOeTS include quicker access to interprofessional health care services, reduced isolation for health professionals (for decision making), timely patient care delivery to people living in geographically isolated areas, and ultimately improved patient outcomes, all with the convenience and safety of being close to family (12). What's more, by 2016–17 the KOeTS had created over $20 million in health system benefits over 11 years, and in 2016–17 had saved $2 million by reducing related medical transportation expenses (12 p10). The KOeTS differs in design from the OTN programs as KO programs encompass Indigenous perspectives of health, rooted in a cultural lens, inclusive of language, history, practices, ceremonies, knowledge, land, and values. For example, Elders play an important role in eHealth and often hold teaching lodges through eHealth to discuss health issues important to the wellness of the community (13). As an example, they may be involved in the design of a new diabetic foot ulcer prevention program and will then use eHealth to hold meetings. Elders are Knowledge Keepers, cultural practitioners, negotiators, and an essential link in sustaining strong kinship relationships that are the roots of healthy communities (13).

Telemedicine – Beyond the Clinic Doors

The link between information communication technologies that support telemedicine, such as KOeTS and the Kuhkenan Network (KNET), and the health of the community arises in the literature; it is seen as resilience and as a means of sustaining the health of the community. Networks like KOeTS and KNET create a digital space for people living in the community and away to keep in contact and nourishes intergenerational communication and the sharing of stories, both of which are important to sustaining health and wellness of individuals and the community (13). First Nation women are using the telemedicine internet platforms (i.e., KNET) for cultural preservation, by using the internet to post photos, news, or stories, as well as to access Indigenous music and authors (13). Information communication technology platforms, as one woman explained, are a means of "sharing our lives in remaining connected with relatives, and sharing our traditional land-based knowledge" (13 p87). While another woman reflected that using the KNET website was a life link to home and family:

> I am located in Southern Ontario attending school and the only means of staying connected to my home community is visiting KNET archives and viewing the photos of community events, feast, elders, etc. Homepages are also a great place to stay connected through the stories and emergency community events, e.g. illness, etc. (13 p87)

KNET also provides space to communicate in their own language: "Using my own language on my KNET homepage … which is good that they have that syllabics fonts on there!" (13 p 88). Sites like Wawatay radio are a means of broadcasting and catching up with community events: "I'm a member of pow wow. Com. I use the website craft section and pow wow announcements for our area" (13 p88). However, the ability for systems like KOeTS and KNET to function as they do means attending to system and structural factors, the pragmatics of fiscal and human resources, and legalities.

KOeTS Taking Care of Details – Human Resources, Social Networking, Security

The effectiveness of First Nation eHealth programs requires attending to system and structural factors (i.e., clinic guidelines on transferring patients out, on-reserve and off-reserve health care coverage, physician billing practices, and so forth). At a 2017 gathering on telemedicine in First Nations communities, the KOeTS manager described some of these challenges as experienced by the KO program. She emphasized the significance of human connection in all KOeTS practices, but noted communication at a distance is not easy for physicians and community members: technology can be slow; calls can be dropped; videoconferencing schedules can be overbooked; and people from away are not readily able to fully appreciate both verbal and nonverbal cues, nor the communities' context, through video screening (12). She also noted human resource challenges, including regional staff supervision and staff turnover (12). As well, technological issues like phone and internet connectivity are a continual concern (12). Billing is also a constant issue as there are not necessarily billing codes for many eHealth practitioner activities (12). Another related issue is the regulation of technology use in health care. Some provinces and territories have regulatory standards that will cover physicians and patients connecting through mobile, tablet, and desktop video solutions; others do not (12). It is evident that as technology becomes more accessible, affordable, and normalized in people's lives, regulatory bodies will have to consider how to address consumer preferences: less expensive and patient-preferred communication technologies, such as Skype and Vidyo, and the associated risks and benefits for patients and practitioners (i.e., protection of personal information, privacy, and confidentiality) (12). The concerns of the KOeTS manager capture the structural issues of telemedicine: how policy and practices on the ground interface (or not) and challenge and impact equity and access to care. KOeTS providers and communities are shifting the conversation of inequitable access to health care as northern First Nation communities take ownership of telemedicine.

Enacting Self-Determination through KOeTS – "Healing from a Distance"

KOeTS programs have all the essential characteristics of self-determination as understood through an Indigenous world view. First, KOeTS is First Nations owned and managed, and it delivers a group of services, including a telecommunications broadband network: KNET (2). The KO's board of directors are the chiefs of six small First Nations (14) whose communities are remote and northern; in addition, several have fly-in access only (14). eHealth programs like KO's exemplify the strength of northern First Nations communities to find their own solutions in a manner that respects Indigenous ways of governing, culture, identity, and traditional knowledge (14). Second, the First Nation principles of ownership, control, access, and possession (OCAP) are respected, and KO communities have ownership and control over their communities' infrastructure (14). Finally, from an OCAP perspective, communities "do for themselves," addressing community priorities, including creating and sustaining local jobs, expanding the capacity of communities to protect and deliver services, and subsequently enhancing the efforts of communities to counteract settler colonialism (14).

Journeying Back into Orbit

Over the last two and a half decades, the evolution of telemedicine has become an integral part of rural and remote health care delivery in northern Ontario. The sophistication, complexity, and contextual nature of telemedicine reveals itself even in this short discussion of the northern Ontario experience of OTN and KOeTS. As we explored the literature, and reached out to various northern networks, to inform the writing, what was revealed was the responsiveness of telemedicine delivery in the North, from traditional Western pathways (i.e., OTN) to the evolution of KOeTS's cultural and linguistic expression of Indigenous health and wellness. The work of non-Indigenous health care and helping providers will need to consider how to reconfigure our contributions as we navigate what Senator Murray Sinclair suggests are rights (human rights) and laws (the legal legacy of the Indian Act) (15) in relation to Indigenous communities' move towards self-determination (i.e., telemedicine programs).

We began our chapter within the clinic walls, in the organized chaos of patient, community, and practice life. As nurses (Michelle, Sally, and Pat), our practice has evolved into faculty and research positions at postsecondary institutions, and we are always striving to sustain our engagement with rural and remote health. As we studied the literature, the voices of patients, families, community members surfaced, sharing not only ideas about the use of telemedicine but also insights into what the health care provider curricula might or should include to allow practitioners to practise in a *good way* with northern and Indigenous peoples and communities (beyond the technology). For example, Indigenous health care providers, alongside patients and families (within the KOeTS catchment areas and throughout the broader Canadian health care system). emphasize that the following key threads should be thoughtfully woven into contemporary health care curricula focused on rural, remote, and Indigenous peoples and communities: *cultural safety and anti-racist and anti-colonial theory, including trauma-informed care* (1,12,16–23). As Dr. Alika Lafontaine and Dr. Cara Bablitz (24) suggest, to work in a good way with Indigenous people means understanding the nuances of equity, power and privilege, and colonialism and racism. It requires a deeper understanding that "innovation in Indigenous health is more than technology such as remote patient monitoring, it is about changing the way people feel about Indigenous patients" (24 p5).

In the mid-1990s, our focus was on managing people from a distance, confining our thoughts to the tasks at hand (managing cancer patients and their response to treatment); our interactions with northern Indigenous people circled around lack of resources, both human and fiscal. There was little discussion of equity, racism, power and privilege, or the frequent positioning of Indigenous people as vulnerable and needing our help and protection. Thinking back now to the generosity of the Elder who came to the clinic with a fishing tackle box, we can see that, in some ways, she was our wakeup call. She provided us an opportunity to rethink the meaning of *working in a good way* with northern Indigenous people and communities. It opened up a space for critical inquiry to question how we understood the needs of Indigenous people, our personal and collective beliefs about Indigenous people's understanding of cancer, and *what goes into the fishing tackle box, necessary for working in a good way*. There is no doubt technology in health care can create access in ways we have yet to fully imagine, but as the discussion of telemedicine evolves, it would serve us well to consider adapting education for a future we can't completely predict (25,26). Table 16.1 provides an initial mapping of emancipatory educational approaches based on the chapter discussion and drawing from Indigenous writers, as well as from critical theorists in the field of contemporary culture and social justice theory in health care. The tackle box has three trays: human rights, laws, and pedagogy. The goal of this chapter was to explore the evolution of telemedicine in remote and northern Indigenous communities. In this short space of writing, we hoped to dig deeply, below the surface of telemedicine as a simple discussion of digital eHealth programing. The chapter began with our reflection on an Elder and the gift of the tackle box, and we have, in some ways, come full circle.

Table 16.1 Working in a good way: The tackle box

Human rights	Focus: Key Indigenous human rights challenges
Right to self-determination	Realign authorities, accountabilities, and resources (27,28), which tie to First Nations, Inuit, and Métis communities' progress towards self-determination and subsequent equity across the health care, education, child welfare, and justice systems. Recognize that Indigenous knowledge "is different and at the same time, it is equal to Western Knowledge. By learning about Indigenous ways of knowing and practices … students will have the opportunity to acknowledge and respect this truth" (29 p9).
Right to culture	Eliminate racism and increase cultural safety (27), as racism is considered by many Indigenous people to be at the heart of inequities and violence.
Right to health	Ensure equitable access to health care (27), which is the path towards healthy people and land.
Laws	**Focus: Making connections between laws and rights**
Indian Act, Treaty rights, systems of segregation, and women's status	Re-examine the Indian Act as race-based legislation that entrenched government control of Indigenous identity, relocated Indigenous people from their homelands onto "reserve lands," and minimized economic and political independence (23). Explore the stipulations for enfranchisement within the Act and what they meant to Indigenous people in relation to "rights" (i.e., voting): stripping people of their "Indian status" and revoking their Treaty rights, and undermining women's roles and status within First Nations societies and their property rights (23). Explore Indigenous and Treaty rights, constitutionally protected rights under section 35 of Canada's Constitutional Act of 1982, inclusive of Indian, Métis, and Inuit peoples in relation to the health and well-being of Indigenous people (23). Support Indigenous people's right for transformational change and the realignment of authorities, accountabilities, and resources in relation to self-determination of Indigenous people and land (27).
Assimilation and cultural genocide	Explore the relationship between the Indian Act and residential schools, the Sixties Scoop generation, and contemporary child welfare (23). Explore the meaning of culture and cultural safety in everyday life from multiple positions (non-Indigenous and Indigenous), the meaning of culture and cultural safety from a health and well-being perspective and an institutional and a professional lens (29).

(*Continued*)

Table 16.1 (continued)

Assimilation and cultural genocide (continued)	Understand and articulate the relationship between the Indian Act, assimilation, cultural genocide, intergenerational trauma, poverty, and overrepresentation of Indigenous children in child welfare in Canada and the need for trauma-informed care (23,27). Understand and articulate the relationship between the Indian Act, assimilation, cultural genocide, and the rupture of Indigenous identity from colonization and racist ideologies (23). Understand and articulate the gendered impact of colonial racism on Indigenous women's health and well-being (23). Understand and articulate racism in the health care experience and health providers' and institutions' role in race-based policies and racist treatment of Indigenous people (23). Understand and articulate implicit bias and racialized health disparities (23). Understand and articulate the relationship between eliminating racism and increasing cultural safety (27).
Telehealth technology	When designing telehealth systems, consider provincial, territorial, and federal jurisdictional barriers (12). Identify challenges, including sustainable funding, human resources, and the availability of training programs at the local level to promote self-determination of communities (12–14). Explore issues of privacy and confidentiality (12–14) Understand how health care legislation shapes the roles and practices of practitioners related to the technologies being suggested (12–14) Understand self-determination (ownership of technology, building capacity within community for trained telehealth providers), sustainable funding for technology, and human resources, and assess technology barriers (bandwidth, etc.) (2,12–14).
Pedagogy	**Focus: Teaching in a good way**
Curricula focuses	Promote cultural safety (anti-racism education and policy are foundational for cultural safety) (17,21,27,28). Eliminate racism (bias and racialized health disparities) (17,21,27,28,30). Examine Indigenous determinants of health, exploring health problems that originate outside the health care system itself (housing, education, employment, poverty, food security, water safety, social supports, early child development, and environment) (17,21,27,28,30). Emphasize trauma-informed care, which is sensitive to how a person's lived experiences can impact their health behaviours and health status. Trauma-informed care considers a person's reactions as a possible result of previous experience or injury, integrating knowledge about trauma into policies, procedures, practices, and setting (17,21,25,27,28,). Understand structural inequities and violence (17,21,27,28,30).

(*Continued*)

Table 16.1 (continued)

Emancipatory pedagogical approaches	**Relational pedagogies:** experiential learning experiences use multiple ways of knowing (empirical, social/political/ethical/aesthetic) to support students to develop professional values and become active, curious, and creative self-directed practitioners who appreciate intrapersonal (what is going on in and between people), interpersonal (what is going on between people and environment), and contextual (what is going on around the people and situation) structures, policies, practices, history, economy, society, governing structures, legislation, and law (31). **Humanism:** the approach involves "learning to recognize and navigate tensions between values (empathy and objectivity, efficiency and quality, standardised and individualized care) … to understand the ways in which power and privilege affect health care and learning interactions" (32 p1). **Critical pedagogy:** it encourages students and teachers to be co-learners in a power-sharing arrangement when navigating the content of learning, inclusive of a range of voices and perspectives; dealing with conflict; and recognizing issues of politics and structural inequities (33). **Dialogic approach to teaching:** the focus is person-centred care: learners and teachers bring their "entire selves" into a non-hierarchical conversation about the human and social aspects of care. It includes patient experiences to deepen and transform learners' perspectives and values by stimulating critical reflection about personal and social identities and ways of knowing, and the effects of structures and processes that organize the delivery of care and interactions (34).
Supporting theoretical perspectives	**Intersectionality** explores how people are affected differentially by structural influences such as sexism, racism, poverty, ability, and place (35). **Anti-colonial perspective** draws attention to history and aims to address and challenge contemporary colonial systems (35). **Identity and social location** explores the complex interplay among individual decisions and choices and life events, community recognition and expectations, societal categorization, classification, and socialization (36).

REFERENCES

1. National Inquiry into Missing and Murdered Indigenous Women and Girls. Reclaiming power and place: the final report of the National Inquiry into Missing and Murdered Indigenous Women and Girls, Vol. 1a [Internet]. Vancouver (BC): National Inquiry into Missing and Murdered Indigenous Women and Girls; 2019 Jun 3 [cited 2019 Jul 3]. Available from: http://www.mmiwg-ffada.ca/wp-content/uploads/2019/06/Final_Report_Vol_1a-1.pdf

2. McMahon R. Digital self-determination: Aboriginal peoples and the network society in Canada [dissertation]. Vancouver (BC): Simon Fraser University, 2013.
3. World Health Organization. Telemedicine opportunities and developments in member states: report on the second global survey on eHealth. Vol. 2 [Internet]. Geneva (CH): World Health Organization; 2010 [cited 2019 Jul 3]. Available from: http://www.who.int/goe/publications/goe_telemedicine_2010.pdf
4. Kalankesh LR, Pourasghar F, Nicholson L, Ahmadi S, Hosseini M. Effect of Telehealth Interventions on Hospitalization Indicators: A Systematic Review. Perspect Health Inf Manag. 2016 Oct 1;13(Fall):1h.
5. Sinclair C. Effectiveness and user acceptance of online chronic disease management interventions in rural and remote settings: systematic review and narrative synthesis. Clin Med Insights Ther. 2015 Oct 11;7(7):43–52.
6. Kotb A, Cameron C, Hsieh S, Wells G. Comparative effectiveness of different forms of telemedicine for individuals with heart failure (HF): a systematic review and network meta-analysis. PLoS One. 2015 Feb 25;10(2):e0118681.
7. Dogba MJ, Dossa AR, Breton E, Gandonou-Migan R. Using information and communication technologies to involve patients and the public in health education in rural and remote areas: a scoping review. BMC Health Serv Res. 2019 Feb 19;19(1):128.
8. Thomas SM, Jeyaraman MM, Hodge WG, Hutnik C, Costella J, Malvankar-Mehta MS. The effectiveness of teleglaucoma versus in-patient examination for glaucoma screening: a systematic review and meta-analysis. PLoS One. 2014 Dec 5;9(12):e113779
9. Ontario Telemedicine Network. OTN annual report 2017/18. Toronto (ON): Ontario Telemedicine Network; 2018.
10. O'Gorman LD, Hogenbirk JC, Warry W. Clinical telemedicine utilization in Ontario over the Ontario Telemedicine Network. Telemed J E Health [Internet]. 2016 Jun [cited 2019 Jul 3];22(6):473–9. Available from: http://www.ncbi.nlm.nih.gov/pubmed/26544163
11. Crawley M. Ontario Telemedicine Network lays off 44 staff. CBC News [Internet]. 2019 May 8 [cited 2019 Jul 3]. Available from: http://www.cbc.ca/news/canada/toronto/doug-ford-ontario-telemedicine-network-1.5126853
12. Exner-Pirot H. Telehealth in northern and Indigenous communities: report from the Telehealth Forum held October 5, 2017 [Internet]. Saskatoon (SK): University of Saskatchewan College of Nursing; 2017 [cited 2019 Jul 3]. Available from: https://nursing.usask.ca/documents/telehealth/2017telehealthreport.pdf
13. Carpenter P, Gibson K, Kakekaspan C, O'Donnell S. How women in remote and rural First Nation communities are using information and communication technologies (ICT). J Rural Community Dev. 2013;8(2):79–97.
14. Beaton B, Campbell P. Settler colonialism and First Nations e-communities in northwestern Ontario. J Community Inform [Internet]. 2014 [cited 2019 Jul 3];10(2):2–11. Available from: http://meeting.knet.ca/mp19/file.php?file=%2F16%2FPublications%2F2014-JoCI-Beaton_Campbell.pdf

15. Sinclair M. Knowing right from law: what you need to know about law school [Internet]. Thunder Bay (ON): Bora Laskin Faculty of Law; 2018 Nov 5 [cited 2010 Jul 3]. Video: 1:06:00 min. Available from: https://www.youtu.be/ellvpPZupTY
16. Truth and Reconciliation Commission of Canada. Honouring the truth, reconciling for the future: summary of the final report of the Truth and Reconciliation Commission of Canada [Internet]. Winnipeg (MB): Truth and Reconciliation Commission of Canada; 2015 [cited 2015 Jul 30]. Available from: http://www.trc.ca/assets/pdf/Honouring_the_Truth_Reconciling_for_the_Future_July_23_2015.pdf
17. Allan B, Smylie J. First Peoples, second class treatment: the role of racism in the health and well-being of Indigenous Peoples in Canada [Internet]. Toronto (ON): Wellesley Institute; 2015 [cited 2019 Jul 3]. Available from: https://www.wellesleyinstitute.com/wp-content/uploads/2015/02/Full-Report-FPSCT-Updated.pdf
18. Paradies Y, Harris R, Anderson I. The impact of racism on Indigenous health in Australia and Aotearoa: towards a research agenda [Internet]. Darwin (AU): Australia Research Centre for Aboriginal Health; 2008 [cited 2019 Jul 3]. Available from: https://dro.deakin.edu.au/eserv/DU:30058493/paradies-impactofracism-2008.pdf
19. Assembly of First Nations. First Nations mental wellness continuum framework [Internet]. Ottawa (ON): Health Canada; 2015 [cited 2019 Jul 3]. Available from: http://www.thunderbirdpf.org/wp-content/uploads/2015/01/24-14-1273-FN-Mental-Wellness-Framework-EN05_low.pdf
20. Greenwood ML, de Leeuw SN. Social determinants of health and the future well-being of Aboriginal children in Canada. Paediatr Child Health. 2012 Aug;17(7):381–4.
21. Reading CL, Wien F. Health inequalities and social determinants of Aboriginal Peoples' health [Internet]. Prince George (BC): National Collaborating Centre for Aboriginal Health; 2009 [cited 2019 Jul 3]. Available from: http://www.nccah-ccnsa.ca/docs/social%20determinates/NCCAH-loppie-Wien_report.pdf
22. Smylie J. The health of Aboriginal Peoples. In: Raphael D, editor. Social determinants of health: Canadian perspectives. Toronto (ON): Canadian Scholars' Press, 2009. p. 280–304.
23. Smylie J, Adomako P, editors. Indigenous children's health report: health assessment in action [Internet]. Toronto (ON): Centre for Research on Inner City Health; 2009 [cited 2019 Jul 3]. Available: http://caid.ca/IndChiHeaRep2009.pdf
24. Canadian Medical Association. CMA health summit 2018: summary report [Internet]. Ottawa (ON): Canadian Medical Association; 2018 [cited 2019 Jul 3]. Available from: https://cmahealthsummit.ca/app/uploads/2019/02/HS-Board-Report_Final.pdf
25. Kelly M, Dornan T. Mapping the landscape or exploring the terrain? Progressing humanism in medical education. Med Educ. 2016 Mar;50(3):273–5. doi: 10.1111/medu.12967

26. Matthews C. Critical pedagogy in health education. Health Educ J. 2013 Nov 25; 73(5):600–9.
27. Richardson L, Murphy T. Bringing reconciliation to healthcare in Canada: wise practices for healthcare leaders [Internet]. Toronto (ON): HealthCareCAN; 2018 [cited 2019 Jul 3]. Available from: http://www.healthcarecan.ca/wp-content/themes/camyno/assets/document/Reports/2018/HCC/EN/TRCC_EN.pdf
28. Blanchet Garneau A, Browne AJ, Varcoe C. Drawing on antiracist approaches toward a critical antidiscriminatory pedagogy for nursing. Nurs Inq. 2018 Jan;25(1). doi: 10.1111/nin.12211
29. Aboriginal Nurses Association of Canada, Canadian Association of Schools of Nursing, Canadian Nurses Association. Cultural competence and cultural safety in nursing education: a framework for First Nations, Inuit and Métis nursing [Internet]. Ottawa (ON): Aboriginal Nurses Association of Canada; 2009 [cited 2010 Jan 3]. Available from: http://www.cna-aiic.ca/~/media/cna/page-content/pdf-en/first_nations_framework_e.pdf
30. Indigenous Physicians Association of Canada, Association of Faculties of Medicine of Canada. First Nations, Inuit, Métis health code competencies: a curriculum framework for undergraduate medical education [Internet]. Ottawa (ON): Indigenous Physicians Association of Canada, Association of Faculties of Medicine of Canada; 2008 [updated 2009 Apr; cited 2019 Jul 3]. Available from: http://www.afmc.ca/sites/default/files/pdf/IPAC-AFMC_Core_Competencies_EN.pdf
31. Hartrick Doane G, Varcoe C. How to nurse: relational inquiry with individuals and families in changing health and healthcare contexts. New York (NY): Lippincott Williams & Williams; 2015.
32. Gaufberg E, Hodges B. Humanism, compassion and the call to caring. Med Educ. 2016 Mar;50(3):264–6.
33. Cavanagh A, Vanstone M, Ritz S. Problems of problem-based learning: Towards transformative critical pedagogy in medical education. Perspect Med Educ. 2019 Feb;8(1):38–42. doi: 10.1007/s40037-018-0489-7
34. Kuper A, Boyd VA, Veinot P, Abdelhalim T, Bell MJ, Feilchenfeld Z, Najeeb U, Piquette D, Rawal S, Wong R, Wright SR, Whitehead CR, Kumagai AK, Richardson L. A dialogic approach to teaching person-centered care in graduate medical education. J Grad Med Educ. 2019 Aug;11(4):460–7.
35. Varcoe C, Browne AJ, Cender LA. Promoting social justice and equality by practicing nursing to address structural inequities and structural violence. In: Kagan PN, Smith MC, Chinn PL, editors. Philosophies and practices of emancipatory nursing: social justice as praxis. New York (NY): Routledge; 2014. p. 266–84.
36. Kirk G, Okazawa-Rey M. Identities and social locations: who am I? who are my people? In: Adams M, Blumenfeld WJ, Castaneda CR, Hackman HW, Peters ML, Zuniga X, editors. Readings for diversity and social justice. New York (NY): Routledge, 2013. p. 51–60.

17 Cultural Safety Training and Education for Health Care Providers: Unsettling Health Care with Inuit in Canada

ALLISON CRAWFORD, CANDICE WADDELL, AND CHRISTINE LUND

Notions of "care" are usually taken for granted in "health care."[1] The idea that medicine, nursing, and other health services could, in fact, contribute to ill health is a much newer understanding and one that has not penetrated deeply or been disseminated widely enough, particularly in the context of the provision of health care for Indigenous peoples in Canada. The calls for action emerging from Canada's Truth and Reconciliation Commission (TRC) specifically locate health as an area for action (1). The TRC urges recognition that "the current state of Aboriginal health in Canada" is a result of past governmental policies, and one of the specific calls to action is a request for changes to health care education:

> 24. We call upon medical and nursing schools in Canada to require all students to take a course dealing with Aboriginal health issues, including the history and legacy of residential schools, the United Nations Declaration on the Rights of Indigenous Peoples, Treaties and Aboriginal rights, and Indigenous teachings and practices. This will require skills-based training in intercultural competency, conflict resolution, human rights, and anti-racism. (1 p3)

Although the work of each author of this chapter started long before the TRC, our focus on health care education, specifically in working with Inuit, is aligned with TRC's call to action for health.

We will discuss the concepts of cultural safety and trauma informed care in the context of health care education, grounded in our own work in Inuit communities in Nunavut, in Ottawa, and nationally. An important part of cultural safety, which will be discussed in more detail below, is locating oneself and the power and privilege intrinsic to particular roles, and recognizing that we each occupy multiple social locations. Allison Crawford is a psychiatrist and medical director of an outreach and telepsychiatry program at the Centre for Addiction and Mental Health, which includes work in northern Ontario and Nunavut. She lived in Iqaluit, Nunavut, from 2009 to 2011 and continues to practise there. She has also been involved in policy consultation with Inuit Tapiriit Kanatami (ITK), the national Inuit land claim organization, and as a scientific adviser working with the Inuit Circumpolar Council on the Sustainable Development Group of the Arctic Council. Candice Waddell is an assistant professor at Brandon University and is involved with First Nations, Inuit, and Métis advocacy, policy development, and education through the Brandon Friendship Centre and the Brandon University Senate Subcommittee on Indigenous Education. She lived in Cape Dorset and Iqaluit, Nunavut, from 2009 to 2015, where she worked as a community psychiatric nurse. Christine Lund is a coordinator with Tungasuvvingat Inuit and is involved with Inuit policy development in Ontario, particularly with children and youth, as well as health promotion. Christine has been working with the Inuit community of Ontario for 12 years. She lived in Iqaluit, Nunavut, from 1980 to 1993, where she studied and then worked as a community social service worker. In addition to the inherent power and privilege involved in our respective health care, academic, and community roles, we each occupy a complex web of social locations that we need to be aware of and acknowledge within our work and professional relationships. Our experiences as part of Inuit communities also made us aware of the history of health care, particularly aspects of health care that contributed to the process of colonization, with impacts that persist today.

Inuit are an Indigenous circumpolar people who inhabit primarily four Arctic regions in Canada: Inuvialuit in the Northwest Territories; Nunatsiavut in Labrador; Nunavik in Quebec; and the territory of Nunavut. Together, these regions are known as Inuit Nunangat, the homeland of Inuit in Canada. There are also Inuit living across Canada outside Inuit Nunangat, primarily in major centres, such as Ottawa, Montreal, Toronto, Edmonton, and Winnipeg. Approximately 72,500 Inuit live in Canada. This young demographic that is one of the fastest growing in Canada, increasing by 32 per cent between 2001 and 2011 (a threefold difference compared with the general Canadian population) (2 p9). Inuit are distinct from First Nations and Métis peoples.

Health outcomes for Inuit often reveal disparities in comparison with the general Canadian population. Although Inuit-specific longitudinal health data are lacking, some identifiable trends capture health status for Inuit, and these are being supplemented by some recent population health surveys in each of the regions, such as the Nunavik Inuit Health Survey 2004, the International Polar Year Adult Inuit Health Survey, and the Nunavut Inuit Child Health Survey, 2007–2008. Life expectancy for those living in Inuit Nunangat is 70.8 years, significantly lower than the national average of 80.6 years (includes non-Inuit) (3). Infant mortality is nearly three times as high, with 14.9 deaths per 1000 compared with 5.2 per 1000 (4). Health inequity is also evident in higher rates of childhood illness (5,6) and in certain illnesses in adulthood, such as tuberculosis (7). Because of the high rates of death by suicide for Inuit youth, mental health is a critical area that has received recent attention. Between 1999 and 2013, 745 deaths were attributed to suicide (8), and among Inuit males ages 15–29 years, the rate of suicide is up to 40 times the national average (8).

There is historical context, now being documented by Inuit, for the current health of Inuit. Many social and health inequities can be traced back to the impacts of colonization and early policies of the Canadian government that resulted in reorganization of Inuit society and cultural loss. The provision and organization of health care was one such policy. The history of the Canadian government's relations with Inuit is addressed in the Royal Commission on Aboriginal Peoples (RCAP), which recognized the distinctness of Inuit from other Aboriginal peoples in Canada, and accepted submissions by Inuit Tapirisat of Canada (1994) and Nunavut Tunngavik (1993) (9). In general, the RCAP found that non-Aboriginal settlers, to further their own economic and political aims, used their power to purposefully destroy Aboriginal ways of life for their own ends (see, for example, 10). The historical treatment of Inuit is unique given its recency and the Canadian government's direct intervention in relocation and resettlment of several groups to the High Arctic. The RCAP concludes that High Arctic relocations constituted "abuse" by the government towards the Inuit people involved. The RCAP report documents additional impacts of contact and colonialism, including settlement, residential schooling, loss of traditional belief systems, loss of traditional relationship with the land, and loss of language.

The Qikiqtani Truth Commission (QTC) was established by the Qikiqtani Inuit Association (the representative organization of the Inuit of the Qikiqtani region of Nunavut) in 2007, with a mandate to investigate historical events "surrounding the alleged dog slaughter, relocations and other decisions made by the Canadian government from 1950 to 1975 that dramatically affected Inuit culture, their economy and their way of life" (11). Like the RCAP, the QTC concluded:

> Since World War Two, the Canadian government has initiated profound social, economic and cultural changes in the North that have had a far-reaching, negative and continuing influence on the lives of Qikiqtani Inuit. The vast majority of these decisions were made without consulting Inuit and the consequences are still felt today. (11)

Although "historical," the QTC emphasizes how these events continue to have impacts at individual, family, and community levels today, resulting in significant, ongoing social suffering. Through the gathering of testimony from across the region, the QTC identified other specific traumatic incidents: settlement, relocations, tuberculosis treatment in the south, killing of qimmit (sled dogs), residential schools, federal day schools, and loss of language and culture. The QTC makes even more explicit use of the terminology of trauma, its historical roots, and its impact across generations, than the RCAP.

One of the important themes to emerge was the role of health care policy and treatment practices in ushering in cultural change and contributing to historical and cultural loss. Testimony by Jaykolasie Killiktee, for example, attests to the impacts of his grandmother's treatment for tuberculosis in a southern sanatorium and eventual death:

> In those days, when my grandmother left on the ship, I think my whole clan – especially our grandfather – was going through stressful times. The only time we could see our grandmother was the next year, or as long as it took to heal. There were no airplanes, no means of mail, no means of telephone, no means of communication with our loved ones. I remember them crying, especially the old ones. It was very traumatic and it had a profound impact on our people … When my grandmother passed away, we were never told if she passed away, or where she passed away. (11)

Other commentators, such as anthropologists, historians, and social scientists have also noted the longstanding impacts of health policy on Inuit in the treatment of tuberculosis (12,13), and on forms of anonymous care that arose out of health bureaucracy (13), such as the use of e-numbers to identify Inuit (13,14). Attention has also been paid to the approach to mental health treatment and suicide prevention, which has also historically involved transport of Inuit to southern treatment centres, and which has privileged biological and medicalized understandings of suicide over social explanations (10,13,15).

Inuit leadership, such as ITK, has brought new emphasis to this *context* of poor health outcomes for Inuit, critically broadening the focus to larger historical and ongoing social inequity. ITK's report on the social determinants of Inuit health asserts:

> This health gap in many respects is a symptom of poor socio-economic conditions in Inuit communities which are characterized by high poverty rates, low levels of education, limited employment opportunities, and inadequate housing conditions. (2 p7)

The report delineates 11 social determinants (16): quality of early childhood development, culture and language, livelihoods, income distribution, housing, personal safety and security, education, food security, availability of health services, mental wellness, and the environment (2 p11).

Similarly, the National Inuit Suicide Prevention Strategy (NISPS), released by ITK in July 2016, takes a holistic approach to conceptualizing high rates of suicide among Inuit, emphasizing the cumulative impacts of historical trauma, cultural discontinuity, community distress, intergenerational trauma, and early life adversity on mental distress and risk for suicide (8). The NISPS promotes a multi-level strategic approach to suicide prevention, with six key strategic priority areas aiming to create social equity through addressing social determinants of health; create cultural continuity through approaches that connect Inuit with their land, culture, and language to foster healing; nurture healthy Inuit children; ensure access to a continuum of mental wellness services; heal unresolved trauma and grief; and mobilize Inuit knowledge for resilience and suicide prevention. Specifically, as part of the priority to create cultural continuity, the NISPS vows to take action to "ensure that health, education, social services, and policing are trauma-informed and culturally safe" (8 p31). Our work occurs within that context of enhancing the cultural safety of health care through the education of health care providers.

What Is Cultural Safety?

The concept of cultural safety has its origins with the Māori of Aotearoa (New Zealand) (17). The cultural safety approach arose in response to "the ongoing and long-term impact of the colonization process on Māori health outcomes" (17, p6). The core principles of cultural safety include that it focuses on health gains and positive outcomes; applies to all relationships within health care; identifies the power relations between those who provide and those who deliver care and empowers service users; and is broad in its application, addressing the relationship of history, political, social, and employment status, housing, education, gender, and personal experience to current health care interactions (18). These principles challenge health providers to examine their practices to recognize power relations and understand their impact as a bearer of their own culture, history, attitudes, and life experiences, and understand how other people may respond to these factors.

There is good reason to think that cultural safety is a useful intervention for health care in other geographic areas, given that racism within medicine continues to be a structural issue (19), particularly with Indigenous communities (20). Brascoupé and Waters (21) provide an overview of the concept and related constructs, and explore its relevance for Indigenous peoples in Canada. They describe that cultural safety "is used to express an approach to health care that recognizes the contemporary conditions of Aboriginal people which result from their post-contact history" (21 p5). Cultural safety is an approach developed to counteract "the resultant power structure [of colonization that] undermined, and continues to undermine, the role of Aboriginal people as partners with health care workers in their own care and treatment" (21 p6). Brascoupé and Waters provide a number of challenges to the concept by noting the ambiguity about what the concept concretely means and the difficulties of creating meaningful partnership, and providing warnings about the focus on individuals with insufficient attention to community and to social determinants of health (21).

Another challenge is beginning to delineate cultural safety from other concepts, such as cultural sensitivity and cultural competence, and determining the contributions each can make; the prevailing distinction is that these represent a spectrum of approaches (22). One useful distinction is that cultural safety changes the emphasis from supplying more knowledge (power) to health providers, as happens with cultural competence, which "leaves the *power* of the interaction in the hands of the professional" (21 p29). In a culturally safe approach, the patient has the power to determine if the interaction has been safe. Many current efforts are being made to operationalize these concepts within the delivery of health care in Canada, with attempts to identify core competencies of culturally safe practice. The Indigenous Physicians Association of Canada (IPAC) and the Association of Faculties of Medicine of Canada have identified core competencies for practitioners working in the area of First Nations, Inuit, and Métis health (23). They provide the following definition of cultural safety:

> Cultural safety refers to a state whereby a provider embraces the skill of self-reflection as a means to advancing a therapeutic encounter with First Nations, Inuit, Métis peoples and other communities including but not limited to visible minorities, gay, lesbian, transgendered communities, and people living with challenges. Self-reflection in this case is underpinned by an understanding of power differentials. (23 p9)

The IPAC competency framework tries to address some concerns with the cultural competence model, such as reducing culture to a set of technical skills, or as a set of "dos and don'ts," and treating cultural groups as homogenous or static entities (23 p9). The IPAC chose cultural safety as the guiding principle of the framework because of the additional emphasis on self-reflection. Other recent consensus guidelines suggest that health professionals should have an understanding of the terms *cultural awareness*, *cultural competence*, and *cultural safety*, and should recognize that First Nations, Inuit, and Métis may have different perspectives about what culturally safe care is. This emphasizes the importance of seeking guidance on community-specific values (24).

The evidence base for cultural safety, and its impact on patient outcomes, is still in its infancy. A scoping review of cultural safety training in Canada, by Guerra and Kurtz (25), identified only 26 such training and education initiatives, of which only 11 were published studies, and few provided formal evaluation of outcomes. Evidence supports the effectiveness of cultural competency training to improve the knowledge, attitudes, and skills of health providers (26) and to have a positive impact on the health outcomes of patients and their satisfaction in health care (27). However, evidence within Indigenous Canadian contexts remains lacking, and there is only one case study of the introduction of cultural safety training for those providers working with Inuit (28).

Cultural Safety Education for Health Care Providers Working with Inuit in Nunavut: An Example

Individually and collectively, we have been involved in other educational initiatives in the areas of cultural safety and trauma informed care, but we present the intervention in Nunavut as an example, outlining the impetus for the course, the process of development and implementation, the evaluation of outcomes, and the lessons learned. Between 2014 and 2015, two of the authors (AC and CW) were involved in developing and implementing a facilitated online educational initiative for mental health nurses working in Nunavut, Canada, supported by a grant from the Department of Health, Government of Nunavut. The demand from mental health nursing staff for this course was identified through a needs assessment process. This need is situated within the context of mental health nursing practice in Nunavut, which is unique given that the large majority of nurses come from outside of Nunavut and most are unfamiliar with the community and culture that they come to practise in. Also, with the large geographic areas and dispersed population in Nunavut, community-based practice can lead to professional isolation and often involves a greater autonomy and scope of practice than in urban settings. Another factor that may have contributed to the expressed need for such a course was the tensions that had emerged between health practitioners and community in some locations (29). Most nurses expressed a desire and willingness to work collaboratively and respectfully with communities but may have felt they needed further skills to do so.

We used a knowledge-to-action (KTA) framework to guide the development of the course curriculum (30). KTA is a dynamic and iterative process that starts with the identification of a problem or need, such as, in this case, knowledge about cultural safety and trauma informed care, and moves towards knowledge creation through inquiry, synthesis, and the creation of knowledge tools. This knowledge is iteratively created and tailored through cycles of assessment, implementation, monitoring of knowledge use, evaluation, sustainment, and adaptation (30). It is critical that knowledge users be central to this development process and to each iterative stage. Given the precepts of cultural safety, we also deemed it crucial to involve Inuit practitioners, knowledge holders, and Elders throughout the process. We were fortunate to have the collaboration of Nunavut Tunngavik Incorporated, the Nunavut land claim organization,[2] and Tuttarviit, an interdepartmental council of the Government of Nunavut comprising people with expertise in Inuit Qaujimajatuqangit (IQ),[3] in addition to Inuit members of the health care team. This involvement included contributing to course design and content, reviewing course material by participating in the course, and providing feedback through interviews and focus groups.

Given the challenges related to the dispersed locations of nursing staff in communities, as well as variable start dates and staff turnover, we decided on an online, self-directed delivery format for the course. The broad goal for the course was to create a climate of respect and safety to ensure that people will seek health care and follow-up, and will experience consideration for their own values and preferences. The following specific learning objectives were identified for participants:

1. Rank cultural safety and trauma-informed care as important aspects of health care practice.
2. Describe the historical, political, and cultural issues that impact the mental health of Inuit in Nunavut.
3. Define some Inuit cultural values and concepts of health and healing.
4. Demonstrate an ability to implement principles of cultural safety and trauma-informed care into practice.
5. Incorporate self-care into health care practice, as measured by use of the curriculum reflection book, and be able to describe effective self-care strategies.

The course format included three components. The first had the five modules, which will be detailed below, covering Inuit social and historical context, Inuit mental health, cultural safety, trauma-informed care (including consideration of historical trauma), and self-care (for health care providers). The second component of the course was self-reflection exercises because cultivating skills in self-reflection is central to cultural safety. The third component was facilitation of the course by a mental health nurse with experience in Nunavut; facilitation involved telephone contact before completion of the course and upon completion of the course. The post-course facilitation included a detailed case study for participant and facilitator to work through to integrate and apply the concepts from the course.

Each module included key concepts, which are outlined here:

1. *Inuit social and historical context* provided an overview of Inuit land occupancy and migration and later contact and colonization, including health care, and introduced some of the impacts as documented through the Qikiqtani Truth Commission. To emphasize Inuit autonomy and resilience, it also covered the process of successful land claims. Current health indicators and social determinants of health were also introduced and linked to

this history. *Reflection* for this module prompted participants to consider the implications of history for current health care practice and the experiences of patients.

2. *Inuit mental health* was included as a topic because the primary intended audience was those working in the area of mental health. Current indicators of mental health, drawn from the Inuit Health Survey, were framed within the context of previous biased and racist ways of framing Inuit expressions of mental distress, such as the "diagnosis" of "Arctic hysteria." It also introduced the concept of social determinants of mental wellness, resilience, strengths-based approaches. The importance of understanding community and individual distress was also introduced. *Reflection* included considering social factors that the participants had witnessed within the community that may have related to mental wellness, and implications for their own practice. Participants also had the opportunity to explore and reflect on the concept of resilience by completing an assessment of their own resilience.
3. *Cultural safety* explored our underlying assumptions about culture and the way these ideas shape how we engage with people across groups and cultures, particularly in our work as health care providers. It also considered health care as a culture. Core concepts included culture, race and ethnicity, cultural biology and neuroscience, approaches to culture within health care, and concepts central to cultural safety, including power, colonialism, othering, and self-reflection. It also included information on Inuit knowledge and values. *Reflection* for this module guided participants through the process of identifying their own culture, their social locations, and their biases, and it provided an opportunity for participants to consider how they could cultivate cultural safety in their practice and attend to the knowledge and values and preferences of Inuit.
4. *Trauma-informed care* was introduced as closely linked with cultural safety, and this module was intended to build on the preceding module. This potential linkage between trauma-informed care and cultural safety is explored in more detail below. Trauma-informed care is used increasingly within health care as a universal precaution to try to minimize the potential traumatic impacts of health care itself, or our potential as providers to re-traumatize those we provide care to or colleagues and members of our team (31). This module covered core trauma-informed principles, including acknowledgement, safety, trust, choice and control, compassion, collaboration, and strength-based understanding. Post-traumatic stress disorder, developmental trauma, and historical trauma were also reviewed. *Reflection* encouraged participants to consider each of the core principles within the context of their own practice.

5. *Self-care* linked the ability to be culturally safe, trauma-informed, and engaged with maintaining one's own self-care. It covered the risks for compassion fatigue and considered how this can impact interactions with clients, and provided an overview of coping practices that can strengthen resilience, including cognitive behavioural techniques. *Reflection* included having participants identify and work through specific experiences from their own practice and evaluate their own coping practices.

An important component of the course was evaluation, to assist in continuing to shape and make the course responsive to both provider and client needs. Evaluation involved a quantitative measure of knowledge and attitude change, qualitative feedback from participants, and observational feedback from the facilitator. Before taking the course, participants completed the Transcultural Self-Efficacy Tool (TSET). The TSET is a validated 83-item questionnaire, developed by Jeffreys and Dogan (32), that measures nursing students' confidence in performing general transcultural nursing skills among diverse clinical populations across three dimension subscales: cognitive (e.g., "how knowledgeable are you about the ways cultural factors may influence nursing care?"), practical (e.g., "how confident are you about interviewing clients of different cultural backgrounds to learn about their values and beliefs?"), and affective (e.g., "how aware are you of your own cultural heritage and belief systems?"). It is not a measure of cultural safety per se, which can be validated only by the client's or patient's experience, but focuses instead on participants' own self-reflection on their efficacy across domains. After completion of the course, participants again completed the TSET and provided qualitative feedback about the course. Facilitators provided additional evaluation by rating the participants' performance on a scale of 1–5 across seven domains of performance integrating core concepts of the course and with an eighth overall rating. The proposal to evaluate the course was reviewed by the Nunavut Ethics Review Board and was granted an exception from full ethics review and approval.

Evaluations were completed by the 18 participants who finished the course and evaluation during the pilot phase. Overall, course satisfaction ratings by participants were high, averaging 4.33/5 overall, with most respondents finding that they were "very" satisfied with the course, would recommend it to other health care providers, and thought that the course would contribute to their health care practice in Nunavut. Facilitator total scores averaged 3.33/5, indicating at least moderate ability of most participants to integrate the content of the course into a practical scenario, with scores highest for "demonstrates knowledge of principles of cultural safety" and "able to integrate principles of trauma-informed care into case discussion and formulation." The item "demonstrated capacity for self-reflection" yielded highly divergent scores (seven participants scoring 5/5 and nine participants scoring 2/5). Participant changes in scores on the TSET were assessed using a paired *t*-test. All tests were two-tailed and performed at an alpha level of 0.05. Scores on the TSET improved significantly after completion of the course, but only on the cognitive ($t = 3.93$, $p = 0.0011$) and practical subscales ($t = 3.22$, $p = 0.0050$), not on the affective subscale ($t = 1.44$, $p = 0.1685$).

The results of the evaluation and our experience implementing the course suggest many strengths of the content and design. Participants were engaged and satisfied and believed that the course had the potential to positively impact their practice. Changes in self-efficacy scores were significant in cognitive and practical domains. However, of interest, the affective scale, which assesses self-awareness (of their own cultural beliefs and biases), acceptance (for example, of a client's refusal of treatment based on cultural beliefs), appreciation (for example, of cultural-specific health care), and recognition (for example, of the impact of values on health care practice), did not significantly change as a result of the course. The course does not seem to impact, at least in participants' *self-appraisal* of, these important domains that are theoretically important for cultural safety. Further, facilitators' findings seem to support something similar. Although facilitators' average ratings of ability to integrate concepts and knowledge were moderate, facilitator ratings of participants' self-awareness were almost dichotomous, suggesting that the group was divided into those with a high degree and those with a low degree of self-reflexivity. The process of evaluation and the discrepancy between self-assessment and facilitator assessment suggest the importance of using facilitation in addition to self-assessment.

These scores begin to suggest two things. First, other pedagogical methods may be needed to change nurses' capacity for cultural safety. Second, the capacity for self-reflection should be more formally assessed during recruitment and hiring because it may be more challenging to change. Other limitations of the course and evaluation, which we are hoping to strengthen and explore in future iterations, are evaluation of practice changes that may result in a more culturally safe environment; this would require direct observation in the nurses' practice environment or the development of simulations to coach and evaluate these skills. Perhaps most importantly, this design did not employ evaluation by patients and clients of these providers. Since it is ultimately the client who determines cultural safety, such interventions could benefit from incorporating client involvement.

Reflections on the Future of Cultural Safety for Health Care Providers Working with Inuit

We recognize that cultural safety is an approach being incorporated by many providers working with Indigenous people and communities globally and across Canada. And while we feel much can be shared and generalized from interventions like ours and others, it is also important to maintain a specificity of approaches so that we do not homogenize (or pan-Indigenize) what should remain unique and responsive to local contexts. In our ongoing work with Inuit in different Canadian contexts, we are exploring the next steps in cultural safety education.

Pedagogical methods and curricula. As the example above highlights, we need to continue to develop methods for enhancing the skills of providers to enact culturally safe environments and interactions. It appears that an online approach, even one that embeds reflection exercises, is able to shift cognitive and practical skills but less effective at shifting the attitudinal aspects of the nursing role. Also, given the interprofessional nature of most health care teams, cultural safety training should include all providers, administrators, and policy-makers involved in the delivery of health care in order to create system change. Our focus has been on individual practitioners, but new approaches should consider cultural safety at the institutional level. There is also an ongoing question about who should create such curricula, with important contributions to be made by those with training in the health care profession (both Inuit and non-Inuit), as well as Inuit knowledge holders and Inuit recipients. As such, the development of curricula is, like cultural safety itself, a relational process in which power should be transparently foregrounded. Approaches will also need to embrace the other aspects of the KTA process, include measures to sustain change, and adapt the pedagogical approach as knowledge and relationships change.

Performing cultural safety. One concern raised within our work so far is the broader focus within health care on competencies. This focus has been critiqued for an over emphasis on the technical aspects of health care provision at the expense of the human elements. When we consider the greater difficulty shifting affective dimensions in our intervention, we have to wonder if people are just learning to mimic accepted skills, rather than engaging in a deeper reflection of their own biases. Concern has also been raised about the negative or unintended consequences of affects like pity or guilt, which can lead to seeing Inuit as weak or victims or to feelings of shame, hopelessness, and apathy (33 p215). More critical attention needs to be given to these affective dimensions, and also to what Ardra Simpson calls the "logics of self-reflexivity" that she feels perpetuate oppression (33 p220).

Cultural humility. A more recent, related concept to cultural safety, cultural humility denotes the stance of the health provider in a culturally safe context. In contrast to the knowing (powerful) learner of cultural competence, cultural humility is "a process of self-reflection to understand personal and systemic biases and to develop and maintain respectful processes and relationships based on mutual trust. Cultural humility involves humbly acknowledging oneself as a learner when it comes to understanding another's experience" (34 para2). This concept can help differentiate between the encounter, judged to be culturally safe (or not) by the recipient of care, from the provider's stance, which can be judged by the provider or patient or other observer. Although we did not explicitly use the construct of cultural humility in our modules, the practices of self-reflection throughout the modules encourage a stance of cultural humility. This will also be incorporated in future iterations of the curriculum.

Trauma-informed care in the context of cultural safety. A promising and important area is critically understanding how cultural safety may fit with trauma-informed care. This is an under-explored area, although others have noted that trauma-informed care is not possible without cultural safety (35 p13). Trauma-informed services take into account an understanding of trauma in all aspects of service delivery and place priority on the individual's safety, choice, and control, creating a treatment culture of nonviolence, learning, and collaboration (35 p12). Further research should focus on the overlapping concepts of these two approaches. Much like with the concept of historical trauma, care should be given to resist characterizing Inuit individuals and communities as "traumatized," rather than as adaptive and resilient, as a strengths-based approach would (see, for example, 36).

Evaluation and outcomes. An exciting area is the development of Inuit-specific evaluation tools, including within the realms of cultural safety and trauma-informed care. This has the potential to make interventions more meaningful and specific to Inuit, and provides a practical way to incorporate Inuit knowledge. As part of these efforts, evaluation by care recipients and at the community level needs to be a priority.

Critical perspectives. In addition to concern about the affective dimensions of cultural safety, and about the potential framing of Inuit as "traumatized victims," other critical perspectives and theories can enhance health care and also redress past failing of health care. Cultural safety, in recognizing the values and knowledge systems (epistemology) and world views (ontologies) of Inuit may not go far enough – these Inuit ways of knowing must be actively incorporated within health care. In fact, cultural safety in Aotearoa is not separated from Māori knowledge but instead is part of an "accepted model of health incorporating taha wairua (spiritual health), taha hinengaro (mental health), taha tinana (physical health) and taha whānau (family health) and … this became widely accepted as the preferred Māori definition of health" (17, p6–7). Other critical perspectives may also productively be brought to bear on critiques of health care, such as from postcolonial theory (19), and with Indigenous health specifically (37). Concepts and goals beyond safety, such as justice, equity, and identity formation (including differences and lack of safety *within* cultural groups) must also be considered (38, for example). The meaning of space and land is one such example, with those living outside of Inuit Nunangat sometimes feeling marginalized, with a different experience of "safe space." Ardra Simpson and others

(33 p227) have also criticized the pressure on the marginalized "other" within culturally safe spaces as bearing the burden of being the representative of their culture rather than being free in space.

Overall, cultural safety is an important minimum standard (and right) in taking action towards reconciliation. However, there is much more to be done to take action to correct the injustices of the past whose effects persist into the present. As Glen Sean Coulthard (39) has decried in *Red Skin, White Masks*, it is no longer sufficient to simply be recognized. The struggle for Indigenous peoples to have their rights recognized within a humanist governmental framework is now being surpassed. Simple recognition that attempts to "reconcile" and accommodate Indigenous identity within existing structures that continue to privilege non-Indigenous people is inadequate. We need to explore new relationalities of ethical reciprocity and mutuality. One of the key differences between cultural safety in the context in which it originated and the new contexts to which it is being generalized is the position of Māori within New Zealand society; Māori have retained a larger degree of power and autonomy in comparison with many other Indigenous groups globally. Similarly, Māori health care is delivered by many Māori providers. Inuit, through land claims progress and through self-governance and strong national leadership at ITK, are also beginning to take increasing ownership over health care. In the coming years, this will provide a fertile context for new possibilities in cultural safety.

NOTES

1 When we use the term *health care*, we are referring to the governmental institution(s) of contemporary, primarily biomedical, health care and not to the broader fields of community-based initiatives and wellness or to traditional Inuit practices.

2 In particular, we would like to thank Ms. Kiah Hatchey who was involved in curriculum development and evaluation. Ms. Hatchey has since moved to another role and was unable to be part of the process of contributing to this chapter.

3 Inuit Qaujimajatuqangit is Inuit values and knowledge. See https://www.gov.nu.ca/culture-and-heritage/information/inuit-qaujimajatuqangit.

REFERENCES

1. Truth and Reconciliation Commission of Canada. Truth and Reconciliation Commission of Canada: calls to action. Winnipeg (MB): Truth and Reconciliation Commission of Canada; 2015.

2. Inuit Tapiriit Kanatami. Social determinants of Inuit health in Canada. Ottawa (ON): Inuit Tapiriit Kanatami; 2014.
3. Statistics Canada. Life expectancy at birth, by sex, five year average, Canada and Inuit regions (2004–2008). CANSIM table #102–0706. Ottawa (ON): Statistics Canada; 2012.
4. Statistics Canada. Live births and infant mortality, by sex, five year average, Canada and Inuit regions (2004–2008). CANSIM table #102–0702. Ottawa (ON): Statistics Canada; 2012.
5. Banerji A. High rates of hospitalization for bronchiolitis in Inuit children on Baffin Island. Int J Circumpolar Health. 2001;60(3):375–9.
6. Egeland GM. The international polar year Nunavut Inuit child health survey 2007–2008: summary report. Montreal (QC): McGill University Centre for Indigenous Peoples' Nutrition and Environment; 2009 Jun.
7. Public Health Agency of Canada. Tuberculosis in Canada, 2012 – pre-release. Ottawa (ON): Minister of Public Works and Government Services Canada; 2013.
8. Inuit Tapiriit Kanatami. National Inuit suicide prevention strategy [Internet]. Ottawa (ON): Inuit Tapiriit Kanatami; 2016 [updated 2016; cited 2016 Jul 30]. Available from: https://www.itk.ca/download/12091/
9. Royal Commission on Aboriginal Peoples. Report of the Royal Commission on Aboriginal Peoples. Vol. 1, Looking forward, looking back. Ottawa (ON): Communication Group Publishing; 1996 Oct.
10. Crawford A. "The trauma experienced by generations past having an effect in their descendants": narrative and historical trauma among Inuit in Nunavut, Canada. Transcult Psychiatry. 2014 Jun;51(3):339–69.
11. Qikiqtani Truth Commission [Internet]. Iqaluit (NU): Qikiqtani Truth Commission; 2015 – . What is the Qikiqtani Truth Commission?; [updated 2016; cited 2016 Nov 30]; What is the main objective of the Qikiqtani Truth Commission?; [updated 2016; cited 2016 Nov 30]. Available from: https://qtcommission.ca/index.php/en/faqs. Jaykolasie Killiktee; [2007?–2010?] [cited 2016 Nov 30]. Available from https://qtcommission.ca/index.php/en/qtpi10
12. Grygier PS. A long way from home: the tuberculosis epidemic among the Inuit. Montreal (QC): McGill-Queen's University Press; 1997.
13. Stevenson L. Life beside itself: imagining care in the Canadian Arctic. Oakland (CA): University of California Press; 2014.
14. Smith DG. The emergence of Eskimo status: an examination of the Eskimo disk list system and its social consequences, 1925–1970. In: Dyck N, Waldram JB, editors. Anthropology, public policy, and Native peoples in Canada. Montreal (QC): McGill-Queen's University Press; 1993. p. 41–74.
15. Tester FJ, McNicoll P. Isumagijaksaq: mindful of the state: social constructions of Inuit suicide. Soc Sci Med. 2004 Jun;58(12):2625–36.
16. World Health Organization [Internet]. Geneva (CH): World Health Organization; [date unknown]. Social determinants of health; [updated 2016; cited 2016 Nov 30]. Available from: http://www.who.int/social_determinants/en/

17. Wepa D, editor. Cultural safety in Aotearoa New Zealand. 2nd ed. Port Melbourne (AU): Cambridge University Press; 2015.
18. Nursing Council of New Zealand. Guidelines for cultural safety, the Treaty of Waitangi and Maori health in nursing education and practice. Wellington (NZ): Nursing Council of New Zealand; 2011.
19. Bleakley A, Brice J, Bligh J. Thinking the post-colonial in medical education. Med Educ. 2008 Mar;42(3):266–70.
20. Allan B, Smylie J. First peoples, second class treatment: The role of racism in the health and well-being of Indigenous peoples in Canada. Toronto (ON): The Wellesley Institute; 2015.
21. Brascoupé S, Waters C. Cultural safety: exploring the applicability of the concept of cultural safety to Aboriginal health and community wellness. Journal de la santé autochtone. 2009 Nov;5(2):6–41.
22. Kirmayer LJ, Fung K, Rousseau C, Lo HT, Menzies P, Guzder J, Ganesan S, Andermann L, McKenzie K. Guidelines for training in cultural psychiatry. Can J Psychiatry. 2012;57(3):S1.
23. Indigenous Physicians Association of Canada; The Association of Faculties of Medicine Canada. First Nations, Inuit, Métis health core competencies: curriculum implementation toolkit for undergraduate education [Internet]. West Vancouver (BC): Indigenous Physicians Association of Canada; The Association of Faculties of Medicine Canada; 2010 Apr [cited 2016 Nov 30]. Available from https://afmc.ca/sites/default/files/pdf/IPAC-AFM_FN_I_M_Health_Curriculum_Implementation_Toolkit_EN.pdf
24. Wilson D, de la Ronde S, Brascoupé S, Apale AN, Barney L, Guthrie B, Harrold E, Horn O, Johnson R, Rattray D, Robinson N; Aboriginal Health Initiative Committee, Alainga-Kango N, Becker G, Senikas V; Special Contributors, Aningmiuq A, Bailey G, Birch D, Cook K, Danforth J, Daoust M, Kitty D, Koebel J, Kornelsen J, Tsatsa Kotwas N, Lawrence A, Mudry A, Senikas V, Turner GT, Van Wagner V, Vides E, Wasekeesikaw FH, Wolfe S. Health professionals working with First Nations, Inuit, and Métis consensus guideline. J Obstet Gynaecol Can. 2013 Jun;35(6):550–8.
25. Guerra O, Kurtz D. Building collaboration: a scoping review of cultural competency and safety education and training for healthcare students and professionals in Canada. Teach Learn Med. 2017 Apr 3;29(2):129–42.
26. Beach MC, Price EG, Gary TL, Robinson KA, Gozu A, Palacio A, Smarth C, Jenckes MW, Feuerstein C, Bass EB, Powe NR, Cooper LA. Cultural competence: a systematic review of health care provider educational interventions. Med Care. 2005 Apr;43(4):356–73.
27. Goode TD, Dunne MC, Bronheim SM. The evidence base for cultural and linguistic competency in health care. New York (NY): Commonwealth Fund; 2006 Oct.
28. James S, O'Brien B, Bourret K, Kango N, Gafvels K, Paradis-Pastori J. Meeting the needs of Nunavut families: a community-based midwifery education program. Rural Remote Health. 2010;10:1355.

29. Hildebrandt A. Nunavut nurse admits to failing to see infant and other allegations. CBC News [Internet]. 2014 Nov 19 [cited 2016 Nov 30]. Available from: http://www.cbc.ca/news/canada/north/nunavut-nurse-admits-to-failing-to-see-infant-and-other-allegations-1.2838235
30. Straus S, Tetroe J, Graham ID. Knowledge Translation in Health Care: Moving from Evidence to Practice. 2nd Edition. London (England): BMJ Books; 2013.
31. Klinic Community Health Centre. Trauma-informed: the trauma toolkit. 2nd ed. [Internet]. Winnipeg (MB): Manitoba Trauma Information and Education Centre; 2013 Oct [updated 2013 Oct; cited 2016 Nov 30]. Available from: http://trauma-informed.ca/wp-content/uploads/2013/10/Trauma-informed_Toolkit.pdf
32. Jeffreys MR, Dogan E. Factor analysis of the transcultural self-efficacy tool (TSET) J Nurs Meas. 2010;18(2):120–39.
33. Simpson A, Smith A, editors. Theorizing Native studies. Durham (NC): Duke University Press; 2014.
34. First Nations Health Authority (BC) [Internet]. East Vancouver (BC): First Nations Health Authority; 2019. Cultural safety & humility; [cited 2019 May 25]. Available from: http://www.fnha.ca/wellness/cultural-humility#learn
35. BC Provincial Mental Health and Substance Use Planning Council. Trauma-informed practice guide [Internet]. [place unknown]: [publisher unknown]; 2012 May [updated 2013 May; cited 2016 Nov 30]. Available from: http://bccewh.bc.ca/wp-content/uploads/2012/05/2013_TIP-Guide.pdf
36. Hatala AR, Desjardins M, Bombay A. Reframing narratives of Aboriginal health inequity: exploring Cree Elder resilience and well-being in contexts of historical trauma. Qual Health Res. 2016 Dec 1;26(14):1911–27.
37. Browne AJ, Smye VL, Varcoe C. The relevance of postcolonial theoretical perspectives to research in Aboriginal health. Can J Nurs Res. 2005 Dec;37(4):16–37.
38. Kuper A, Veinot P, Leavitt J, Levitt S, Li A, Goguen J, Schreiber M, Richardson L, Whitehead CR. Epistemology, culture, justice and power: non-bioscientific knowledge for medical training. Med Educ. 2016 Nov 1;51(2):158–73.
39. Coulthard GS. Red skin, white masks: rejecting the colonial politics of recognition. Minneapolis (MN): University of Minnesota Press; 2014.

18 Integrating Traditional Healing and Northern Health Care: Indigenous Conceptions of Living Well

CINDY PELTIER

It is imperative to open this discussion with the declaration that I have entered into a sacred research partnership only with the Manitoulin Anishinaabek communities who agreed to participate in my research. Any knowledge that I share about other Indigenous peoples is limited to information obtained from the academic literature. In avoiding a pan-Indigenous approach, I draw upon some of the parallels in knowledge shared by Anishinaabe Elders I have interviewed and the recorded knowledge of Inuit and the Cree found within the literature. This chapter is by no means an exhaustive review of literature on Indigenous healing. Instead, it presents understandings of Indigenous healing and what it means to live well from the perspectives of the *Tununirmiut* (north) and *Uqqurmiut* (south) Baffin Inuit Elders, the *Whapmagoostui Iyiyuu'ch*, and *Eeyou Istchee* Cree of the James Bay region in northern Quebec, as well as the Anishinaabek of Manitoulin Island in northeastern Ontario. While Manitoulin Island would not be considered to be Canada's hinterland, its communities are rural and with their being located in northern Ontario (1,2), access to certain health resources remains a challenge (2,3). It is through these perspectives that I examine issues impacting Indigenous healing in three northern regions of Canada.

Indigenous ways of knowing reflect how Indigenous peoples come to learn about the world. For Indigenous peoples, this learning is procured through relationships, languages, histories, spiritualities, and their world views (4,5). Indigenous conceptions of wellness and healing are also based in relationality, language, and cosmology. King, Smith, and Gracey (6) acknowledge that much of the research on the health of Indigenous peoples has focused on non-Indigenous conceptions of health and disease. Biomedical or conventional models of health are often limited to a focus on the physical domain and may be ill-equipped to address Indigenous understandings of wellness and the root causes of poor health – namely, the Indigenous determinants of health (7). Indigenous health equity requires a broader, more holistic understanding of wellness, which includes the mental, emotional, and spiritual domains (5,8). Hence, it is necessary to begin this discussion with how Anishinaabe, Inuit, and Cree nations conceive of wellness and healing.

Ootoova et al. (9) interviewed the *Tununirmiut* (north Baffin) and *Uqqurmiut* (south Baffin) Elders of Nunavut to chronicle knowledge of traditional Inuit healing. Inuit Elders shared their conception of health, which centres on developing a strong mind and resilient body. For these Elders, it is understood that physical or bodily health is dependent on a healthy mind, where this body-mind connection appears to be a function of both holism and relationality:

> The body is hence to be put in close relation with all human experiences including quality of interpersonal relationships, quality of the relations to the environment and game, and quality of relations to the deceased and the spirits. (9 p1)

For Inuit, healing encompasses more than the eradication of disease and extends the notion of healing to the larger social, physical, and spiritual environments. Inuit elders note two conditions for successful healing: the removal of an "offensive element" from the person's body, and "rehabilitation of the sick person" within community and among human or spiritual ancestors (9 p2). The works of Ootoova et al. (9) and Boulanger et al. (10) concur that "Inuit notions of health are holistic, and, contrary to western medicine, do not focus on the absence of illness or injuries" (10 p87). Specifically, health and healing can encompass activities like harvesting berries for a variety of purposes, including sustenance and healing, but that participation in land-based activities also contributes to personal, family, and community well-being.

Tagalik (11) also interviewed Inuit Elders to gain insight into *Inuit Qaujimajatuqangit* or Inuit world view. Those Elders interviewed placed emphasis on holism but also on interconnectedness and reciprocity in their conception of what it means to live a good life. Inuit live by *maligait* or big laws, which describe the contribution of skills and knowledge for the common good, respect for all living beings, maintenance of balance, and preparation for a better future (11). In Inuit cultures, there are also parental teachings, called *inunnguiniq*, which instil that living a good life involves contentment, harmony, and respectful relationships with others. These teachings also promote problem solving as a means to overcome obstacles. Imbalance is a collective problem of the family and community, and not solely that of an individual. Inuit describe the healing process or *anniatpalauqmataajuq* whereby harmony can be regained by talking or letting it out (11). These Inuit Elders see a strong need for healing from the impacts of colonization through this process of "letting it out." This type of healing requires effective intergenerational communication, which facilitates both healing and transferring traditional Inuit knowledge between generations (11,12). While there may be a tendency in Western cultures to think of healing and living well as individualistic pursuits, for many Indigenous nations, including Inuit, living well is a lifelong process guided by relationships with others and is ultimately for the greater good of all.

The Cree of the James Bay region have a similar conception of health and well-being. Adelson shares that the Cree term *miyupimaatisiiun* in its best English translation means "being alive well" (13 p61). As it does for Inuit, the Cree conception of living well extends beyond the domain of physical health. The *Whapmagoostui Iyiyuu'ch*, the Cree of Whapmagoostui, connect "being alive well" to life on the land and Cree identity. Living a Cree way of life is central to their understanding of what it means to be *miyupimaatisiiun* – "all that the *Iyiyuu* [the Cree of northern Quebec] was and had been before he [the Cree in general] used and integrated the white man's way of life into his own life" (13 p62). Relationality is central to the Cree understanding of wellness. As such, in avoiding starvation and working to stay warm in their harsh, northern climate, the Cree accept collective responsibility for one another but also encourage self-sufficiency for *miyupimaatisiiun* (13).

Cree scholar Michael Anthony Hart (14) further describes the importance of the collective in his description of *mino-pimatisiwin*, which goes beyond an individual's experience of living well to include sharing with and respect for fellow community members. The term *mino-pimatisiwin* involves the individual's experience within a greater social environment. Hart (14) states that colonization has left an imprint on the individual, community, and nation that requires collective healing. In her doctoral work, Radu (15) shares the relational perspective of the Cree of Eeyou Istchee and *miyupimaatisiiun*, where culture-based healing "in the bush" involves reconnecting youth with land and with Elders through positive intergenerational relationships to find purpose and meaning. Similar to the Cree understandings of Adelson's *miyupimaatisiiun*, and Hart's *mino-pimatisiwin*, Anishinaabe *minobimaadiziwin* or "the way of a good life" encompasses a number of these parallel understandings that are central for Indigenous healing (5,8,16).

Peltier (5,8) describes Anishinaabe *minobimaadiziwin* from the perspective of the Elders on Manitoulin Island as balance and the ability to live well physically, mentally, emotionally, and spiritually. They shared that people must work at maintaining a state of equilibrium in all four of these elements to achieve *minobimaadiziwin* and that this is a constant process. The four elements of a person's being are seen as highly interconnected, and a change in one area will reflect changes in the other areas of a person's life. *Minobimaadiziwin* was further described as a path of living well, which is dependent on personal choice and not without challenges or obstacles to overcome (5,8,17). This notion of *minobimaadiziwin* as a "path of life beset with obstacles and a state of unhealthiness" (17 p454) has been attributed by other scholars to colonialism and its impacts on the contemporary life of the Manitoulin Anishinaabek (17). Similar to both Inuit and Cree understandings of living a good life, the Manitoulin Anishinaabek believe *minobimaadiziwin* depends on using the heart to guide one's actions in treating others with respect, love, and kindness (8).

It is evident that Inuit *maligait* and *inunnguiniq*, Cree *miyupimaatisiiun/mino-pimatisiwin*, and Anishinaabe *minobimaadiziwin* share parallel teachings for living well. There is acknowledgement that wellness extends beyond the physical domain to include the mind (i.e., mental), the heart (i.e., emotional), and the interconnectedness with all living (i.e., physical) and non-living beings in Creation (i.e., spiritual). There is a common understanding that wellness is only maintained with balance in these areas and that living well entails respect for all things, which is both a personal and a collective responsibility. Anishinaabe anthropologist Sonya Atalay's work (18) illustrates a multidimensional understanding of wellness that is experienced through the work of repatriation of the tangible (i.e., ancestral remains) and intangible (i.e., songs, language, traditional ecological knowledge, and stories) aspects of cultural heritage. Her work examines how reclamation and repatriation contribute to both personal and community health and well-being, beyond just the physical (18). These parallel understandings and how they relate to living well will be reflected upon in the following discussion of Indigenous healing.

Anishinaabe, Inuit, and Cree Perspectives of Healing: A Means for Living Well

The concept of Indigenous healing has often been misunderstood, it has been difficult to define, and through Indigenous resurgence efforts, it is evolving (18–22). Perhaps one of the most quoted definitions for this phenomenon comes from the Report of the Royal Commission on Aboriginal Peoples (23 p325):

> Traditional healing has been defined as practices designed to promote mental, physical and spiritual well-being that are based on beliefs which go back to the time before the spread of Western "scientific" bio-medicine. When Aboriginal Peoples in Canada talk about traditional healing, they include a wide range of activities, from physical cures using herbal medicines and other remedies, to the promotion of psychological and spiritual well-being using ceremony, counseling and the accumulated wisdom of Elders.

With respect to the Indigenous conceptions of living well, this definition can be appreciated for its attempt at an understanding of Indigenous healing beyond the physical realm. The works of Martin-Hill (20,24) caution that Indigenous healing should not be disconnected from the family and community contexts – it is all-encompassing and part of a way of life for Indigenous peoples. Hence, Indigenous healing should never be perceived as an isolated phenomenon whose goal is a cure for illness. Instead, it should be perceived as a means to wellness. Peltier (8) has shared that any discussion of Indigenous healing should occur within a context that acknowledges the impacts of colonization. This chapter will take a strengths-based approach to discussing the impacts of colonization and will focus on the agency required for Indigenous people's wellness.

In an effort to facilitate this discussion of Indigenous healing, the experience of the Manitoulin Anishinaabek is presented as a case study along with connections made to relevant literature on Inuit and Cree traditional medicine and healing. Figure 18.1 adapted from Peltier (8) provides a frame for understanding proximal, intermediate, and distal determinants of contemporary Indigenous

Figure 18.1 Determinants of Indigenous healing

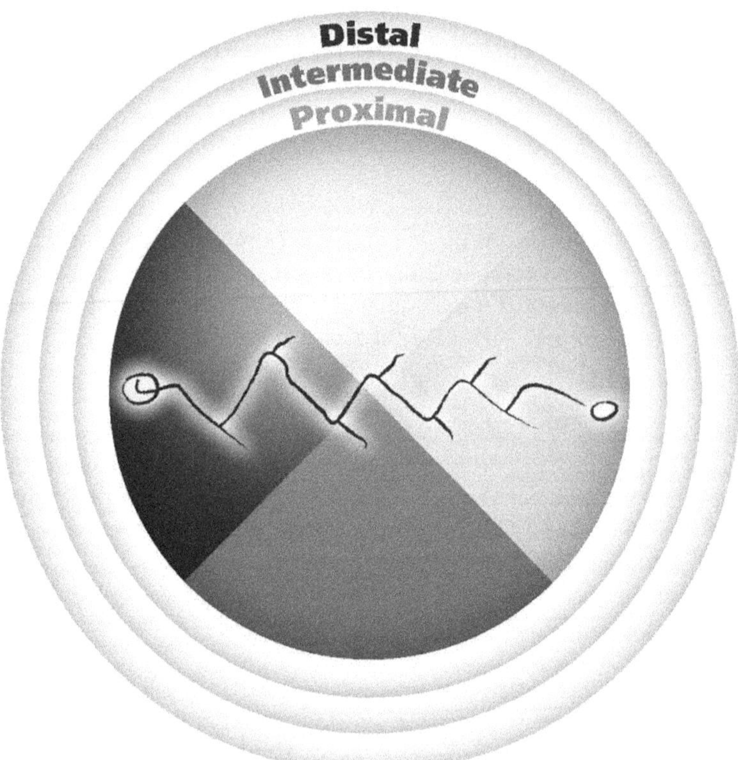

Figure source: Cindy Peltier

healing. This discussion will begin at the centre of the model and will work outwards to the distal level. Each level will offer a perspective of Indigenous healing informed by Anishinaabe, Inuit, and Cree nations.

The centre of the model represents Anishinaabe, Inuit, and Cree interpretations of Indigenous healing. For many Indigenous peoples, these forms of healing involve a spiritual component, which some describe as spiritual intervention manifested in various ways. For instance, healers may have prior knowledge of things not yet verbally communicated to them. There is often no scientific explanation for how Indigenous healing works, but Indigenous peoples often refer to this as the work of the spirits. This spiritual component of healing is thought to be the source of healing (8). One healer interviewed in Peltier (8 p246) describes this spiritual intervention as the Great Mystery:

> It goes in line with our traditional ways. The spirits did it, I didn't. That's the whole part of the healing besides the medicine that we incorporate into that type of situation. We call it the Great Mystery. We don't know how it works, but we know if we do these certain ceremonies, if we say these certain prayers, and give this certain medicine that it works. It's all based on our tribal and traditional ways. This Great Mystery was given to us by the Great Spirit. We still have people that can count on and use that regularly.

The acknowledgement of this spiritual intervention is what some consider the component of Indigenous healing that facilitates Anishinaabe *minobimaadiziwin*. The cosmologies of Inuit peoples also involve the understanding that healing exists within social, natural, and supernatural realms. Healing and treating illnesses can involve relationships with other people, animals, the land, and spirits. In treating illness, a cure may encompass a physical recovery, but equally important is the attainment of emotional and spiritual well-being fostered through relationality (9,25–27). Similarly, the Cree acknowledge this spiritual component of healing in the language they use to describe medicine people and their capacities. For example, the Cree term *otsapaheak* means one who has the ability to see into the future for healing purposes (28). In their comparative analysis of Western and Cree healing practices, Morse et al. (29) describe the spiritual aspects of Cree healing in which the healer mediates between the patient and the spirit helpers to facilitate the process of healing.

Indigenous healing is described by the Anishinaabe of Manitoulin as a holistic concept wherein the mental, emotional, spiritual, and physical wellness of the person are supported. This type of healing promotes *minobimaadiziwin* through a conscious effort to work within all aspects of a person's being. Hence, Indigenous healing is an active method of healing in which the commitment and participation of the person seeking healing is expected (8). This Anishinaabe healer shared her active, holistic view of healing:

> There's a role for you to be part of your healing journey where you need to [work on] some of those areas yourself. In the spiritual aspect, acknowledging your spiritual helpers and doing your own spiritual offerings. In terms of emotions, what are [you] doing to release some of the grief associated with illness or imbalance. Looking at the physical aspect, what are you doing to retain that physical wellness [by] exercising, walking and being as active as possible? In the mental, try to the best of your ability to think *naa naa gideh ehn dum, naa naa gdeh ehn mowin* [taking the time to use your heart/feelings to think in a logical way about all factors in order to come up with your decisions] which is thinking holistically, in our language. We use our mental capacity to think before we do things that could actually create the imbalance in our lives. (8 p250)

Ootoova et al. (9) describe the Inuit holistic view of health and the interconnections between the mind, body, and *tarneq* (soul) or spirit. These authors' views concur with the notion of imbalance implied in the comment above, where weakness in one area of a person's being will create weakness in another (8,9,27,30). Morse et al. (29) also frame Cree healing as a holistic and balanced process where the role of the healer involves caring (i.e., emotional), curing (i.e., physical and spiritual), and counselling (i.e., mental) aspects of healing. Other studies have used the medicine wheel to frame the concept of balance and restoring Cree wellness (31,32). These and other studies acknowledge relationality, the participatory role of the person or community in maintaining balance, and connections to the land or land-based practices (10,15,27,31–33) in the Cree and Inuit understandings of healing.

Indigenous healing is also understood as being preventive and as having a protective function that maintains wellness. Within this understanding, medicine carries a more holistic function than would be commonly understood in the pharmaceutical or biomedical context. This Anishinaabe healer emphasizes the importance of integrating Indigenous healing into daily life for maintaining *minobimaadiziwin*:

> [Indigenous healing] addresses all of you, physically, mentally, emotionally and spiritually. It helps to put that into your daily life and you are encouraged to use it all of the time. Anishinaabe medicine is about incorporating or using it as a preventative tool. It will help with detoxifying in the spring, or getting yourself ready in the fall for the cold and flu season, and boosting up your immune system. It's about putting that into your daily life instead of waiting until you get sick. (8 p254)

For many Indigenous peoples, food is viewed as a medicine. Borré (26) studied the use of seal in *Tununirmiut* (north Baffin Island) Inuit healing practices. Seal was found to be an essential component in maintaining wellness within both the *tiimuit* (body) and the *tarneq* (soul). For this reason, seal products are recommended as preventive medicine. Specifically, seal products are used to maintain good physical and mental health in women and to promote endurance and strength in men (26). For other Inuit of Nunangat, consuming food attained through direct relationships with the land, like berries (10) and country foods (27), has preventive and protective healing purposes, beyond purely physical benefits. The Cree also believe that consuming *iyimiichim* (food procured from animals through trapping, hunting, or fishing) is one way to preserve *miyupimaatisiiun* and can facilitate healing. For instance, caribou fat is highly regarded for both sustenance and ceremonial purposes (13). This understanding of food as medicine and the high regard for animals are based in relational and spiritual connections.

Ceremonial healing practices are also regarded as a form of protection. In the Cree healing practices described by Morse et al. (29), smudging is used in purification ceremonies to open spiritual channels, but it also has a protective function for the healer. The healers in Peltier (8) share why preventive and protective factors are necessary not only for the person seeking healing from cancer but also for the healers themselves:

> Part of the protocol is to know if they have taken chemotherapy. Sometimes when we're working on people we ingest what we draw out. If they had chemotherapy or radiation they have to make that known, otherwise it will make me sick. I try and go before they have treatments. After treatment, juniper helps to clear that out of the body …
>
> Sometimes that radiation hinders us from doing what we need to do with the person after they have the radiation and the chemotherapy. That is a poison to us also and [it's] the nature of what we do, we take that into us. But our spirits won't allow us to do that … When there's chemo and things, we kind of back off and we still pray for them and we still do the ceremonies and help them as much as we can … I'm not saying that ours is the only way. But in some cases, collaboration, we do what we can and they do the therapies and whatever. We have good results with that. (8 p272)

The latter comment alludes to relationships at the proximal level of the model, which are discussed in the next section. Collaborative relationships between practitioners of Indigenous healing and conventional medicine are necessary for patient agency and will support Indigenous peoples' wellness but also support the reclamation of Indigenous healing practices. This and other challenges are addressed in the following sections on proximal, intermediate, and distal determinants of Indigenous healing.

Proximal Determinants of Indigenous Healing

The proximal level of the model concerns the notion of relationships and relationality with respect to Indigenous healing. One precept of Indigenous healing is that it never occurs in isolation (28) but involves relationships with family, community, health practitioners, and beings within the spiritual realm. Informants in Peltier (8) agree that the support and care provided through family and community relationships, especially in times of healing, is essential for the realization of Anishinaabe *minobimaadiziwin*. The Manitoulin Anishinaabek conveyed how Indigenous healing assists in achieving *minobimaadiziwin* at the end of physical life when a person's spirit is entering the Western doorway or "getting ready to go home" (8 p164). For the Manitoulin Anishinaabek, visiting has always been a means of providing comfort, information, and support, but it also has great spiritual significance for those who are preparing to go through the Western doorway. Many informants in Peltier (8) believed that the visiting and caring provided during this time is something that Anishinaabe families do without question:

> [The] *bimaadiziwin* or Anishinaabe approach to palliative care, becomes a very family, community approach at that time. The community is coming in to take care of family who is taking care of their loved one. That in itself, is *bimaadiziwin*; taking care of our family and community … In taking care of the family, we're feeding them; we're giving them rest time; and being emotionally supportive, or listening. We are trying to keep those loved ones in a balanced place, despite the grieving … When you come into our homes, our people automatically feed you and to refuse is sometimes an insult. What the people are doing when they feed you is giving life. They're acknowledging the spirit of who you are as a person … People visit at that palliative stage and the person welcomes that. You hear, "Oh, they're so happy that you came to visit" because it's a spiritual visit, physically you're there but it's a spiritual visit of giving each other life. (8 p173)

Some Anishinaabek fear that our communities are suffering by moving away from these particular practices of Anishinaabe *minobimaadiziwin* (8). Family and community relationships, and the social interactions that foster these relationships, such as visiting and storytelling, have been recognized as contributing factors to well-being for Anishinaabe, Inuit, and Cree peoples (8,9,10,11,13,14,27,32). In fact, the work of Kral (34) and Kral et al. (12), attribute the high suicide rates in Inuit communities, in part, to colonialism, specifically the government's intervention on Inuit family and community life, as well as the interference with *Inuit Qaujimajatuqangit* (Inuit traditional healing practices). Indigenous people rely on maintaining relationships for living well. It is not the quantity but the quality of those relationships that matters most. Morse et al. (29) discussed Indigenous patients' dissatisfaction with the conventional health care system and attributed this to the quality of relationships with physicians and nurses. Conventional health care practitioner-patient relationships were characterized as a siloed, top-down, time-sensitive approach to care. In contrast, these authors described the care a Cree healer provides as fostering autonomy, as participatory, and as providing holistic health care.

Intermediate Determinants of Indigenous Healing

The intermediate level of the model focuses on access to Indigenous healing. Peltier (8) notes several challenges, based in colonialism, that Manitoulin Anishinaabek face in accessing Indigenous healing. For instance, many of the Western practitioners interviewed by Peltier (8) acknowledge their ignorance of Indigenous healing. Moreover, the Manitoulin Anishinaabek report lack of agency with respect to the use of Indigenous healing in a health care setting. This healer noted what she believed to be the greatest impediment to Indigenous healing:

> I think the biggest barrier is the belief, *debwenmowin* [to believe in the truth]. Historical factors have caused our people not to believe in our ways. We have a high number of people that don't believe in it. It goes back to *debwenmowin*. Sometimes people don't believe in our own people at the local level. Or, they don't want anybody to know that they actually believe in it so they hide it. It went underground, *bi zha gwen ma, zha gwen ma nishnabena* [learned shame, shamed Anishinaabe] they don't want anybody to know ... we are ashamed. (8 p261)

Rather than focusing on barriers, this discussion frames these issues as opportunities, taking a strengths-based approach aimed at promoting agency for living well.

Several authors, including Jacklin and Warry (2), have argued that an understanding of colonialism is essential for overall health improvement and health equity, and I would add, for Anishinaabe *minobimaadiziwin*. This understanding can be obtained through a cultural safety approach, which provides the opportunity to include knowledge concerning Indigenous healing as a legitimate option for living well. Cultural safety is a pedagogical approach that brings awareness of structural and colonial forces to promote change within health care institutions and systems (35,36). It is through this lens of cultural safety that health care and education systems can address the history of colonization *and* the ongoing process of colonization. Cultural safety pedagogies should be aimed at decolonizing Indigenous healing to facilitate its integration or "braiding" with conventional healing methods for a more comprehensive, holistic health care model that contributes to Anishinaabe *minobimaadiziwin* (8), Inuit *maligait* and *inunnguiniq*, and Cree *miyupimaatisiiun*.

Distal Determinants of Indigenous Healing

The distal level of the model concerns the broader concepts of colonialism, self-determination, and cultural continuity, and their implications for Indigenous healing. In the context of Indigenous health, colonialism is understood to be the "cause of causes" (37 p1) and a root cause of health inequity (7,35). Cultural continuity has been understood to mean "being who we are" (38 p3) and, for the purposes of this discussion, can be thought of as maintaining an Indigenous way of life whether based in an Inuit, Cree, or Anishinaabe perspective. In this way, Indigenous healing can be conceived of as a form of decolonization for Indigenous peoples. For many, participation in Indigenous healing provides an opportunity to relearn or to reclaim Indigenous teachings (8,18,27,39) lost or "left by the trail" (39 p93), and there are now options to integrate Indigenous healing with conventional biomedicine in some health care centres.

Peltier (8) refers to the movement toward braiding or integrating contemporary biomedicine with Indigenous healing as a means of restoring wellness or Anishinaabe *minobimaadiziwin*. Successful models of braiding are being implemented in northern Ontario Aboriginal Health Access Centres. The availability of Indigenous healing has been increased through traditional medicine programs offered within these Aboriginal Health Access Centres and in other provincial health services in Canada (40). This healer who is employed with an Aboriginal Health Access Centre articulates how the structure of the institution can facilitate braiding:

> [Indigenous healing] is the centrepiece of everything ... when you look at the structure of the building the healing room is at the centre and everything else is around it – the western practitioners, the nutritionists, but traditional [medicine], it's the centre piece ... One of the things I like about this is the opportunity to educate ... One day I was making cough syrup and the doctors were very curious and wanting to know ... It's nice that it gives the doctors an opportunity to see and witness how the medicines are working.[1]

Similarly, there is a movement towards reclaiming Indigenous healing practices through birthing centres and midwifery among Inuit (41,42) and the *Eeyou Istchee* Cree of James Bay in northern Quebec (43). Research into the reclamation of birthing practices has seen positive outcomes extending to the wider community with respect to healing, restoring pride, fostering family and community relationships, and capacity building. Reclamation of Indigenous healing is also evident in diabetes research. For instance, type 2 diabetes research with an ethnobotanical focus also supports the effective integration of traditional medicinal plant knowledge with conventional medicine for Inuit (10,30) and *Eeyou Istchee* Cree (44–46), where diabetes prevalence is high.

Conclusion

Indigenous scholars have emphasized the importance of reclaiming the original teachings and the use of Indigenous healing as a means of decolonization, self-determination, and wellness (18,27,47). Manitowabi and Shawande (17) shared that achieving Anishinaabe *minobimaadiziwin* requires that people consistently "mitigate these powerful and contemporary forces undermining the [Anishinaabe] of life" (17 p454), implying that decolonization, self-determination, and wellness are works in progress. In her work on decolonizing botanical Anishinaabe teachings, Wendy Geniusz refers to *biskaabiiyang* an Anishinaabe concept meaning coming back or a "returning to ourselves" (47 p9). In this vein, *biskaabiiyang*, in part, reflects our collective effort as Indigenous peoples to reclaim our own methods of healing as a resource to mitigate colonial forces. In doing so, *biskaabiiyang* also fosters a level of cultural continuity that affords Indigenous people the agency to "be who they are" (38 p3). The objective in reclaiming Indigenous healing practices is then twofold. First, it can lend to current health care models a more holistic approach that responds to Indigenous concepts of wellness, fostering Inuit *maligait*, *inunnguiniq*, Cree *miyupimaatisiiun*, and Anishinaabe *minobimaadiziwin*. Second, the reclamation of Indigenous healing can foster Indigenous self-determination in which solutions to promoting equity in health will germinate within Indigenous communities for Indigenous peoples.

NOTE

1 This quotation is from a participant denoted as IHP06A (participant from the Indigenous health perspective) within Peltier (6). The source is the participant theme files but was not included in the final dissertation.

REFERENCES

1. Williams A, Kulig J. Health and place in rural Canada. In: Kulig J, Williams A, editors. Health in rural Canada. Vancouver (BC): UBC Press; 2012. p. 1–19.
2. Jacklin K, Warry W. Decolonizing First Nations health. In: Kulig J, Williams A, editors. Health in rural Canada. Vancouver (BC): UBC Press; 2012. p. 373–89.

3. Hout S, Ho H, Ko A, Lam S, Tactay P, MacLachlan J, Raanaas RK. Identifying barriers to health care delivery and access in the circumpolar North: important insights for health professionals. Int J Circumpolar Health [Internet]. 2019 Jan [cited 2019 Mar 25];78(1):1–8. Available from: https://doi.org/10.1080/22423982.2019.1571385
4. Wilson S. Research is ceremony: Indigenous research methods. Halifax (NS): Fernwood Publishing; 2008.
5. Peltier C. An application of Two-Eyed Seeing: Indigenous research methods with participatory action research. Int J Qual Methods [Internet]. 2018 Nov [cited 2019 Mar 20];17:1–12. Available from: https://doi.org/10.1177%2F1609406918812346
6. King M, Smith A, Gracey M. Indigenous health part 2: the underlying causes of the health gap. Lancet [Internet]. 2009 Jul [cited 2019 Mar 20];374(9683):76–85. Available from: http://www.thelancet.com/action/showPdf?pii=S0140-6736%2809%2960827-8
7. Reading C. Structural determinants of Aboriginal peoples' health. In: Greenwood M, de Leeuw S, Lindsay N, Reading C, editors. Determinants of Indigenous peoples' health in Canada: beyond the social. Toronto (ON): Canadian Scholars' Press; 2015. p. 3–15.
8. Peltier C. The lived experience of Anishinaabe people with cancer: a focus on Indigenous healing, Western medicine and minobimaadiziwin [dissertation]. Sudbury (ON): Laurentian University; 2015.
9. Ootoova I, Atagutsiak TQ, Ijjangiaq T, Pitseolak J, Joamie A, Joamie A, Papatsie M. Interviewing Inuit Elders. Vol. 5: perspectives on traditional health [Internet]. Iqaluit (NU): Nunavut Arctic College Library; 2001 [cited 2018 Jun 30]. Available from: http://www.tradition-orale.ca/english/pdf/Perspectives-On-Traditional-Health-E.pdf
10. Boulanger-Lapointe N, Gerin-Lajoie J, Siegwart Collier L, Desrosiers S, Spiech C, Henry GHR, Hermanutz L, Levesque E, Cuerrier A. Berry plants and berry picking in Inuit Nunangat: traditions in a changing socio-ecological landscape. Hum Ecol [Internet]. 2019 Feb [cited 2019 Mar 25];47(1):81–93. Available from: https://doi.org/10.1007/s10745-018-0044-5
11. Tagalik S. Inuit knowledge systems, elders, and determinants of health. In: Greenwood M, de Leeuw S, Lindsay NM, Reading C, editors. Determinants of Indigenous peoples' health in Canada: beyond the social. Toronto (ON): Canadian Scholars' Press; 2015. p. 25–32.
12. Kral MJ, Idlout L, Minore JB, Dyck RJ, Kirmayer LJ. Unikkaartuit: meanings of well-being, unhappiness, health, and community change among Inuit in Nunavut, Canada. Am J Community Psychol [Internet]. 2011 Mar [cited 2019 Mar 29];48:426–38. Available from: https://doi.org/10.1007/s10464-011-9431-4
13. Adelson N. "Being alive well" health and the politics of Cree well-being. Toronto (ON): University of Toronto Press; 2000.
14. Hart MA. Seeking mino-pimatisiwin: an Aboriginal approach to healing. Halifax (NS): Fernwood Publishing; 2002.

15. Radu I. Miyupimaatisiiun in Eeyou Istchee: healing and decolonization in Chisasibi [dissertation]. Montreal (QC): Concordia University; 2015.
16. Rheault D. Anishinaabe mino-bimaadiziwin (the way of a good life): an examination of Anishinaabe philosophy, ethics and traditional knowledge [Internet]. Peterborough (ON): Debwewin Press; 1999 [cited 2019 Mar 29]. Available from: http://eaglefeather.org/series/Native%20American%20Series/Anishinaabe%20Tradition%20D%27Arcy%20Rheault.pdf
17. Manitowabi D, Shawande M. The meaning of Anishinabe healing and wellbeing on Manitoulin Island. J Indig Wellbeing [Internet]. 2011 [cited 2019 Mar 29];9(2):441–58. Available from: https://journalindigenouswellbeing.com/the-meaning-of-anishinabe-healing-and-wellbeing-on-manitoulin-island/
18. Atalay S. Braiding strands of wellness: how repatriation contributes to healing through embodied practice and storywork. Public Hist [Internet]. 2019 Feb [cited 2019 Mar 28];41(1):78–89. Available from: http://tph.ucpress.edu/content/41/1/78.full.pdf+html
19. Broome B, Broome R. Native Americans: traditional healing. Urol Nurs. 2007; 27(2):161–73.
20. Martin-Hill D. Traditional medicine in contemporary contexts: protecting and respecting Indigenous knowledge and medicine [Internet]. Ottawa (ON): National Aboriginal Health Organization; 2003 [cited 2019 Mar 29]. Available from: https://epub.sub.uni-hamburg.de/epub/volltexte/2013/15417/pdf/research_tradition.pdf
21. Struthers R, Eschiti VS, Patchell B. Traditional indigenous healing: part I. Complement Ther Nurs Midwifery. 2004;10:141–9.
22. Waldram JB, Herring A, Young TK. Aboriginal health in Canada. 2nd ed. Toronto (ON): University of Toronto Press; 2006. Chapter 9, Aboriginal healing in the contemporary context; p. 236–61.
23. Royal Commission on Aboriginal Peoples. Report of the Royal Commission on Aboriginal Peoples. Ottawa (ON): Royal Commission on Aboriginal Peoples; 1996.
24. Martin-Hill D. Traditional medicine and restoration of wellness strategies. Int J Indig Health [Internet]. 2009 [cited 2019 Mar 29];5(1):26–42. Available from: https://jps.library.utoronto.ca/index.php/ijih/article/view/28976/23904
25. Tester FJ, McNicoll P. "Why don't they get it?" Talk of medicine as science. St. Luke's Hospital, Panniqtuuq, Baffin Island. Soc Hist Med. 2006;19(1):87–106.
26. Borré K. The healing power of the seal: the meaning of Intuit health practice and belief. Arctic Anthropol.1994;31(1):1–15.
27. Robertson S, Ljubicic G. Nunamii'luni quvianaqtuq (it is a happy moment to be on the land): feelings, freedom and the spatial political ontology of well-being in Gjoa Haven and Tikiranajuk, Nunavut. Environ Plan D [Internet]. 2019 Jan [cited 2019 Mar 29];37(3):1–19. Available from: https://journals.sagepub.com/doi/abs/10.1177/0263775818821129
28. Robbins JA, Dewar J. Traditional Indigenous approaches to healing and the modern welfare of traditional knowledge, spirituality and lands: a critical

reflection on practices and policies taken from the Canadian Indigenous example. Int Indig Policy J. 2011;2(4):1–17.

29. Morse JM, Young DE, Swartz L. Cree Indian healing practices and western health care: A comparative analysis. Soc Sci Med. 1991;32(12):1361–6.
30. Black PL, Arnason JT, Cuerrier A. Medicinal plants used by the Inuit of Qikiqtaaluk (Baffin Island, Nunavut). Botany. 2008;86:157–63.
31. Danto D, Walsh R. Mental health perceptions and practices of a Cree community in northern Ontario: A qualitative study. Int J Ment Health Addict [Internet]. 2017 Aug [cited 2019 Mar 29];15(4):725–37. Available from: https://link.springer.com/article/10.1007/s11469-017-9791-6
32. Gesink D, Whiskeyjack L, Guimond T. Perspectives on restoring health shared by Cree women, Alberta, Canada. Health Promot Int [Internet]. 2018 Jan [cited 2019 Mar 29]. Available from: https://academic.oup.com/heapro/advance-article/doi/10.1093/heapro/dax099/4788355
33. Walsh R, Danto D, Sommerfeld J. Land-based intervention: a qualitative study of the knowledge and practices associated with one approach to mental health in a Cree community. Int J Ment Health Addict [Internet]. 2018 Oct [cited 2019 Mar 29]. Available from: https://doi.org/10.1007/s11469-018-9996-3
34. Kral MJ. Postcolonial suicide among Inuit in Arctic Canada. Cult Med Psychiatry. 2012 Jun;36(2):306–25.
35. Allan B, Smylie J. First Peoples, second class treatment: the role of racism in the health and well-being of Indigenous peoples in Canada [Internet]. Toronto (ON): Wellesley Institute; 2015 [cited 2018 Jun 30]. Available from: http://www.wellesleyinstitute.com/wp-content/uploads/2015/02/Full-Report-FPSCT-Updated.pdf
36. Metzl J, Hansen H. Structural competency: theorizing a new medical engagement with stigma and inequality. Soc Sci Med. 2014;103:126–33.
37. Czyzewski K. Colonialism as a broader social determinant of health. Int Indig Policy J. 2011;2(1):Article 5.
38. Oster RT, Grier A, Lightning R, Mayan MJ, Toth EL. Cultural continuity, traditional Indigenous language, and diabetes in Alberta First Nations: a mixed methods study. Int J Equity Health. 2014;13:1–11.
39. Benton-Banai E. The Mishomis book: the voice of the Ojibway. Minneapolis (MN): University of Minnesota Press; 1988.
40. Drost JL. Developing the alliances to expand traditional Indigenous healing practices within Alberta Health Services. J Altern Complement Med [Internet]. 2019 Mar [cited 2019 Mar 29]:25(S1):69–77. Available from: https://doi.org/10.1089/acm.2018.0387
41. Van Wagner V, Epoo B, Nastapoka J, Harney E. Reclaiming birth, health and community: midwifery in the Inuit villages of Nunavik, Canada. J Midwifery Women's Health. 2007;52(4):384–91.
42. Douglas VK. The Rankin Inlet Birthing Centre: community midwifery in the Inuit context. Int J Circumpolar Health [Internet]. 2012 Mar [cited 2019 Mar 29]: 70(2):178–85. Available from: https://doi.org/10.3402/ijch.v70i2.17803

43. Duff T, Little J. Bringing traditional midwives back to Cree communities in Quebec. CBC News [Internet]. 2016 Aug 6 [cited 2018 Jun 30]. Available from: http://www.cbc.ca/news/canada/north/cree-birth-midwifery-program-1.3708035
44. Nistor Baldea LA, Martineau LC, Benhaddou-Andaloussi A, Arnason JT, Levy E, Haddad PS. Inhibition of intestinal glucose absorption by anti-diabetic medicinal plants derived from the James Bay Cree traditional pharmacopeia. J Ethnopharmacol 2010 Nov 11;132(2):473–82.
45. Shang N, Guerrero-Analco J, Musallam L, Saleem A, Muhammad A, Walshe-Roussel B, Cuerrier A, Arnason JT, Haddad PS. Adipogenic constituents from the bark of Larix laricina du Roi (K. Koch; Pinaceae), an important medicinal plant used traditionally by the Cree of Eeyou Istchee (Quebec, Canada) for the treatment of type 2 diabetes symptoms. J Ethnopharmacol. 2012 Jun 14;141(3):1051–7.
46. Leduc C, Coonishish J, Haddad P, Cuerrier A. Plants used by the Cree Nation of Eeyou Istchee (Quebec, Canada) for the treatment of diabetes: a novel approach in quantitative ethnobotany. J Ethnopharmacol. 2006;105:55–63.
47. Geniusz WM. Our knowledge is not primitive: Decolonizing botanical Anishinaabe teachings. Syracuse (NY): Syracuse University Press; 2009.

19 Health and Health Care Research Ethics: Health Research Ethics in Northern Canada

FERN BRUNGER AND BRITTANY CHUBBS

Research engaging Canada's northern communities poses particular challenges for research ethics. The vast geography means that research ethics boards may not have sufficient knowledge of local contexts to appropriately review the researchers' assessment of the potential risks and benefits of research. To compound the problem of context sensitivity, guidelines for ethical research involving Indigenous communities in Canada are not always easily applicable. In Canada, the Tri-Council Policy Statement: Ethical Conduct for Research Involving Humans (here called the TCPS), which guides research involving human subjects, was revised in 2010 to include a chapter on research involving First Nations, Inuit, and Métis communities in Canada (1). Based on an earlier set of recommendations created for health research involving Indigenous communities in Canada (2), the TCPS contains prescriptions for creating effective collaborations with communities before engaging in research. However, the guidelines may be difficult to implement in complex communities where there is no clear authority or where a politically defined territory does not map neatly onto group identity. Questions of who controls the research agenda, what it means to be over-researched as a group, and who has the authority to effectively represent a group may be particularly difficult to ask and answer.

This chapter outlines the contemporary Canadian structure of health research ethics review, with particular attention to research involving Indigenous communities. The perspectives in this chapter emerge from research conducted with researchers, members of research ethics boards, and community members engaged in research with the Inuit of southern Labrador (the "Southern Inuit").[1] The research was conducted in collaboration with the NunatuKavut Community Council. The NunatuKavut Research Ethics Project established a system of research oversight for the Southern Inuit and, over a five-year period, performed a critical examination of that process to make recommendations for best practices. We set out to examine how best to implement Canadian policy guidelines for community consultation, consent, or collaboration (1) in a community with complex identities and authority structures.[2] Drawing on examples derived from that research, this chapter examines challenges with and strategies for oversight of health research involving northern and remote Indigenous communities, focusing on questions of authority and representation in complex communities.

The Challenge of Authentic Representational Review

To examine and strategize around the challenges of health research ethics review in Canada's North, we need to begin by distinguishing between three types of research review processes: research ethics boards (REBs), governmental or Indigenous community research advisory committees (RACs), and hospital- or health-region-based operational review committees (ORCs).

REBs – called institutional review boards in the United States and research ethics committees in the United Kingdom – review the ethics of the research, ensuring compliance with provincial or territorial and federal laws or policies. In Canada, the three major public funders (Canadian Institutes of Health Research, Social Sciences and Humanities Research Council of Canada, and the Natural Sciences and Engineering Research Council of Canada) have the joint policy mentioned above: the TCPS (1). Researchers and their institutions must adhere to the policy as a condition of funding. REBs ensure compliance with the TCPS. These committees[3] are affiliated with the institution of the researcher (typically a university, but sometimes a health institution and very often both).

RACs are formal bodies appointed by governments or Indigenous community authorities to review proposed research for its appropriateness and acceptability to the community. RACs review and approve – or decline – research, which may or may not have already been approved by an REB, to ensure compatibility with the resources, values, social-cultural-economic context, and priorities of the jurisdiction. For communities in which there is a correspondence between membership, land, and political authority, the RAC may be formed by a territorial government (e.g., 3) or an Indigenous government (e.g., 4). In other cases, the RAC may take the form of an institutional REB located in the primary research institution through which researchers apply to work in that geographical, political, or cultural context (e.g., the Aurora Research Institute (5) governs research involving the Northwest Territories and the Inuvialuit Settlement Region). By contrast, an Indigenous RAC may represent a collective of Indigenous communities that are members of a nation with oversight of lands and people across political jurisdictions (e.g., 6,7). In yet another model, where the association between nationhood and political or geographical region is complex or not formally recognized by outsiders, an RAC may represent members of a collective that is united through insider recognition of nationhood. For example, research involving the Southern Inuit of Labrador is under the oversight of the NunatuKavut Community Council's RAC (8,9). Not all Indigenous RACs use the phrase *research advisory committee.* The name or descriptor varies across communities; for example, such bodies may be referred to as community REBs.

Each region in northern Canada has some combination of the above models in their processes for research review and approval, and these processes vary tremendously from jurisdiction to jurisdiction.[4] Moreover, existing processes may be refined or radically altered over time, as political or economic landscapes shift. Some communities and types of research may require separate applications for specific licences (e.g., access to archaeological sites, compared to accessing traditional knowledge, compared to retrieving patient health information). Approval may take the form of letters of no objection, letters of support, letters of community consent, or certificates of approval, depending on the RAC's policies and the type of research. Some RACs have formal processes for creating and signing researcher-community agreements; others do not. Some RACs meet regularly; others meet rarely. Therefore, researchers must consult with the relevant northern government or Indigenous community officials for advice on the research approval process and must allot ample time (in some cases, months) for review and approval to take place.

Regardless of their structure, northern and Indigenous RACs play a gatekeeping role, allowing only those research projects that meet the community's research needs, resources, values, and ethical standards to access their peoples and their knowledge (19 p88). By asserting oversight of and authority over the ethics of research that will involve them, northern governments and Indigenous groups ensure that only research that is appropriate to the community's values, needs, and resources will be accepted.

ORCs within health care, educational, and other institutions may review research to ensure that it is compatible with institutional values and available resources, including human resources (1 article 8.3). For example, researchers who want to access patients or providers within a particular hospital apply for review and approval from the hospital, which determines whether the research is feasible and whether the costs (for example, drain on resources) is balanced with the benefits of the research. They ensure that proposed research involving patients in their region or resources in their institutions is within their capacity to facilitate. Similarly, research involving students or teachers requires the permission of the school board, school principal, or both, before research can be undertaken. Sometimes, the operational review is one aspect of the work of a hospital or health region REB. In other cases, the work of research ethics and operational review may be delegated to separate committees; for example, one based in a university and the other in a hospital.

The Challenge of Context Sensitivity

In Canada, as elsewhere, there have been increasing calls for centralized systems of research ethics review, with the aim of avoiding the inefficiencies of multiple reviews (20–22). However, this poses a dilemma: health research being conducted in rural and remote areas must be reviewed in a way that accounts for the particular contexts of rural and remote research sites. Context sensitivity is a crucial part of the system of checks and balances that REBs must undergo in the process of ethics review. For example, the standard across Canada, reflected in the TCPS, is to ensure that local issues and values are taken into account in the review of research ("Sensitivity to context is a key issue in the application of the core principles of this Policy to the ethics review of research involving multiple institutions and/or REBs" [1 article 8.2]). The dilemma is that REBs are often geographically and culturally very distant from rural and remote research sites, posing challenges to a context-sensitive review.

REPRESENTATIONAL REVIEW

While it would seem intuitive that northern and Indigenous representation on (southern-based) REBs would be an ideal solution to respond to gaps where northern/ Indigenous communities have scarce resources, a representation approach has drawbacks that must be considered. In a representation model, a southern university- or hospital-based REB expands its membership to include representatives from those geographical areas or populations not deemed to be sufficiently represented on the REB. The purpose of expanding REB membership in this way is to ensure sensitivity to the unique contexts of different areas and populations. However, the model raises problems of representation, specifically in terms of authority and legitimacy. Using the example of Newfoundland and Labrador – a province that, by its small size, would seem to be one of the easiest places to effectively implement a representation model of community oversight of health research – the pitfalls of such an approach are quickly evident. For example, an individual from the Miawpukek First Nation residing in the southern community of Conne River on the island portion of Newfoundland and Labrador may constitute an "Indigenous" representative, but that individual would not necessarily be qualified to represent the needs and priorities of research conducted with the Inuit of northern Labrador. The inclusion of multiple additional members to represent the province's range of Indigenous communities (Inuit, Southern Inuit, and Innu First Nations from two very different geographical areas of Labrador, as well as the Mi'kmaq from both the Qalipu and the Miawpukek First Nations of the island portion of the province) might minimize these issues, but would not eliminate them entirely, and would lead to additional problems related to meeting quorum. Similarly, including a northern representative from the Labrador-based regional health authority on the centralized (southern) review committee to ensure attention to northern health needs (that is, beyond the Indigenous populations) would not be effective in terms of authentic representation.

Moreover, application of the representational review model would not alleviate the need for additional northern Indigenous community review, as well as operational review by health regions. Two functions are important for effective and authentic northern/Indigenous community review: (1) prioritizing research needs for the community, and (2) avoiding community or organization research fatigue. Fulfilling these roles requires having sufficient oversight and authority to ensure that research that *may be important and ethical but is not of immediate or high priority* for resource-stretched communities is not accepted if the community deems it does not have the capacity to effectively engage at that time (8,23). Similarly, when health regions review research for its appropriateness in terms of local human and infrastructural resources, they have a comprehensive knowledge of all research being conducted within the health institutions of their region; they can recognize both gaps and overlaps in research. Gaps may then represent areas in which further research is required while overlaps may represent inefficiencies that can be addressed to avoid wasting the time and effort of health stakeholders. For reasons of representation, efficiency, and authenticity, then, it would not be entirely helpful to rely on community representation on a southern-based REB.

AD HOC ADVISERS

Another potential model to ensure local community oversight of research is the use of ad hoc advisers. Ad hoc advisers are used by REBs when there is a lack of specific expertise or knowledge necessary to determine the ethical acceptability of a particular research proposal (1 article 6.5). Ad hoc advisers tend to be used in instances where REBs lack methodological or disciplinary expertise; however, they are occasionally used when participant or community representation is required to determine the ethical acceptability of research within the context in which it will be conducted. Ad hoc advisers alter neither the composition nor the representation of the REB, as they are not true REB members. As such, they are not counted in the REB's quorum and cannot vote during REB decision making. Their input, however, may be considered in, and thus inform, the decision making of the REB.

Applying this model, a southern-based REB could have a roster of regional or community-based researchers or lay members from stakeholder Indigenous communities to call upon when context-specific knowledge is required. This model of research oversight presents issues similar to the representational review model in that it does not obviate the need for Indigenous community oversight and review. While the ad hoc model is more feasible than the representational review model, given the lesser practical demands it places on community volunteers, it is still not as effective as a fourth option – supporting the effective functioning of Indigenous review committees by recognizing and bolstering the authority of and expertise of these committees.

Strategy

Research institutions and funders should support and facilitate the work of northern and Indigenous RACs to ensure that effective community-based oversight and review of research is in place. Strategies might include, for example, fee-for-service arrangements by research institutions (as pharmaceutical companies do with REBs) and revising the policies of Canada's major funding councils to enable 10 per cent of administrative costs to go directly to communities to support the material and human resources required for effective research oversight and review (23).

The Challenge of Role Demarcation between REBs, RACs, and Other Research Review Processes

The distinction between reviews for research ethics, Indigenous community appropriateness, and health care institutional resources can be confusing, particularly when compounded by reviews for environmental safety, educational access, or other levels of screening. Our research in Labrador indicated that researchers may receive contradictory information and, until a process that is widely accepted across all types of research review within a jurisdiction is established, frustrations and delays in research review can result (23).

For example, the distinction between the roles and responsibilities of a hospital-based organization review committee and an REB was a source of confusion for researchers during the implementation of Newfoundland and Labrador's Health Research Ethics Authority Act in 2011 (24). Before the implementation of that legislation (24), which created a centralized Health REB (HREB) system, the province's northern health region had maintained its own REB. That REB had included representation from the Inuit, Southern Inuit, and Innu First Nations groups. Under the newly legislated province-wide HREB system, the northern REB was transformed into a health regional ORC – its mandate was to review for resource appropriateness to the health region, not for research ethics. This change left a wide geographical area of the province without effective ethics review: members of the southern-based centralized HREB had little knowledge of the context of the region's northern or Indigenous communities. Therefore, in the first months following the transition to the centralized HREB system, the health region's newly minted ORC felt obliged to continue to function as an REB as a way of addressing the gap in context-sensitive ethics review.

Research conducted through the NunatuKavut Research Ethics Project revealed that at the heart of the early confusion was the question of whether a health region's ORC can request changes to a researcher's protocol, particularly where such changes contradict the direction given to the researcher by the REB. The question was sparked by one particular event in which a consent form was deemed to be inappropriately worded for the context of the rural and remote research site. A process of negotiation between the HREB and northern ORC took place over six months, through which the roles of the HREB in relation to the northern ORC were debated and increasingly refined and defined. The examination of that process in the context of the NunatuKavut Research Ethics Project and through a provincial Indigenous ethics workshop (25) led to a clearly delineated role demarcation between operational review and ethics review for the province.

Strategy

Operational review by a hospital's or health region's ORC examines resource use, the impact on the health care organization, and access to confidential information. The specific task of the ORC is to determine whether the method, process, and dissemination, or any other aspect of the research, is appropriate to the local context, including both resources and values. In addition, health institutions may use the operational review process to catalogue all research activities within the institution. During the operational review process, context-specific details may be identified that the researcher or southern-based REB members had no awareness of, and researchers may be asked to alter their protocol.

Review by a northern government or Indigenous community examines the appropriateness to the community context (values, culture, ways of life, and so on), resources available for the community to be effectively engaged (in light of community priorities for research), potential harms and benefits to the community, and adherence to the OCAP principles (ownership, control, access, and possession) (26) or other locally described principles.

If an REB has approved a protocol (including the consent), then that protocol should remain unchanged *except for* where a governmental or Indigenous community RAC or a health institutional ORC has deemed that some aspect of the research is not appropriate to the context or that it is unduly potentially harmful to local participants. For example, a community-based review may reveal that a consent must be provided in an additional language to reflect the demographics of the population being recruited. Or it may request that patient records on a particular health condition not be included in the research because of inevitable stigma to and loss of health resources for the subset of patients involved. In these examples, the researcher must also apply to the HREB to have the protocol amendment or consent amendment approved. Importantly, genuine engagement by a community in health research means that a need for an amendment could happen during research – in that sense, community consent to research is, like individual consent to research, an ongoing negotiation.

Which Review Is Conducted First?

Our research revealed that navigating multiple reviews (research ethics, northern government or Indigenous community research review, and hospital operational review) was a confusing experience for communities, researchers, and REBs. Conflicting messages were given and received about which review should happen first. For example, is REB approval required to approach a northern government or Indigenous community for review and approval? Or is that northern/Indigenous research review and approval a prerequisite for REB approval?

In Newfoundland and Labrador, the HREB had begun with the approach of delaying ethics review until it received confirmation of Indigenous community support for the research. However, analysis of this approach made it clear that the approach was unjust: community members were reviewing research that had not yet undergone REB review and revision for ethics considerations, and so the northern RAC reviewers were, in fact, performing the bulk of the ethics review. To remedy the situation, we switched the order; we had the REB do its work and had the researcher address the changes before the submission to the community RAC. This significantly reduced the workload of the community RAC but introduced two new problems. First, community RACs were concerned that research that had already been through REB approve had progressed too far without sufficient community review and consent. Second, with this approach, any changes requested by the community then would have to be returned to the REB as an amendment before final approval, adding an additional step for the researcher and the REB. However, as the priority lay with lightening the burden for the community RAC, and given the minimal additional effort required of the REB and researcher, the deliberative approach illustrated in Figure 19.1 was felt to be the most appropriate.

Through negotiations with Indigenous community councils and governments of Labrador, the process finally established by the HREB is a deliberative one, whereby the order in which reviews are done is directed and determined by the Indigenous community. However, final HREB approval (required for funding, as well as for data collection to commence) is not granted until proof of RAC approval is obtained. For researchers whose studies involve multiple Indigenous RACs, this means that the HREB itself must be flexible and ready to accommodate different approaches to which review comes first within a single application to the HREB.

Figure 19.1 Process for research institution (REB), community (RAC), and operational (ORC) reviews of health research involving Indigenous communities

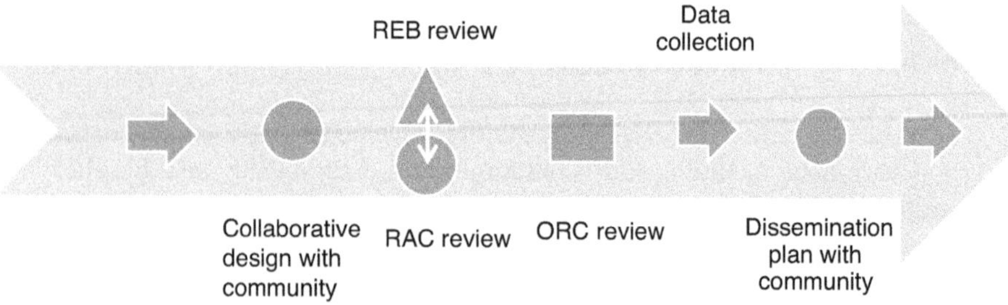

Figure source: Fern Brunger

Strategy

Research ethics that emphasize the principle of justice in resource allocation and the primacy of community control over research require an iterative approach between Indigenous community review and REB review. This means that, depending on the Indigenous community's needs or expectations, the northern or Indigenous RAC can either request HREB review and approval in principle first or require it as a second step following RAC approval.

Whose Authority Counts? The Politics of Risk and Representation in Research Ethics

Scholars of research ethics have long recognized that there are problems of representation and authority to speak on behalf of a group, given intra-group politics and power differentials, even within a relatively cohesive community (27–32). The challenges of consent in a "non-cohesive" community are even more complex. There are concerns about censorship if community consent were needed when studying a powerful group (for example, if a subgroup of powerful leaders wanted to silence research that was supported by the majority of community members and pointed to exploitation of the majority by those leaders). And the use of community categories themselves for seeking consent may problematically reify the categories (33). Scholars of research ethics continue to examine and refine decolonizing practices for research involving Indigenous communities (34–39).

The TCPS requirement for consultation extends only to those Indigenous community governments with authority, where the definition of authority is dependent on land rights "recognized" by the colonizers (1 article 9.3). It narrows the formal authority to Inuit with a mandate under a recognized land claims agreement and First Nations with adopted ethical codes and research protocols and inherent right to self-government recognized in federal government policy (1 article 9.6). Virtually no guidance is provided to research involving the Métis and urban, rural, and non-status Indian communities that compose more than 50 per cent of Indigenous peoples in Canada. More importantly, there is no guidance for community consultation where a community has self-identified as having authority over specific lands in the absence of "official" recognition by outsiders in the form of a treaty or a recognized land claim.

Our research indicated that the distinction between what counts as collaboration, compared to consultation, compared to community consent was at the heart of the complexity around navigating whose authority counts. Researchers and REBs understandably do not always appreciate the distinction between a community collaborator's letter of support-in-principle, a letter of support from an Indigenous appointed official, and a letter of RAC approval following a formal community review and approval process. Challenges include determining the nature and extent of Indigenous community involvement when the research includes, but does not specifically target, Indigenous patients; determining when and how an RAC can decline research by outsiders in cases where the impetus for the research came from community members who have collaborated with the researcher in co-designing a study; and determining whether, in cases where research is driven by appointed community leaders and approved by an RAC, smaller communities within the jurisdiction of the RAC have the right to decline participation (8).

Strategy

Our research indicated that simplification of community-researcher negotiation of research to a "community consent" model, reducing the process to something akin to individual consent on a larger scale, is inappropriate and misleading to both communities and researchers. The complexities of navigating community engagement and Indigenous RAC approval requires careful negotiation of the complexities of authority and representation within the context and according to the nature of the research and of the researcher-community relationship. Researchers and REBs must explicitly attend to the politics of risk – the ways in which collective identity and research risks are co-constructed (8) – and then, from that process, determine whose authority counts for that study at that time, given that particular researcher-community relationship.

Key to effective community negotiation of research is the development of a thorough researcher-community agreement. Models for these vary, but key elements include (1) a lay summary of objectives; (2) descriptions of direct and indirect potential harms and benefits to the community at large; (3) descriptions of direct and indirect potential harms and benefits to individual sub-communities or subgroups within the broader collective; (4) expectations of how community leaders and members will be engaged in design, data collection, and knowledge translation; (5) copies of any data collection tools, consents, or other study documents; (6) identification of who will be data guardians; and (7) a detailed plan for knowledge dissemination, including (a) whether and how community members have the right to veto or respond to statements made about the community, and (b) plans for local dissemination of results in lay language and in an accessible format.

Summary

Effective and authentic governance of research in Canada's North requires careful attention to the intersection of power, identity/representation, and risk. The process of decolonization, which at least in Canada has been determined to be integral to the ethics of research involving Indigenous communities, requires the ongoing scrutiny and disruption of relations of power that inhibit community control of research. But that is not sufficient. We need also to disrupt normative assumptions about the binary relationships of power that shape the way we imagine and do research ethics: at a minimum, the following binaries deserve scrutiny and disruption: researcher-researched (or colonizer-colonized), health institution–community, researcher-REB, north-south, and central-peripheral. Most obviously, researchers are sometimes also community members, and members of REBs may be community members and researchers. Communities (as with REBs, research institutions, and health institutions) are multifaceted and have complex relations of power and differences both among and between them in terms of geography, cultural capital, values, and health research goals. Attention to the spaces in which power, identity/representation, and risk intersect will enable an approach to research ethics that is just and accounts for the uniqueness of Canada's North.

NOTES

1 This research was supported by the Canadian Institutes of Health Research (operating grant #106542): F. Brunger (PI), J. Bull, J. Graham, D. Pullman, D. Wall, C. Weijer (Co-Investigators), *The Labrador Inuit-Métis Research Ethics Project: An Experiment in Aboriginal Governance of Health Research in Complex Communities*. This research benefited from the guidance of the Labrador Aboriginal Health Research Committee which was assisted by the Canadian Institutes of Health Research–funded Atlantic Aboriginal Health Research Program. The NunatuKavut Community Council partnered in this study and provided in-kind support for the

Labrador-based research. Ethics approval was obtained from Memorial University's Interdisciplinary Committee for the Ethics of Human Research (ICEHR 2010 /11-036-ME). Community approval was obtained from the NunatuKavut Research Advisory Committee. We wish to thank all those participants who gave of their time to inform us about ethical research relationships.

2 For a complete description of the methodology, please see (23).

3 We use the terms *committee* and *board* interchangeably as they are both used within the Canadian REB system to mean the group of individual scientists, ethicists, lawyers, and community representatives who meet to review research involving humans that takes place within the jurisdiction or under the auspices of that institution.

4 See, for example, for Yukon (3,10,11); for Northwest Territories and the Inuvialuit Settlement Region (5); for Nunavut (12,13); Nunavik does not have a local formal licensing board for research, but researchers should consult with the Nunavik Research Centre (14); for the Assembly of First Nations in Quebec and Labrador (15); for Nunatsiavut (16). Importantly, the Inuit Tapiriit Kanatami's (ITK) National Inuit Strategy on Research (6) describes the ITK's coordinated approach to research ethics for all Inuit in Canada and should be consulted for research involving members of the Inuvialuit Settlement Region (Northwest Territories), Nunavut, Nunavik (northern Quebec), and Nunatsiavut (Northern Labrador). Additional information for the governance of research ethics involving Canada's northern Indigenous communities can be found at First Nations Information Governance Centre (17) and the Association of Canadian Universities for Northern Studies (18).

REFERENCES

1. Canadian Institutes of Health Research, Natural Sciences and Engineering Research Council of Canada, Social Sciences, Humanities Research Council of Canada. Tri-council policy statement: ethical conduct for research involving humans. 2nd ed. Ottawa (ON): Secretariat on Responsible Conduct of Research; 2014.
2. Canadian Institutes of Health Research, Natural Sciences and Engineering Research Council of Canada, Social Sciences, Humanities Research Council of Canada. Tri-council policy statement: ethical conduct for research involving humans. Ottawa (ON): Secretariat on Responsible Conduct of Research; 2007.
3. Cultural Services Branch, Department of Tourism and Culture, Government of Yukon. Guidebook on scientific research in Yukon [Internet]. Whitehorse (YK): Yukon Tourism and Culture; 2013 Jul 31 [revised 2008 Apr; cited 2019 Jun 3]. Available from: https://yukon.ca/sites/yukon.ca/files/tc/tc-guidebook-scientific-research-2013.pdf

4. Nunatsiavut Research Centre [Internet]. Nain (NL): Nunatsiavut Government. Nunatsiavut Government research application; 2015; [cited 2017 Feb 6]. Available from: https://nunatsiavutresearchcentre.com/application/
5. Aurora Research Institute. Doing research in the Northwest Territories: a guide of researchers [Internet]. Inuvik (NT): Aurora Research Institute; 2019 Jan [1996; revised 2011 Feb; cited 2019 Jun 3]. Available from: http://nwtresearch.com/sites/default/files/ari_guide_to_research_2019.pdf
6. Inuit Tapiriit Kanatami. National Inuit strategy on research. Ottawa (ON): Inuit Tapiriit Kanatami; 2018 [cited 2019 Jun 3]. Available from: https://www.itk.ca/wp-content/uploads/2020/10/ITK-National-Inuit-Strategy-on-Research.pdf
7. Mi'kmaq Ethics Watch. Mi'kmaw research principles and protocols [Internet]. Sydney (NS): Unama'ki College of Cape Breton University; 2015 [cited 2015 Sep 5]. Available from: http://mikmaki.ca/wp-content/uploads/2016/07/Mikmaw-Research-Principles.pdf
8. Brunger F, Russell T. Risk and representation in research ethics: the NunatuKavut experience. J Empir Res Hum Res Ethics. 2015 Oct;10(4):368–79.
9. NunatuKavut Community Council [Internet]. Application for research with NunatuKavut; 2013 [rev 2014 Jul; cited 2015 Sep 5]. Available from: https://nunatukavut.ca/departments/research-education-culture/
10. Vice-Present, Research. AR-03 research ethics policy [Internet]. Whitehorse (YK): Yukon University; 2009 [revised 2014 Oct; cited 2019 Jun 3]. Available from: http://www.yukoncollege.yk.ca/sites/default/files/inline-files/AR-03_Research_Ethics_Policy_-_October_2014_0.pdf
11. Arctic Institute of Community-Based Research for Northern Health and Well-Being [Internet]. Whitehorse (YK): Arctic Institute of Community-Based Research for Northern Health and Well-Being; 2019. Community-based research [cited 2019 Jun 3]. Available from: http://www.aicbr.ca/community-based-research
12. Nunavut Research Institute (NRI) [Internet]. Iqaluit (NU): Nunavut Research Institute. Research licensing applications; 2015 [cited 2021 Mar 1]. Available from: https://www.nri.nu.ca/research-licensing-applications
13. Nunavut Arctic College. Obtaining a research license under Nunavut's Scientists Act: a guide for applicants [Internet]. Iqaluit (NU): Nunavut Arctic College; 2018 Dec [cited 2019 Jun 3]. Available from: http://www.nri.nu.ca/sites/default/files/public/licence_application_guidelines20182.pdf
14. An Indigenous political organization representing the Inuit of Nunavik since 1978 [Internet]. Kuujjuaq (QC): Makivik Corporation. Nunavik Research Centre; 2019 [cited 2019 Jun 3]. Available from: http://www.makivik.org/nunavik-research-centre/
15. Assembly of First Nations Quebec-Labrador. First Nations in Quebec and Labrador's research protocol, 2014 [Internet]. Wendake (QC): Assembly of First Nations Quebec-Labrador; 2014 [cited 2019 Jun 3]. Available from http://cssspnql.com/docs/default-source/centre-de-documentation/protocole_recherche_en_web.pdf

16. Nunatsiavut Research Centre [Internet]. Nain (NL): Nunatsiavut Government. Nunatsiavut Government research advisory committee; 2021 [cited 2021 Mar 1]. Available from: https://nunatsiavutresearchcentre.com/ngrac/
17. Our data. Our stories. Our future [Internet]. Akwesasne (ON): First Nations Information Governance Centre. About FNIGC; 2019 [cited 2019 Jun 3]. Available from: https://fnigc.ca/about-fnigc/
18. Association of Canadian Universities for Northern Studies. Ethical principles for the conduct of research in the North [Internet]. Ottawa (ON): Association of Canadian Universities for Northern Studies; 2003 [cited 2019 Jun 3] Available from: https://acuns.ca/wp-content/uploads/2010/09/EthicsEnglishmarch2003.pdf
19. Battiste M, editor. Reclaiming Indigenous voice and vision. Vancouver (BC): UBC Press; 2000.
20. Zawati MH, Junker A, Knoppers BM, Rahimzadeh V. Streamlining review of research involving humans: Canadian models. J Med Genet. 2015 Aug;52(8):566–9.
21. Enzle ME, Schmaltz R. Ethics review of multi-centre clinical trials in Canada. Health Law Rev. 2005;(13):51–7.
22. Matheson LA, Huber AM, Warner A, Rosenberg AM. Ethics application protocols for multicentre clinical studies in Canada: a paediatric rheumatology experience. Paediatr Child Health. 2012 Jun;17(6):313–16.
23. Brunger F, Wall D. "What do they really mean by partnerships?" Questioning the unquestionable good in ethics guidelines promoting community engagement in Indigenous health Research. Qual Health Res. 2016 Nov;26(13):1862–77.
24. Government of Newfoundland and Labrador [Internet]. St. John's (NL): Queen's Printer. Health Research Ethics Authority Act, SNL2006 chapter H-1.2; 2013 [amended 2011; cited 2015 Feb 27]. Available from: http://assembly.nl.ca/Legislation/sr/statutes/h01-2.htm
25. Brunger FR, Schiff R, Morton-Ninomiya, M, Bull J. Animating the concept of ethical space: the Labrador Aboriginal Health Research Committee ethics workshop. Int J Indig Health. 2014;10(1):3–15.
26. Schnarch B. Ownership, control, access, and possession (OCAP) or self-determination applied to research. J Aborig Health. 2004;1(1):80–95.
27. Burgess MM, Brunger F. Collective effects of medical research. In: McDonald M, editor. The governance of health research involving human subjects (HRIHS). Ottawa (ON): Law Commission of Canada; 2000. p. 117–52.
28. Glass KC, Kaufert J. Research ethics review and Aboriginal community values: can the two be reconciled? J Empir Res Hum Res Ethics. 2007 Jun;2(2):25–40.
29. Kaufert J, Commanda L, Elias B, Grey R, KueYoung T, Masuzumi B. Evolving participation of Aboriginal communities in health research ethics review: the impact of the Inuvik workshop. Int J Circumpolar Health. 1999 Apr;58(2):134–44.
30. Macaulay AC, Delormier T, McComber AM, Cross EJ, Potvin LP, Paradis G, Kirby RL, Saad-Haddad C, Desrosiers S. Participatory research with native community

of Kahnawake creates innovative code of research ethics. Can J Public Health. 1998 Mar–Apr;89(2):105–8.

31. Weijer C, Goldsand G, Emanuel EJ. Protecting communities in research: current guidelines and limits of extrapolation. Nat Genet. 1999 Nov;23(3):275–80.
32. Weijer C. Protecting communities in research: philosophical and pragmatic challenges. Camb Q Healthc Ethics. 1999;8(4):501–13.
33. Brunger F, Weijer C. Politics, risk, and community in the ICBG-Chiapas case. In: Lavery VJ, Wahl ER, Grady C, Emanuel EJ, editors. Ethical issues in international biomedical research: a casebook. New York (NY): Oxford University Press; 2007. p. 35–42.
34. Battiste M. Research ethics for protecting Indigenous knowledge and heritage: Institutional and researcher responsibilities. In: Denzin NK, Lincoln YS, Tuhiwai Smith L, editors. Handbook of critical and Indigenous methodologies. Thousand Oaks (CA): Sage; 2008. p. 497–510.
35. Kovach M. Emerging from the margins: Indigenous methodologies. In: Brown L, Strega S, editors. Research as resistance: revisiting critical, Indigenous, and anti-oppressive approaches. Toronto (ON): Canadian Scholars' Press; 2015. p. 43–64.
36. Stiegman ML, Castleden H. Leashes and lies: navigating the colonial tensions of institutional ethics of research involving Indigenous peoples in Canada. Int Indig Policy J. 2015;6(3):2.
37. Morton Ninomiya ME, Pollock NJ. Reconciling community-based Indigenous research and academic practices: Knowing principles is not always enough. Soc Sci Med. 2017 Jan;172:28–36.
38. Riddell JK, Salamanca A, Pepler DJ, Cardinal S, McIvor O. Laying the groundwork: a practical guide for ethical research with Indigenous communities. Int Indig Policy J [Internet]. 2017 [cited 2021 Mar 1];8(2). Available from: https://ir.lib.uwo.ca/iipj/vol8/iss2/6
39. Sylvestre P, Castleden H, Martin D, McNally M. "Thank you very much … you can leave our community now.": geographies of responsibility, relational ethics, acts of refusal, and the conflicting requirements of academic localities in Indigenous research. ACME: Int E-J Crit Geog [Internet]. 2018 [cited 2021 Mar 1];17(3). Available from: https://www.acme-journal.org/index.php/acme/article/view/1327

20 Patchy and Southern Centric: Rewriting Health Policies for Northern and Indigenous Canadians

JOSÉE G. LAVOIE, DEREK KORNELSEN, AND YVONNE BOYER

Introduction

Although Canada is a vast country, four-fifths of its population lives near the US border. It is not surprising, then, that most policies, whether related to resource exploitation or health care, are driven by the needs of populations, corporations, and governments in the "south."[1] This approach reflects priorities and service delivery mechanisms that poorly serve the interest of Canadians living in rural, remote, and northern environments.

Canada's North, the *northern hinterland* as defined by Statistics Canada (1), is a collection of hundreds of relatively small communities, peppered over large tracts of land. Indigenous communities are located in areas of spiritual and cultural significance that are also used for food harvesting. In some cases (on the west coast for example), these settlements preceded colonial encroachment (2). In other, and in fact most, cases, these settlements emerged as a result of colonial activities, which included Treaty signing; the creation of Métis settlements, First Nation reserves, and Inuit permanent communities, which forced settlement to facilitate the expansion of the post–World War II welfare state; and the imposition of colonial policies (3). Still, for the most part, First Nations, Métis, and Inuit communities emerged in areas of historical, cultural, spiritual, and economic significance, at a time when rivers and the sea were the main means of transportation. A shift to land-based transportation resulted in a rerouting of economic activities, which now largely bypass many Indigenous communities.

In contrast to Indigenous peoples' experience, many, if not most, non-Indigenous northern communities emerged as a result of economic activities (mainly resource extraction) and can and do collapse when these activities wane. This difference is of fundamental importance since many Indigenous communities have become economically, politically, and geographically marginalized and remote through the economic development of settler societies and the infrastructures that have been put in place to serve them.

In this chapter, we define the Canadian North to include Canada's three territories (Yukon, the Northwest Territories, and Nunavut) and the northern part of seven provinces. We draw from other northern contexts, including the US state of Alaska; Greenland, which is an autonomous constituent country within the Kingdom of Denmark; the northern Scandinavian countries of Sweden, Norway, and Finland, the last of which is home to Indigenous Sámi; and northern Russia, which is also the home of Indigenous Sámi and of numerous other Indigenous populations (Aleuts, Alyutors, Chelkans, Chukchis, Chulyms, Chuvans, Dolgans, Enets, Siberian Yupik, Inuit, Evenks, Evens, Itelmens, Kamchadals, Kereks, Khanty, Koryaks, Kumandins, Mansi, Nanai, Negidals, Nenets, Nganasans, Nivkhs, Oroks, Orochs, Selkups, Shors, Soyots, Taz, Telengits, Teleuts, Tofalars or Tofa, Tubalars, Tozhu, Udege, Ulchs, Veps, and Yukaghirs) (4).

Although this chapter focuses on northern contexts, in Canada, important policies remain largely driven by Ottawa. The territories retain substantial autonomy on matters of territorial jurisdiction (including health care) that are nevertheless constrained by limited budgets; a considerable amount of care (tertiary and specialized care and, in some cases, primary and secondary care as well) is accessed by territorial residents in southern provinces. For northern Indigenous peoples living in Quebec and Newfoundland and Labrador, policies are defined in the provincial capitals. The same is true for all countries cited above, including Greenland, which remains largely influenced by Denmark-defined health policies. Like Canadian territorial residents, Greenlanders also have to travel, in their case to Copenhagen, to access tertiary and specialized care (5).

Bringing together findings from two different studies, the Policy Synthesis Project and a project focusing on a health policy review of Organisation for Economic Co-operation and Development (OECD) countries, this chapter focuses on the policy framework that currently informs northern and northern Indigenous health service delivery. We draw from the experience of other circumpolar countries to provide a framework for the analysis of health policies. Our analysis highlights complexities, innovations, and areas requiring more attention. We conclude by proposing promising northern-centric policy options.

Locating Ourselves

I, Josée Lavoie, am of French-Quebec ancestry. I grew up in northern Quebec communities where resource extraction was the dominant economy. My family was engaged in Quiet Revolution developments, with a focus on bringing congression-led and private hospitals into the newly created Quebec public health care system. When I was growing up, access to care in rural and remote communities was the centre of my discussions with my father. The same issues remain a core interest today. It was this interest that led me to make the Nunavik health care system the focus of my master's thesis; to move to Rankin Inlet (then part of the Northwest Territories) in 1990 to work for the Keewatin Regional Health Board and learn from that perspective about the federal policy of devolution of responsibilities (including health care) to the territories; and to work for and learn from Saskatchewan First Nation health organizations (Peter Ballantyne Cree Nation, the Prince Albert Grand Council) that are managing their own on-reserve health care systems. The same interest took me to Tromsö, Norway; motivated me to apply to the Fulbright Arctic Initiative Scholarship program; and is now leading me to learn from the Southcentral Foundation in Alaska as a Fulbright Arctic scholar.

I, Yvonne Boyer, am a Métis mother and grandmother who grew up in Moose Jaw, Saskatchewan. My Métis ancestry comes from Saskatchewan and the Red River. I spent much of my life as a nurse working in small rural hospitals. The experiences I had working in the hospitals were the grounding for my work as a lawyer. As a result, my academic focus has been on studying the intersect between health and the law. I have dedicated my career to advocating for Indigenous health practices and Treaty rights to health and to addressing racism and discrimination against First Nations, Métis, and Inuit peoples in health care policies and systems.

I, Derek Kornelsen, identify as a non-Indigenous settler in Canada. My ancestors were Mennonites and arrived in Canada from Europe in the late eighteenth and early nineteenth centuries. It was only in my early adult life that I began to learn about the past and present practices of colonization in Canada. I became interested in *decolonization* after spending a number of years working in Winnipeg's inner city with Indigenous youth and adults. Here, I recognized that typical non-Indigenous systems tend to pathologize Indigenous peoples while imposing "solutions" that perpetuate colonial world views and control and that undermine Indigenous self-determination and well-being. This led me to pursue graduate studies focused on understanding the philosophical foundations of Western and Indigenous political, legal, and social systems with an aim to better understand how to decolonize colonial systems. Since then, I've been fortunate to develop professional and personal relationships with Indigenous individuals and communities, focusing our work mainly on how "resource development" impacts Indigenous peoples' lands, rights, and well-being and using this knowledge to decolonize policy and practice at the local, provincial or territorial, and national levels. I am incredibly grateful to the communities and individuals who have taken the time to teach me so much and have trusted me with their friendship.

Method

The Policy Synthesis Project was a desk review of Canadian federal, provincial, and territorial legislation and policies containing Indigenous-specific provisions (6). The information for this project was compiled over one year (March 2007–April 2008). Internet key word searches included the following terms and combinations of these words: Aboriginal, First Nation(s), Inuit, Métis or Métis, Indian, *Amérindiens*, reserve, health, and medical. Key websites explored included the Parliamentary Library; Health Canada;[2] the Public Health Agency of Canada; Indigenous and Northern Affairs Canada; Department of Justice Canada; Statistics Canada; the Aboriginal Canada Portal (now archived); provincial and territorial websites, including any ministries/departments responsible for Indigenous affairs or health; and Indigenous organizations.

The health policy review of OECD countries focused on health services for vulnerable and marginalized populations. The information collated for this chapter was obtained from the policy documents of English-speaking countries and countries with policy documents that have been translated into English. For non-English-speaking countries or countries with no English translation for policy documents, we obtained information from peer-review articles and from recognized organizations. In some cases, Google Translate was also used. A literature review was conducted by a computer-generated search of a number of key words, including mental illness; homeless/homelessness/rooflessness; drug and alcohol misuse; injection/intravenous drug users; marginalization; access; policy; HIV/AIDS; ethnic/visible minorities; margin; and social exclusion. The key words were entered into a database search of CINHAL; Medline; PsycINFO; PubMed Central; Science Direct; and Biomed Central Open Access. Finally, grey literature, including current reports, policy, and unpublished documents from health organizations were searched. This information was supplemented with a more in-depth analysis of policies in place in Norway to meet the needs of vulnerable populations (7) and supplemented by 15 interviews with service providers and decision makers. Norway was chosen because it is the only Scandinavian country to have an explicit Sámi policy.[3] In this chapter, the international analysis is used to position Canada's experience within a larger, international context.

Findings

Paradigms at Play

Internationally, northern Indigenous health policies have been informed by either of two, at times complementary, at times contradictory, paradigms. A first paradigm focuses on equity and responsiveness. Within this paradigm, debates have emerged as to the best way to ensure equity and responsiveness in health care. Some have advocated for parallel (vertical-equity-informed) services to ensure equity and responsiveness in health services. For example, countries like Canada and the United States developed parallel health services specifically to serve the needs of First Nations and Inuit (10,11). Critiques of this approach have argued that separate services will invariably be under-resourced (12). Instead, Scandinavian countries such as Norway have focused on integrated services (7) but fail to monitor their performance on achieving equity.

The second paradigm privileges a definition of Indigenous self-determination that requires self-administration. This paradigm echoes the language embedded in international covenants with their focus on cultural protection and revitalization. For example, the United Nations Declaration on the Rights of Indigenous Peoples Article 23 deems that "Indigenous peoples have the right to determine and develop priorities and strategies for exercising their right to development" (13 p9). In particular, Indigenous peoples have the right to be actively involved in developing and determining health, housing, and other economic and social programs affecting them and, as far as possible, to administer such programs through their own institutions (13). In addition, the United Nations framework of treaties and covenants guarantees equality rights, self-determination of peoples, respect for human rights, and fundamental freedoms for all without distinction as to race, sex, language, religion, and conditions of economic and social progress and development. These are basic rights that all human beings share. Health is also a basic human right, appearing in a variety of United Nations instruments or conventions that compose the United Nations framework. The right to health encompasses the right to a culturally appropriate health care system. As with other human rights, the right to health is particularly concerned with the disadvantaged, the marginalized, and the vulnerable while confirming standards of equality and non-discrimination. State obligations to fulfil the right to health are monitored by human rights bodies. Canada, as signatory to a number of international treaties and covenants, has acknowledged the importance of health to the well-being of Indigenous peoples and recognized Indigenous peoples have a right to health, based on international law (14). To date, most attempts at operationalizing this paradigm have focused primarily on Indigenous control of community-based primary health care services.

In Canada and other countries, both paradigms are currently at play in Indigenous health discourses, and many leaders and scholars make use of both simultaneously in their arguments. This is not necessarily problematic, at this time, when health inequities continue to be prevalent in most communities and countries. However, the arguments are often conflated. This is problematic because Indigenous rights are not an outcome of health or other inequities.

Rather, these Indigenous rights are recognized and affirmed by section 35 (1) of the Constitution Act, 1982 as inherent "Aboriginal rights"[4] or negotiated "treaty rights" (14,15). In countries where health inequities are either not prevalent or simply not documented (Scandinavian countries come to mind), the legitimacy of Indigenous rights is challenged by the prevailing commitment to the "equity and responsiveness" paradigm. While the equity and responsiveness paradigm is also relevant in northern, non-Indigenous contexts, community-level self-determination is Indigenous-specific.

Northern and Indigenous Systems Designs

From an international perspective, jurisdictions have approached northern Indigenous health system designs based on geography and history, but also on demographic factors. Table 20.1 provides an overview of Indigenous and northern health systems designs, highlighting demographic factors.

There are a few key points to be made, based on the above. First, ensuring access to services that are responsive to Indigenous needs in Indigenous-centric systems, where Indigenous peoples are a majority, is less of a concern. In such contexts, which tend to be northern-based, the democratic process alone can reasonably be expected to ensure that decisions are northern centric and responsive to Indigenous needs. The same cannot be assumed of southern-centric contexts.

In integrated systems in which northern Indigenous peoples are a relatively small minority, equity oversight is necessary and requires a strong regulatory and monitoring system. We note that very little information exists on northern Indigenous peoples' access to health services in Russia, although a recent report suggests that "many indigenous peoples are today deprived of ... access [to health services] due to a policy of dismantling public services in remote settlements" (4 p33). The OECD's review of the Russian health care system suggests an emerging regulatory oversight now nested in the Federal Service for Supervision of Consumer Protection and Welfare (*Rospotrebnadzor*) and the Federal Service in Surveillance in Health Care and Social Development (16). This regulatory system focuses on quality of care but is silent on Indigenous or northern access to health services. Likewise, Scandinavian countries' regulatory systems focus on equitable access for Sámi, if not fully fluent in the local Scandinavian language. There is no monitoring of equitable access to health services focusing on the needs of Sámi (7), this despite documented evidence of discrimination and racism (17,18).

In contrast, ensuring that parallel services can be responsive and contribute to better outcomes requires appropriate funding, investments in quality improvement processes, and integration of services within the larger health care system. This is poorly developed in Canada (health information systems, prejudice, jurisdiction, underfunding, see 19,20).

Table 20.1 Indigenous and northern health systems designs

Model	Demographic context	Description	Jurisdictions
Northern-centric systems	Located in northern jurisdictions	Systems located in areas where northern concerns predominate political decision making	Canada's territories, Alaska, Greenland
Southern-centric systems	Located in jurisdictions in which a relatively small portion of the population lives in northern contexts	Systems located in areas where northern concerns are likely to be overshadowed by southern concerns; northern-based regional authorities can mitigate limitations to some extent	Canada's provinces, Scandinavian countries
Indigenous-centric systems	Jurisdictions in which Indigenous people are the majority	Health system design more integrated, with few provisions for cultural protection	Nunavut and Greenland
Integrated systems	Jurisdictions in which Indigenous population is small and arguably more vulnerable	Few provisions to ensure that services are culturally appropriate	Sweden, Norway, Finland, and Russia
Parallel systems	"In-between" jurisdictions, in which Indigenous populations constitute between 25% and 60% of the overall populations	In Yukon and Alaska, parallel services exist; Northwest Territories adopted some policy-specific provisions to address specific issues	Canada's federally funded on-reserve health services in the provinces and, to a lesser extent, Alaska, and Yukon*

*The Alaska Native Tribal Health Consortium manages its own first-, second-, and third-level health care system, and is considered a model worldwide (https://anthc.org). Yukon communities can compete for funding along with other urban Indigenous non-government organizations to provide selected primary prevention programs.

Ensuring equitable access to health services in most health systems requires state constitutional protection of Indigenous rights, especially in countries where Indigenous peoples are small minorities. For northern populations, ensuring equitable access requires the adoption of northern-centric policies promoting the implementation of models of care adapted to northern communities' priorities and needs. The following section discusses the policy framework that currently exists in Canada.

Canada's Northern and Indigenous Health Policies

Canada's northern health policy landscape is unique in that it includes the three territories, the northern portion of seven provinces (Prince Edward Island, Nova Scotia, and New Brunswick do not have northern jurisdictions), and Indigenous Services Canada, which since 2018 has replaced in name but not yet in structure and approaches the First Nations and Inuit Health Branch of Health Canada (FNIHB; 21). This 14th health care system, which cuts across some territorial and all provincial health care systems, is the only health care system in Canada operating primarily in rural and remote communities.[5] This section discusses legislative and policy options in these jurisdictions, and then discusses their relevance to access to health care in the north.

FEDERAL JURISDICTION

The 1867 British North America Act (also known as the Constitution Act, 1867) created the federal dominion. The Constitution Act, 1867 defined "Indians and lands reserved for Indians" as an area of federal jurisdiction and health services as an area of provincial jurisdiction. As shown in Table 20.2, the language was, however, broad, leaving considerable room for interpretation.

Broadly speaking, the current interpretation of these provisions is that the federal government is responsible for matters related to those recognized as "Indians" under the Indian Act and Inuit.[6] Since the 2016 Daniels' decision (24), Métis and non-status Indians are recognized as Indians under section 91(24) of the Constitution Act. As this decision has yet to shift the application of policies, the discussion that follows will highlight implementation as it exists at the time of writing.

The federal government's engagement in health care delivery was and remains, according to the federal government, not an obligation defined in the Constitution or the Treaties but rather a matter of policy. According to the federal government's policy, services are provided for humanitarian reasons only, to compliment services provided by the provinces and territories (25; also see 26 p178–81). This interpretation of obligations is, however, not shared by

Table 20.2 Areas of exclusive jurisdiction, 1867

Areas of federal jurisdiction	Areas of provincial jurisdiction
91(24) Indians, and Lands reserved for the Indians.	92(7) The Establishment, Maintenance, and Management of Hospitals, Asylums, Charities, and Eleemosynary Institutions in and for the Province, other than Marine Hospitals.

First Nations. First Nations signatories of Treaties 6, 8, 10, and 11 negotiated access to health care services (6). Only Treaty 6 shows written evidence of these discussions; however, in oral negotiations health was discussed and the interpretation of this provision remains a matter of debate (15). More recently, the 1979 Indian Health Policy was adopted largely to appease First Nations' unrest following a federal attempt in 1978 to limit access to a key program, the Non-Insured Health Benefit (NIHB) program, to only those living in poverty (27). Rather than being humanitarian policy, access to the NIHB program has long been defended by First Nations as a matter of inherent Aboriginal rights and negotiated Treaty rights. The 1979 Indian Health Policy is a two-page document that highlights the importance of community development, the relationship of the federal government with Indian communities, and the Canadian health care system as the three pillars, but that makes no commitment or statement of obligations (28).

The current federal legislative and policy framework remains remarkably limited, with no federal legislation defining federal obligations towards Indigenous peoples living in the territories or the provinces. Indigenous Services Canada now funds services previously funded or provided by FNIHB. These services, which include community-based health services on First Nations reserves across all provinces and in the Yukon, are provided outside of any legislative or policy obligations. The services funded or provided remained largely undefined until the production of the first Program Compendium in 2003 (29), a resource that has been periodically updated since (30). The compendium includes mainly primary and secondary prevention programs, and a basic level of primary care provided by nurses with an expanded scope of practice in selected remote and larger northern communities (nursing stations). This resource is the closest to a definition of *obligations* in existence. We are not aware of provincial defined obligations to northern jurisdictions. Finally, the lack of coordination between the federal government and provincial jurisdictions has been well documented and results in poorer outcomes (for examples, see 31,32).

PROVINCIAL AND TERRITORIAL RESPONSIBILITIES

Until the late 1980s, the federal government oversaw the provisions of health services in Yukon and the Northwest Territories. At the time, Nunavut was still part of the Northwest Territories. The idea of devolving the responsibility of managing health care to the territories had been progressively happening since the 1970s (33). From a legislative and policy context, territorial health care systems are somewhat younger than provincial systems. From a service delivery perspective, small populations and low densities limit the viability of providing specialized care in the territories. North-south corridors of referral thus exist, as shown in Table 20.3. These grew largely from flight corridors (34 p44).

Table 20.3 Jurisdictional implications of accessing a full complement of health care services, depending on residence

Northern jurisdiction	North-south referral pattern	Crossing jurisdictions
Yukon (YK)	Communities to Whitehorse, YK, to Vancouver, BC	Territorial-provincial
Northwest Territories (NWT)	Yellowknife, NWT, to Edmonton, AB	Territorial-provincial
Nunavut: Kitikmeot	Edmonton, AB	Territorial-provincial
Nunavut: Kivalliq	Winnipeg, MB	Territorial-provincial
Nunavut: Qikiqtaaluk	Ottawa, ON	Territorial-provincial
Northern British Columbia*	Vancouver, BC	Federal-provincial for on-reserve residents
Northern Alberta*	Edmonton, AB	Federal-provincial for on-reserve residents
Northern Saskatchewan*	Prince Albert to Saskatoon or Regina, SK	None
Northern Manitoba†	Winnipeg, MB	Federal-provincial for on-reserve residents
Northern Ontario‡	Sioux Lookout, Thunder Bay, Sudbury, Toronto, or Ottawa	Federal-provincial for on-reserve residents
Northern Quebec‡	Montreal, QC	James Bay and Northern Quebec Agreement-provincial; federal-provincial for Innu
Labrador	St Johns, NL	Federal-provincial for Innu; Nunatsiavut/NunatuKavut governments to provincial for Inuit

Source: Based on (1).

* Defined as north of the 54th parallel † Defined as north of the 53rd parallel ‡ Defined as north of the 49th parallel

While most Canadians think of medicare as a national program that applies across all jurisdictions, the Canada Health Act (1984), in fact, does not apply on First Nation reserves. The Canada Health Act (1984) is an act of parliament that specifies the conditions and criteria (public administration; comprehensiveness; universality; portability; and accessibility of insured benefits, which include hospital care and access to family physicians and specialists) with which the provincial and territorial health insurance programs (known as medicare) must conform to receive federal transfers of payment under the Canada Health

Transfer (35). While provisions of the Canada Health Act imply access to insured benefits (hospital care, access to family physicians and specialists) for all Canadians, including northerners, the Act provides no guidance on how jurisdictions are to resolve cross-jurisdictional service provision.

Territorial residents who require access to medical services not available in the territories are referred to a provincial point of care where these services can be accessed without charge. Provincial authorities track these services and invoice territorial health departments. No such mechanism exists for First Nations who manage their own health services on reserve. First Nation communities receive funding for health services delivered on reserve only for residents recognized as "Indians" under the Indian Act who live on reserve. When non-status residents, non-Indigenous residents, and those living off-reserve use on-reserve health services, the First Nation is not compensated for the services.[7] Thus, underfunded health services (36) are stretched even further, creating responsiveness and sustainability issues.

When looking at territorial and provincial health legislative frameworks, we note some jurisdictions (Northwest Territories, BC, Saskatchewan,[8] Manitoba, Ontario, Quebec, and Newfoundland and Labrador) have in place a regionalized model of health care planning and delivery. Provinces with such regional health authority (HA) systems have northern-centric HAs (Northern Health in BC; Athabasca, Keewatin Yatthé, and Mamawetan Churchill River in Saskatchewan; Northern in Manitoba; North East and North West in Ontario; Nord-du-Québec, Terres-Cries-de-la-Baie-James, and Nunavik in QC; Labrador-Grenfell Health in Labrador) where priorities in health care planning and delivery are more likely to reflect northern and Indigenous priorities. Generally, provincial health authority legislation does not require Indigenous representation on the boards (23). Ontario is a notable exception. The boundaries defined for these authorities may or may not coincide with tribal/nation boundaries, thus creating another dimension of jurisdictional complexities (6). Notable exceptions are the Terres-Cries-de-la-Baie-James and Nunavik HAs in Quebec, both created as a result of the 1974 James Bay and Northern Agreement, an agreement often referred to as the first modern treaty.

Existing noteworthy health legislation includes those containing specific provisions to clarify these territories' and provinces' responsibilities in Indigenous health. These are, however, quite limited and focus on jurisdiction. For example, legislation in Alberta is said to apply to Métis settlements. Alberta, Saskatchewan, and Ontario legislation specifically state that the minister may opt to enter into an agreement with Canada or First Nations for the delivery of health services, thereby clearly indicating that the provisions of services is outside the province's mandate. Health legislation in Yukon, Quebec, and Newfoundland and Labrador contains provisions related to existing self-government agreements, thereby clarifying the territory's and provinces' roles and responsibilities in health only in the areas included in these self-government agreements.

A few pieces of legislation scattered across Canada recognize Indigenous healing knowledges and practices. Ontario extends this exemption to traditional healers. British Columbia, Alberta, Saskatchewan, Manitoba, and Ontario exempt the use of tobacco for ceremonial purposes from being regulated under their tobacco legislation (6). Yukon is the only jurisdiction in which health legislation recognizes the need to respect traditional healing practices. Quebec, Ontario, and Manitoba recognize that Indigenous midwives should be exempted from control specified under the Code of Professions. Article 6.1 of the Nunavut Consolidation of Midwifery Profession Act (37) states that only registered midwives can practise midwifery (although instructional content of the midwifery course must contain content based on traditional Inuit knowledge, skills, and judgment). What this means is that Inuit midwives who have been traditionally trained by Indigenous methods and who have not completed the midwifery education regulated by Nunavut may be found guilty, fined, and imprisoned "for a term not exceeding three months" (37 article 4). Considering the practice of midwifery is an inherent Aboriginal right that is protected by the Constitution Act, 1982, this and other similar legislation fails to consider the Indigenous inherent right to health and may be in direct contravention of Canada's Constitution.

Discussion: Existing and Proposed Innovations in Northern and Remote Regions

A recent review of the literature on innovations in northern and remote regions, which included 383 articles, suggests that the literature is generally optimistic, highlighting innovations in organizational structure of health services, use of telehealth and eHealth, medical transportation, and public health challenges. Sadly, the literature focused primarily on foreign initiatives (38). In the Canadian context, effective innovations need to address equitable access to a full continuum of care, often across jurisdictions. From northern and Indigenous standpoints, the Canadian health care map more readily resembles an unassembled puzzle with numerous missing pieces. At a system's level, progress requires the creation of a northern and Indigenous-centric system supported by legislation and policies. Despite a paucity of supportive policies, some innovations are noteworthy.

Innovation 1: Aligning Indigenous and Provincial Health Authorities' Territories

As noted above, the northern Quebec Terres-Cries-de-la-Baie-James and Nunavik HAs are the only regional HAs, that we know of, created with respect for Indigenous nationhood. They are an outcome of the James Bay and Northern

Quebec Agreement, designed specifically to meet the needs of James Bay Cree and Nunavik Inuit, respectively. They are a by-product of federal-provincial-Indigenous negotiations yet were integrated into the Quebec health care governance system on par with other health authorities. These two health authorities are able to represent the interests of Cree and Inuit populations at provincial policy and implementation tables, thereby ensuring that the needs of northern Cree and Inuit are known and considered in Quebec policy development.

Innovation 2: Welcoming Indigenous Peoples to Northern Cross-Jurisdictional Tables

In BC, the First Nations Health Authority (FNHA) is now resourced to plan, manage, deliver, and fund health services previously provided by the federal government. This provides the FNHA substantial leverage to address jurisdictional and health services gaps in First Nation and other settings, including the North. Although the innovation is relatively new and hasn't yet had the opportunity to demonstrate its full potential, it remains a promising model for other jurisdictions (39). Quebec Nunavik Inuit and James Bay Cree have been managing their own local health services since the late 1970s through a tripartite (federal-provincial-Indigenous governments) agreement.

Innovation 3: Apply Principles in Policy Development That Include the Constitutional Supremacy of Aboriginal and Treaty Rights

To initiate new government health policies, certain principles must be acknowledged and discussed. National linkages must be created that bridge the divide between federal, provincial, and territorial governments and Indigenous peoples. An example is the *First Nations Health Blueprint for British Columbia* (40), which was created in 2005 to improve access and quality of health services for all Indigenous peoples through a collaborative approach that included the Canadian governments and the national Aboriginal organizations (representing their constituents). The following key principles were noted:

- Health is holistic in nature.
- The distinctiveness of the constitutionally recognized Indigenous groups must be acknowledged, with partnerships built on inclusion.
- A funding source is required, and the *Blueprint* must be reviewed in a timely manner to ensure accountability and goal attainment.

Integral to the framework are several approaches that were fundamental to the *Blueprint*, such as building on Indigenous knowledge, women's participation, the determinants of health, engagement and inclusivity, sustainability and accountability, and a description of current mandates.

To put the frameworks into action, a distinction-based approach was implemented that addressed the specific needs of First Nations, Métis, and Inuit. The 2005 *Blueprint* called for a 10-year transformative plan (the federal self-government agreements were cognizant of the timelines) and called for the recognition of the constitutionally protected rights of Aboriginal peoples in Canada. The *Blueprint* did not confine itself to health necessities but looked at policy developments from a collaborative, holistic perspective – confirming that there are no quick fixes.

These three innovations indicate areas of significant progress. In addition to these, we propose a broader, over-arching innovation to further guide northern policy development across Canada.

Proposed Innovation: Using a "Whole Approach" (Whole of Indigenous and non-Indigenous Government Approach)

Collaborative efforts must address the needs of both Indigenous peoples and government to move forward. We propose that certain key principles must be reflected and adhered to while developing, changing, and influencing policy:

- Every Indigenous person born in Canada has a powerful set of constitutionally protected rights through section 35 of the Constitution Act, 1982.
- Health care policies must reflect the constitutional rights as expressed in section 35.
- These constitutional rights include (among others) the inherent right to self-determination, self-government, and control over one's own living circumstances and quality of life (41).
- Root causes of ill health (colonization, southern-centric policies, legislative policies, guardian and ward theories, etc.) must be addressed, rejected, and replaced with policies that reflect the fiduciary relationship between the federal and provincial and territorial governments and Indigenous people (42 p20).
- A collaborative approach that includes the whole of government (federal, provincial, territorial, municipal, and Indigenous) and all three constitutionally recognized Indigenous groups, with acknowledgment of the distinctions within each group. This approach is required to establish the political will to affect change and implement policy reform and constitutionalized Indigenous health care.
- A holistic approach must be engaged that considers all determinants of health and all aspects of health; that connects every person to their family, community, and nation through a cycle of interdependence; and that is

cognizant of the requirement that self-determination includes the ability to determine timelines.
- An evidence-based approach must be used to advance Indigenous health.

While there is a significant and growing body of work by First Nations scholars and organizations outlining their particular perspectives on health and wellness, less is known to date about Métis and Inuit perspectives. More research must be conducted to develop Inuit- and Métis-specific programs and approaches. However, important studies are emerging, such as the *Social Determinants of Inuit Health in Canada* (43) and *Land, Family and Identity: Contextualizing Métis Health and Well-Being* (44). These provide a pathway towards the developments of Inuit- and Métis-centric programs, policies, and strategies.

Proposed Innovation: A Canada Health Act for the New Millennium and for All Canadians

The Canada Health Act remains focused on guaranteed access to high-cost, curative care: insured services include hospital, family physician, and specialist care. Provincial and territorial authorities have expanded this list to include a complement of other public health and preventive services, in the hope of shifting the use of health services towards prevention. Despite recorded worst outcomes in rural and northern communities, which correlate in part with poorer access to care, southern-centric delivery models informed by stringent scope of practice regulations limit opportunities for northern-centric innovations. It is time to reopen the Canada Health Act and embed guarantees of access for all Canadians.

Conclusion

Health care delivery in northern contexts is challenged by jurisdiction, geography, climate, low population density, and, in some, policies that have been developed with a southern-centric and urban-context focus. In the Canadian context, the interplay of multiple jurisdictional authorities adds additional barriers and complexities. Indigenous peoples living in these environments face additional challenges when trying to access health services, which are exacerbated when they need specialized care only available in urban centres, where jurisdictional, linguistic, cultural, and contextual misunderstandings and prejudice can undermine the quality of care.

This chapter has focused on the legislative and policy framework that currently informs northern health service delivery, highlighting innovations, complexities, and areas requiring more attention. We conclude with a suggestion for a broad strategic vision to create a new policy framework for the future for First

Nations, Métis, and Inuit peoples – one that uses an interdisciplinary approach with the law to address barriers and challenges in the current system. Intertwined with this recommendation is the need to reopen the Canada Health Act to include commitments to access to care that considers northern context and speaks to these needs directly. It is our reflection that northern and Indigenous northern health remains an afterthought in the current Canadian health care systems and that outcomes can only improve with legislative and policy renewal.

NOTES

1 In this chapter, we use the word *south* to refer mainly to the national and provincial capitals, which we argue more readily take into consideration the needs of populations at proximity.

2 The First Nations and Inuit Health Branch of Health Canada, and Indigenous and Northern Affairs Canada were dismantled in 2019 and replaced by Indigenous Services Canada and Crown-Indigenous Relations and Northern Affairs Canada. We use the name of the departments as they existed at the time of our searches (websites and document authorships survived past the creation of the new departments).

3 Scandinavian countries have largely side-stepped issues of Indigenous rights and focused on a narrative of the equality of all citizens. At this point, Norway is the only Scandinavian country to have a Sámi policy, which recognizes some of the rights of Sámi reindeer herders, who live on the most northern tip of Norway (8,9).

4 At the request of First Nation, Métis, and Inuit organizations, the term *Aboriginal* is slowing being replaced by *Indigenous* in government interactions and documents. In this chapter, we use the word *Aboriginal* when speaking of the Canadian Constitution and of associated Aboriginal rights, where the term is entrenched. We opt to use the term *Indigenous* in all other instances.

5 While regional health authorities have emerged in most provinces to facilitate more localized decision making over priorities and system design, these regions are part of provincial health care systems that remain southern centric in their policies and approaches (22).

6 For the determination of constitutional jurisdiction, Inuit are included within the term *Indians* in section 91(24). See Reference re Whether the Term "Indians" in s.91(24) of the B.N.A. Act 1867, includes Eskimo Inhabitants of Quebec, [1939] SCR 104. See also Leslie (23).

7 This is true for all communities except those served by a nursing stations, which are funded on the basis of population in their catchment area.

8 In 2017, Saskatchewan consolidated its provincial health authorities into a single Saskatchewan Health Authority. Excluded from this consolidation were the Indigenous-led health authorities such as the Northern Intertribal Health Authority and the Athabasca Health Authority.

REFERENCES

1. du Plessis V, Beshiri R, Bollman RD, Clemenson H. Definitions of "rural." Ottawa (ON): Statistics Canada; 2002. (Agriculture and rural series working paper; no. 61).
2. Kelm M-E. Colonizing bodies: Aboriginal health and healing in British Columbia 1900–50. Vancouver (BC): UBS Press; 1998.
3. Damas D. Arctic migrants/Arctic villagers: the transformation of Inuit settlement in the central Arctic. Montreal (QC): McGill-Queens University Press; 2002.
4. Rohr J. Indigenous peoples in the Russian Federation. Copenhagen (DK): International Work Group for Indigenous Affairs; 2014.
5. Bjerregaard P, Mulvad G. The best of two worlds: how the Greenland Board of Nutrition has handled conflicting evidence about diet and health. Int J Circumpolar Health. 2012;71:18588.
6. Lavoie JG, Gervais L, Toner J, Bergeron O, Thomas G. Aboriginal health policies in Canada: the policy synthesis project. Prince George (BC): National Collaborating Centre for Aboriginal Health; 2013.
7. Lavoie JG. Policy and practice options for equitable access to primary healthcare for Indigenous peoples in British Columbia and Norway. Int Indig Policy J. 2014;5(1):1–17.
8. Norwegian Ministry of Labour and Social Inclusion. Summary of Sami policy. Oslo (NO): Norwegian Ministry of Labour and Social Inclusion; 2008. White Paper No. 28 (2007–2008).
9. Semb AJ. How norms affect policy – the case of Sami policy in Norway. Int J on Minor Group Rights. 2001;8:177–222.
10. Adams A. The road not taken: how tribes choose between tribal and Indian health service management of health care resources. Am Indian Cult Res J. 2000;24(3):21–38.
11. Lavoie JG, O'Neil JD, Reading J. Community healing and Aboriginal self-government. In: Belanger YD, editor. Aboriginal self-government in Canada: current trends and issues. 3rd ed. Saskatoon (SK): Purich Publishing; 2009. p. 172–205.
12. Titmuss RM. Essays on "the welfare state." 2nd ed. London (GB): Unwin University Books; 1963.
13. United Nations. United Nations declaration on the rights of Indigenous peoples. Geneva (CH): United Nations; 2007.
14. Boyer Y. Moving Aboriginal health forward: discarding Canada's legal barriers. Saskatoon (SK): Purich Publishing; 2014.
15. Rotman LL. Defining parameters: Aboriginal rights, treaty rights, and the Sparrow justificatory test. Alta Law Rev. 1997;149:163–4.
16. Organisation for Economic Development and Co-operation. OECD reviews of health systems: Russian Federation 2012. Paris (FR): Organisation for Economic Development and Co-operation; 2012.

17. Hansen KL, Melhus M, Lund E. Ethnicity, self-reported health, discrimination and socio-economic status: a study of Sami and non-Sami Norwegian populations. Int J Circumpolar Health. 2010;69(2):111–28.
18. Hansen KL. Ethnic discrimination and bullying in the Sami and non-Sami populations in Norway: the SAMINOR study [dissertation]. Tromso (NO): Universitetet i Tromsø; 2011.
19. Lavoie JG, Boulton A, Dwyer J. Analysing contractual environments: lessons from Indigenous health in Canada, Australia and New Zealand. Public Adm. 2010;88(3):665–79.
20. Lavoie JG. Policy silences: why Canada needs a national First Nations, Inuit and Métis health policy. Int J Circumpolar Health. 2013;72:22690.
21. Indigenous Services Canada [Internet]. Ottawa (ON): Indigenous Services Canada; 2019. Indigenous Services Canada; [modified 2021 Mar 10; cited 2019]. https://www.canada.ca/en/indigenous-services-canada.html
22. Lavoie JG, Kornelsen D, Boyer Y, Wylie L. Lost in maps: regionalization and Indigenous Health Services. Healthc Pap. 2016;16(1):63–73.
23. Leslie JF. Indian Act: an historical perspective. Can Parliam Rev. 2002;(25)2.
24. Canada. Canada (Indian Affairs and Northern Development), 2016 SCC 12, [2016] 1 SCR 99.
25. Lux MK. Separate beds: a history of Indian hospitals in Canada, 1920s–1980s. Toronto (ON): University of Toronto Press; 2016.
26. Waldram JB, Herring DA, Young TK. Aboriginal health in Canada: historical, cultural and epidemiological perspectives. 2nd ed. Toronto (ON): University of Toronto Press; 2006.
27. National Health and Welfare Canada. Policy directive for the provision of uninsured medical and dental benefits to status Indians and Inuit. Ottawa (ON): Department of Health and Welfare Canada; 1978.
28. Indigenous Services Canada. Indian health policy, 1979. Ottawa (ON): Indigenous Services Canada; 1979.
29. Health Canada First Nation and Inuit Health Branch. First Nations and Inuit health program compendium. Ottawa (ON): Health Canada; 2003.
30. Health Canada First Nation and Inuit Health Branch. First Nations and Inuit health program compendium 2011/2012. Ottawa (ON): Health Canada; 2012.
31. Jordan's Principle Working Group. Without denial, delay, or disruption: ensuring First Nations children's access to equitable services through Jordan's Principle. Ottawa (ON): Assembly of First Nations; 2015.
32. Lavoie JG, Kaufert JM, Browne AJ, Mah S, O'Neil JD. Negotiating barriers, navigating the maze: First Nation peoples' experience of medical relocation. Can Public Admin. 2015;58(2):295–314.
33. Weller GR. The devolution of healthcare to Canada's north. In: Dacks G, editor. Devolution and constitutional development in the Canadian North. Ottawa (ON): Carlton University Press; 1990. p. 121–56.

34. Marchildon GP, Torgenson R. Nunavut: a health system profile. Montreal (QC): McGill-Queen's University Press; 2013.
35. Canada Health Act. RSC, 1985, c C-6.
36. Lavoie JG, Forget EL, Browne AJ. Caught at the crossroad: First Nations, health care, and the legacy of the Indian Act. Pimatisiwin. 2010;8(1):83–100.
37. Nunavut. Consolidation of Midwifery Profession Act, SNu 2008, c18.
38. Mitton C, Dionne F, Masucci L, Wong S, Law S. Innovations in health service organization and delivery in northern rural and remote regions: a review of the literature. Int J Circumpolar Health. 2011;70(5):460–72.
39. O'Neil JD, Gallagher J, Wylie L, Bingham B, Lavoie JG, Alcock D, Johnson H. Transforming First Nations' health governance in British Columbia. Int J Health Governance. 2016;21(4):229–44.
40. British Columbia First Nations Leadership Council. First Nations Health Blueprint for British Columbia. Prince George (BC): 2005.
41. Asch M. Aboriginal self-government and the construction of Canadian constitutional identity. Alta Law Rev. 1992;30:465–75.
42. Rotman LL. Parallel paths: fiduciary doctrine and the Crown-Native relationship in Canada. Toronto (ON): University of Toronto Press; 1996.
43. Inuit Tapariit Kanatami. Social determinants of Inuit health in Canada. Ottawa (ON): Inuit Tapariit Kanatami; 2004.
44. Macdougall, B. Land, family and identity: contextualizing Métis health and well-being. Prince George (BC): National Collaborating Centre for Aboriginal Health; 2017.

Conclusions: Achieving Health Equity in Northern Canada

REBECCA SCHIFF AND HELLE MØLLER

From the knowledge and wisdom presented in this book, what have we learned about health and health care in northern Canada? As demonstrated, one of the most compelling issues, which has a profound impact on northerners, is that old and new forms of colonial programs and policies continue to create health and health care disparities in the North.

In this conclusion, we return to our original question: why focus on northern health and health care? Sections I and II presented critical components of our response to this question: we must recognize the health and health care inequities experienced in the North and appropriately frame these inequities to develop and support responses and solutions that are embedded in the unique strengths and resilience of northerners. As the chapters in Section I demonstrate, we have compelling evidence that the dimensions of health and wellness among northerners continue to be disproportionately affected by the social and ecological determinants of health (SEDoH) and Indigenous social determinants of health (ISDoH), and that northerners experience these effects in ways that are different from their southern counterparts.

We know, from chapter 1 by Fiona Walton, that northern residents have been harmed by unequal access and colonial approaches to education that ignore the histories, contemporary circumstances, and cultures of Indigenous northerners. We know, from Schiff and Schembri in chapter 2 and Kauppi and colleagues in chapter 3, that northerners experience substandard access to core needs such as food and housing, largely because of policy environments that obscure the ability to achieve self-determination and favour southern approaches to the provision of these resources. We learned from these chapters and from Orr and Larcombe in chapter 4 that such disparities in SEDoH have resulted in disproportionate rates of infectious and chronic diseases. In chapter 5, Healey and colleagues illustrated how Inuit women (in their critical roles as mothers, partners, sisters, aunts, extended family, and friends) experience significant mental health inequities and effects of domestic violence, issues that are partly caused by ISDoH that must be addressed by policies and programs rooted in the perspectives and knowledge of northern Indigenous women. In chapter 6, to close Section I, Jones and Johnston demonstrated the ways in which resource development and inequity in the disadvantages and benefits of resource development continue to significantly affect the health of people, and particularly Indigenous people, living in northern Canada.

The chapters in Section II built on this narrative, demonstrating how northerners' health disparities are compounded by inequitable and culturally unsafe health care systems. Raymond Pong (chapter 7) and Helle Møller (chapter 8) outlined the historic challenges in attracting and retaining health care professionals, how colonialism has shaped the provision of nursing and medical care, and how the lack of health care providers has impacted northern health. The chapters by Cidro and Sinclair (chapter 9) and Beatty and McKay (chapter 10) showed us that current systems of care are inadequate and inequitable for those at the beginning (mothers and infants) and those nearing the end (Elders and those in long-term care) of life and that more support and recognition are needed for contextually relevant Indigenous approaches to caregiving. Azaad Kassam (chapter 11) and Josephine Tan (chapter 13) continued this emphasis on the need for contextually relevant and culturally safe mental health care, underscoring the fact that care should be rooted in northern perspectives and values, and build on the strengths of northern residents. Section II highlighted another critically important health and health care issue in the North, presented by Cunsolo and colleagues in chapter 12: the disproportionate environmental effects that climate change is having on northern health care systems. In our ongoing efforts to achieve health equity, we must confront and grapple with the realities of climate change and what that change means for our health and health care systems.

Perhaps more important than what we have learned about the current state of health and health care is what we have learned about the path to achieving health equity in the North. Many of the chapters in Section I and II provide some promising approaches and solutions, such as improvements in the provision of northern education described by Walton, the promises of community-led and bottom-up approaches to decolonizing food systems described by Schiff and Schembri, the possibilities of new recruitment and retention approaches described by Pong and Møller, the potential of Indigenous-designed and Indigenous-led suicide prevention strategies described by Tan, and the immeasurable importance of repatriating birthing to the North as discussed by Cidro and Sinclair.

The chapters in Section III took a deeper dive into the path forward – reiterating the need to focus on strengths-based, northern-led, culturally safe design of health care policy and programs. In chapter 14, Matheson and colleagues demonstrated that current research consistently points to the need for strengths-based, participatory approaches to program development for northern Indigenous youth. As they indicate, supporting the health of northern youth will require us to "to recognize the factors that promote resilience and wellness, and to incorporate an understanding of the contradictions, complexity, and self-determination of the lives of Indigenous peoples as the driver for change." We learned in chapter 15 from Mushquash and colleagues about the possibilities for Indigenous-designed frameworks for mental health care to respond to some of the recommendations made by Kassam in Section II. Focusing on the fast-moving developments and potential for Indigenous-led telehealth and telemedicine networks, in chapter 16, Spadoni and colleagues also highlighted some of the tools we can use to partially address the health care inequities described in Section II. Crawford and colleagues in chapter 17 responded to role of health care providers in the persistence of health inequities. They demonstrated the potential for cultural safety training to address the ongoing systemic and structural racism experienced by northern Indigenous peoples in their health care systems. In chapter 18, Cindy Peltier reiterated the incredible importance of "reclaiming the original teachings and the use of Indigenous healing as a means of decolonization, self-determination, and wellness," and that current health care models for northern Indigenous communities must take a more holistic approach that is grounded in Indigenous culture and self-determination.

Researchers, from both academic and non-academic institutions, are of course implicated in all the previous and ongoing work on northern health and health care. In chapter 19, Brunger and Chubbs reminded us that we must take incredible care in the design and ethical review of research with northern Indigenous communities to ensure that we do not replicate and reinforce colonial frameworks and relationships in the research process and knowledge products. In chapter 20, the final chapter, Lavoie and colleagues brought us again to the discussion of colonialism and the impact of southern bias on the health of northerners. Health policy has a decisive and fundamental role in shaping the ways in which health resources are provided and accessed in the North. The current landscape of Canadian health policy is mired, however, in a complexity of jurisdictional issues and plagued by southern-centric decision makers. While acknowledging the complexity of the northern health care legislative and policy environments, they also presented us with possibilities to eradicate colonialist policy frameworks and develop new strategies rooted in the values, vision, leadership, and needs of northerners.

The chapters in this book have provided a broad overview of what we (as editors and authors) identified as some of the current and important topics in northern health and health care. Authors presented some innovative models for improving health care delivery and new approaches to improving the SEDoH that are grounded in principles of self-determination for northern and northern Indigenous communities.

As we recommended earlier in this book, the future of health care in the North should not attempt to replicate southern models but rather respond to unique northern contexts and embrace northern strengths. With a focus on continuous improvement, northern health care models should evolve to consider the unique combinations of travel-in, travel-out, and remote technology that can provide the most effective and culturally safe care for northerners. This combination will look different for different communities, depending on their size, geography, culture, and resources – and therefore, the future of northern health care must be rooted in self-determination and the involvement of northerners in directing the evolution of their health care systems.

Important and innovative work is being done that can inform the future of northern health care and could be explored in further research, action, and knowledge dissemination/mobilization and policymaking venues. For example, Indigenous control of health care services in Inuit and northern First Nations continues to expand but requires ongoing commitment from the federal government to principles of self-determination (1,2) and to a willingness to meaningfully address the Truth and Reconciliation Commission's calls for action (3,4). Telehealth and telemedicine are rapidly expanding areas of health research and development, with improvements in service applications and delivery in both Indigenous and non-Indigenous northern communities (5,6). Innovative work is also being done to improve northern housing (7); develop new approaches to bringing specialized services to communities (5,6,8,9); revise health-related travel support programs (10); address occupational health concerns (11); repatriate birthing to the North through increased access to midwifery services (12); improve supports for people living with developmental disabilities, address oral health inequities, and improve water treatment facilities (13); and address a broad spectrum of environmental contamination and environmental health concerns (14). These developments require consideration when reflecting and acting on northern health issues.

We – meaning the broad collective of northern health practitioners and researchers – will also need to monitor Canada's continued progress on the Truth and Reconciliation Commission's 94 calls to action (4) and Canada's (recently implemented) Arctic and Northern Policy (14), which includes pillars focused on northern health but still lacks detail regarding implementation. Keeping up with these innovations and changes in northern health policy, health care delivery, and SEDoH status will require constant monitoring. Most importantly, we must continue to scrutinize changes to health status, health policy, and programs that address the SEDoH, to ensure that northerners – and their cultures, values, strengths, and leadership – are at the centre of the ongoing work to achieve social justice and health equity in the North.

REFERENCES

1. Lavoie JG, Dwyer J. Implementing Indigenous community control in health care: lessons from Canada. Aust Health Rev. 2016 Aug 26;40(4):453–8.
2. College of Family Physicians of Canada, Indigenous Physicians Association of Canada, Society of Rural Physicians of Canada. Indigenous health in Canada requires stronger commitment by the federal government [Internet]. Mississauga (ON): College of Family Physicians of Canada; 2019 [cited 2020 Jan 6]. Available from: http://www.cfpc.ca/uploadedFiles/Publications/News_Releases/News_Items/News-Release-More-commitment-for-Indigenous-Health.pdf
3. Jewel W, Mosby I. Calls to action accountability: a status update on reconciliation [Internet]. Toronto (ON): Yellowhead Institute; 2019 Dec 17 [cited 2020 Jun 20]. Available from: https://yellowheadinstitute.org/2019/12/17/calls-to-action-accountability-a-status-update-on-reconciliation/
4. Crown-Indigenous Relations and Northern Affairs Canada [Internet]. Ottawa (ON): Government of Canada. Learn how the Government of Canada is responding to the Truth and Reconciliation Commission's Calls to Action 18 to 24; 2019 Sep 5 [cited 2020 Jul 14]. Available from: http://www.rcaanc-cirnac.gc.ca/eng/1524499024614/1557512659251
5. Indigenous Services Canada [Internet]. Ottawa (ON): Government of Canada. Government of Canada supports Nishnawbe Aski Nation's Mental Health and Addictions Program for Northern Ontario First Nations; 2020 Jul 10 [cited 2020 Jul 15, 2020]. Available from: http://www.canada.ca/en/indigenous-services-canada/news/2020/07/government-of-canada-supports-nishnawbe-aski-nations-mental-health-and-addictions-program-for-northern-ontario-first-nations.html
6. Yanor, F. COVID-19 prompts telehealth boon for rural and remote patients and practitioners in B.C. Star [Internet]. 2020 Apr 24 [cited 2020 Jul 15]. Available from: http://www.thestar.com/news/canada/2020/04/24/covid-19-prompts-telehealth-boon-for-rural-and-remote-patients-and-practitioners-in-bc.html
7. Indigenous Services Canada [Internet]. Ottawa (ON): Government of Canada. Indigenous Homes Innovation Initiative brings together Indigenous innovators and mentors to further develop Indigenous-led housing ideas; 2020 Jan 20 [cited 2020 Jul15]. Available from: http://www.canada.ca/en/indigenous-services-canada/news/2020/01/indigenous-homes-innovation-initiative-brings-together-indigenous-innovators-and-mentors-to-further-develop-indigenous-led-housing-ideas.html
8. Taylor D. Building capacity for Elder exercise programming in northwestern Ontario's remote and rural Indigenous communities [Internet]. Thunder Bay (ON): North West Regional Rehabilitative Care Program; 2019 Apr 1 [cited 2020 Jun 20]. Available from: https://static1.squarespace.com/static/5ab122ecb98a78aa0833a6e4/t/5cca0117a4222f229eb7cc13/1556742424899/Elder+Exercise+Program+Final+Report.pdf

9. Community Therapy Assistant Project Team. Dialogue on community therapy assistant: engagement sessions summary report [Internet]. Thunder Bay (ON): North West Local Health Integrated Network Regional Rehabilitative Care Program; 2020 Apr 30 [cited 2020 Jun 20]. Available from: https://static1.squarespace.com/static/5ab122ecb98a78aa0833a6e4/t/5eecc14c12519764086a84bd/1592574286721/Community+Therapy+Assistant+Community+Needs+Assessment+-April+2020.pdf
10. BayToday Staff. NDP bill to improve Northern Health Travel Grant passes second reading. Sudbury.com [Internet]. 2019 Dec 7 [cited 2020 Jul 14]. Available from: http://www.sudbury.com/local-news/ndp-bill-to-improve-northern-health-travel-grant-passes-second-reading-1947863
11. Northern Safety Association [Internet]. Yellowknife (NT): Northern Safety Association. About the NSA; [2020 Aug 14]. Available from: https://www.nsa-nt.ca/about-the-nsa
12. World Health Organization [Internet]. Geneva (CH): World Health Organization. Bringing midwifery back to a northern Canadian community; 2020 Jan 31 [cited 2020 Jun 20]. Available from: http://www.who.int/news-room/feature-stories/detail/bringing-midwifery-back-to-a-northern-canadian-community
13. Beaumont, H. What would it look like to take the First Nations water crisis seriously? Walrus [Internet]; 2019 Oct 18 [updated 2020 Feb 13; cited 2020 Jul 15]. Available from: https://thewalrus.ca/what-would-it-look-like-to-take-the-first-nations-water-crisis-seriously/
14. Crown-Indigenous Relations and Northern Affairs Canada [Internet]. Ottawa (ON): Government of Canada. Canada's Arctic and northern policy framework; [modified 2019 Nov 18; cited 2019 Dec 17]. Available from: http://www.rcaanc-cirnac.gc.ca/eng/1560523306861/1560523330587

Contributors

Hymie Anisman – professor, Department of Neuroscience, Carleton University, Ottawa, Ontario

Ajani Asokumar – doctoral student, Department of Neuroscience, Carleton University, Ottawa, Ontario

Bonita Beatty – associate professor, Department of Indigenous Studies, University of Saskatchewan, Saskatoon, Saskatchewan

Yvonne Boyer – adjunct professor, Faculty of Law, University of Ottawa, Ottawa, Ontario; adjunct professor, Johnson Shoyama Graduate School of Public Policy, University of Regina, Regina, Saskatchewan

Fern Brunger – professor, Centre for Bioethics and Faculty of Medicine, Memorial University of Newfoundland, St. John's, Newfoundland and Labrador

Brittany Chubbs – PGY-2 resident, Department of Psychiatry, University of Alberta, Edmonton, Alberta

Jaime Cidro – associate vice-president, Research and Innovation; Canada Research Chair in Health and Culture; director, MDP, Indigenous Development; professor, Department of Anthropology, University of Winnipeg, Winnipeg, Manitoba

Allison Crawford – assistant professor, Department of Psychiatry, University of Toronto, Toronto, Ontario; associate chief of virtual mental health and outreach, Centre for Addiction and Mental Health, Toronto, Ontario

Ashlee Cunsolo – dean, School of Arctic and Subarctic Studies, Labrador Institute of Memorial University, Happy Valley-Goose Bay, Newfoundland and Labrador

Sally Dampier – professor (retired), Nursing Program, Confederation College, Thunder Bay, Ontario

Alexandra S. Drawson – clinical psychologist, St. Joseph's Care Group Mental Health Outpatient Program; adjunct professor, Department of Psychology, Lakehead University, Thunder Bay, Ontario

Emily Faries – associate professor (retired), Department of Indigenous Studies, University of Sudbury, Sudbury, Ontario

Janet Gordon – chief operating officer, Sioux Lookout First Nations Health Authority, Sioux Lookout, Ontario

Sherilee Harper – Canada Research Chair (Tier II) in Climate Change and Health, and associate professor, School of Public Health, University of Alberta, Edmonton, Alberta

Gwen Healey Akearok – executive and scientific director, Qaujigiartiit Health Research Centre, Iqaluit, Nunavut

Inuit Mental Health Adaptation to Climate Change Team

Lesley Johnston – PhD candidate, School of Public Health Sciences, University of Waterloo, Waterloo, Ontario

Jen Jones – lead consultant, Jen Jones Consulting, Whitehorse, Yukon

Azaad Kassam – assistant professor, Department of Psychiatry, University of Ottawa, Ottawa, Ontario; assistant professor, Department of Psychiatry, Northern Ontario School of Medicine, Thunder Bay, Ontario; psychiatrist, Pinecrest-Queensway Community Health Centre, Ottawa, Ontario; psychiatrist, Timmins and District Hospital, Timmins, Ontario; lead, Culture and Psychiatry Initiative, University of Ottawa, Ottawa, Ontario

Carol Kauppi – professor, School of Social Work, and director, Centre for Research in Social Justice and Policy, Laurentian University, Sudbury, Ontario

Theresa Koonoo – territorial community health representative coordinator, Government of Nunavut, Iqaluit, Nunavut

Derek Kornelsen – adjunct assistant professor, Department of Geography and Planning, Queen's University, Kingston, Ontario; president, Rootstalk Resources, Winnipeg, Manitoba

Linda Larcombe – associate professor, Max Rady Faculty of Health Sciences, University of Manitoba, Winnipeg, Manitoba

Josée G. Lavoie – professor, Rady Faculty of Health Sciences, University of Manitoba, Winnipeg, Manitoba

Christine Lund – senior policy advisor, Pauktuutit Inuit Women of Canada, Ottawa, Ontario

Emily MacLeod – assistant professor, Department of Nursing, Cape Breton University, Cape Breton Island, Nova Scotia

Kimberly Matheson – professor, Neuroscience, and joint research chair, Culture and Gender Mental Health, Carleton University and University of Ottawa – Institute of Mental Health Research, Ottawa, Ontario

Josephine McKay – special projects and operations manager, Peter Ballantyne Cree Nation Health Services, Prince Albert, Saskatchewan

Lynn M. Meadows – associate professor emerita, Department of Community Health Sciences, University of Calgary, Calgary, Alberta

Kathy Michael – published posthumously

Helle Møller – associate professor, Department of Health Sciences, Lakehead University, Thunder Bay, Ontario

Phyllis Montgomery – professor, School of Nursing, Laurentian University, Sudbury, Ontario

Sharolyn Mossey – assistant professor, School of Nursing, Laurentian University, Sudbury, Ontario

Christopher Mushquash – Canada Research Chair in Indigenous Mental Health and Addiction, and professor, Department of Psychology, Lakehead University and Northern Ontario School of Medicine, Thunder Bay, Ontario; psychologist, Dilico Anishinabek Family Care, Fort William First Nation, Ontario; director, Centre for Rural and Northern Health Research,

Thunder Bay, Ontario; associate vice president research, Thunder Bay Regional Health Sciences Centre, Thunder Bay, Ontario; chief scientist, Thunder Bay Regional Health Research Institute, Thunder Bay, Ontario

Pamela Orr – professor, Departments of Internal Medicine, Medical Microbiology and Infectious Diseases, and Community Health Sciences, University of Manitoba, Winnipeg, Manitoba

Henri Pallard – professor emeritus, Department of Law and Justice, and director, International Centre for Interdisciplinary Research in Law, Laurentian University, Sudbury, Ontario

Cindy Peltier – associate professor, Faculty of Arts and Science and Faculty of Education and Professional Studies – Schulich School of Education, Nipissing University, North Bay, Ontario

Raymond W. Pong – professor emeritus and director emeritus, Centre for Rural and Northern Health Research, Laurentian University, Sudbury, Ontario

Victoria Schembri – master's of health sciences student, Department of Health Sciences, Lakehead University, Thunder Bay, Ontario

Rebecca Schiff – professor and chair, Department of Health Sciences, Lakehead University, Thunder Bay, Ontario

Patricia Sevean – professor emeriti, Department of Nursing, Lakehead University, Thunder Bay, Ontario

Inez Shiwak – Inuit researcher, Rigolet, Nunatsiavut, Labrador

Stephanie Sinclair – doula research coordinator, First Nations Health and Social Secretariat of Manitoba, Winnipeg, Manitoba

Michelle Spadoni – associate professor, School of Nursing, Lakehead University, Thunder Bay, Ontario

Josephine Tan – associate professor, Department of Psychology, Lakehead University, Thunder Bay, Ontario

Elaine Toombs – clinical psychologist, Dilico Anishinabek Family Care, Fort William First Nation, Ontario

Candice Waddell – associate professor, Department of Psychiatric Nursing, Brandon University, Brandon, Manitoba

Fiona Walton – 3M National Teaching Fellow and retired member, Faculty of Education, University of Prince Edward Island, Charlottetown, Prince Edward Island

Michele Wood – health researcher/evaluator, Department of Health and Social Development, Nunatsiavut Government, Happy Valley-Goose Bay, Newfoundland and Labrador

Index

Page numbers in **bold** and *italics* denote tables and figures, respectively. Page numbers with suffix n denote notes.

Milton Keynes UK
Ingram Content Group UK Ltd.
UKHW012229190424
441406UK00003B/289

9 781487 521790